MRI of Degenerative Disease of the Spine

Paola D'Aprile • Alfredo Tarantino

MRI of Degenerative Disease of the Spine

A Case-Based Atlas

Second Edition

Springer

Paola D'Aprile
Radiology - Neuroradiology
Ospedale San Paolo
Bari
Italy

Alfredo Tarantino
Radiology - Neuroradiology
Ospedale San Paolo
Bari
Italy

ISBN 978-3-030-73706-1 ISBN 978-3-030-73707-8 (eBook)
https://doi.org/10.1007/978-3-030-73707-8

This Springer imprint is published by the registered company Springer Nature Switzerland AG
The registered company address is: Gewerbestrasse 11, 6330 Cham, Switzerland

Foreword

Five years after the first edition of the successful seminal book of Paola D'Aprile and Alfredo Tarantino, "MRI of degenerative disease of the spine", this second edition of the atlas, with a few new cases added, remains an up-to-date reference book for all the physicians involved in the diagnosis and treatment of spine diseases.

The twin book *MRI of the Rheumatic Spine* is an almost indispensable integration to master all the intriguing aspects of the pathology of this relevant and delicate anatomical component of our body. However, no matter of the many progresses made by the impressive improvements of the imaging modalities, mainly MRI that have opened the spine and spinal cord to noninvasive, thorough investigation as CT did in the seventies for the brain, we must admit that no equivalent progresses have been made in treating the multiform clinical, structural and morphological aspects of the different diseases of the spine.

We are still limited, for the treatment of the majority of the degenerative diseases, to surgical invasive procedures, though very effective, from the less invasive vertebroplasty to the more aggressive spine fixation, or disc and vertebral bone replacements.

The expectations created by a different biological, genetical and molecular approach have been disappointing. Cooperative promising multicentre research projects such as EURODISC 2005, GENODISC 2013 and DISCKOMICE 2016 have not yet produced significant results in the noninvasive, medical replacement treatment (stem cells?) that could be the future of this relevant aspect of Medicine. Imaging, and MRI in particular, could have a significant role in clinical trials, to check and follow therapy-related changes.

For the time being, the experience gained up to now in the diagnosis (and understanding) of degenerative disease of the spine is completely and perfectly exposed in this second edition of the book. Young trainees in radiology and neuroradiologists, as well as mature radiologists, orthopaedic surgeons, neurosurgeons and clinicians will find in this book, an indispensable guide to approach this complex field.

Giuseppe Scotti
Medical School
University San Raffaele
Milan, Italy

Preface

Five years after the first publication, the second edition of this book is borne.

In this edition we wanted to widen and deepen the topic of the degenerative pathology of the spine, keeping on sharing our knowledge on the aspects of magnetic resonance imaging (MRI).

Spine degenerative disease includes a series of arthrosic degenerative processes, which affect mechanical supports, resulting from a natural aging/worn process.

As known, degenerative pathology is extremely widespread in the population and has a great socio-economic impact.

Degenerative changes can be localized in the anterior vertebral compartment (vertebral-disc unit) and in the posterior vertebral compartment (interapophyseal joints, spinal ligaments and para-vertebral muscles), so in the diagnostic process with MR, it is very important to check carefully all anatomic elements of the spine as well as muscular and ligamentous supports.

The main clinical onset of this disease is pain which is more often localized in the lumbar region and can also cause impaired mobility.

Magnetic resonance is the gold standard imaging for the study of degenerative disease of the spine for its accuracy and diagnostic efficacy, but the appropriate use of MRI sequences is fundamental to an accurate diagnosis.

MR study protocol includes T2-weighted images with fat saturation, since more sensitive to the pattern of oedema, also with administration of contrast medium in some cases, for more accurate assessment of the inflammatory stage of the disease.

It is very important to make a correlation between the clinical data and the results of the MR in order to find out the cause of the pain and consequently identify therapeutic "targets" and specific therapeutic procedures.

In conclusion, this case-based atlas aims at showing less common aspects of the degenerative disease highlighted with the MR mainly in their active inflammatory phase. Moreover, in this new edition, we have widened the casistry and added an important new chapter on postoperative spine.

Thanks to its "case-based" structure, this book offers an easy-to-use but thorough handbook for radiologists, neuroradiologists, orthopaedists, neurosurgeons, rheumatologists as well as students.

Bari, Italy — Paola D'Aprile
Bari, Italy — Alfredo Tarantino

Acknowledgements

We thank all the technical and nursing stuff at the MRI, without whose cooperation and dedication we would not have been able to work peacefully and in harmony, respecting the patient, always trying to give affirmative and appropriate answers to all those who have chosen to undergo neuroradiological examinations in our department.

A special thanks, with respect, gratitude and friendship, goes to Dr. Randy Jinkins for his teachings and for giving us the passion and interest to the spine.

We thank Luca Salamanno for the technical management of images.

We thank Springer Milan, in particular Antonella Cerri and Corinna Parravicini for showing trust in our project.

We also like to thank all those who will read this book with the hope that it will be a little help and comparison in the daily research of the diagnosis.

Bari, Italy — Paola D'Aprile
Bari, Italy — Alfredo Tarantino

Contents

Part I

Clinical and Technical Aspects

Biomechanics of the Spine

1

1.1 Spine Stability

The spine is a multiarticular structure composed of motion segments (MS) whose correct function has stability as prerequisite.

A number of definitions of stability exist in literature.

The American Academy of Orthopedic Surgeons defined it as "the capacity of the vertebrae of remaining cohesive in all physiological body movements" [1].

White and Panjabi considered the clinical stability as "the ability of the spine under physiologic loads to limit patterns of displacement to not damage or irritate the spinal cord and nerve roots and to prevent incapacitating deformity or pain caused by structural changes" [2].

Spinal stability is a fundamental property for the protection of nervous elements, the active generation of forces in the body trunk and the transfer of them between the upper and lower limbs, the prevention of the early biomechanical deterioration of its own components and the reduction of energy expenditure during muscle action.

The key feature of the biomechanics and stability of the spine is the highly nonlinear load/displacement ratio, the effort required for movement significantly changing in its various phases [3].

In every MS, the initial part of range of motion (ROM), on either side of neutral posture, meets a scarce resistance and requires a relatively low effort, because of the general laxity status of ligaments and joint capsules. This part of motion, referred to as neutral zone (NZ), is replaced by the elastic zone (EZ) where the ligaments, capsules, fascias and tendons in tension require more effort per unit of displacement nearing the ends of ROM.

In this way, two opposed needs are met, reducing the muscle effort near the neutral posture and ensuring stability at the end of joint excursion.

Each vertebra can perform, with respect to adjacent vertebrae, three translations and three rotations in relation to each of the x-, y-, z-cartesian axes of space and various combinations of main and coupled movements.

Each movement has its ROM, NZ and EZ.

Stability implies an appropriate relationship between NZ and EZ even within a normal ROM.

The stabilization of the spine is guaranteed by a stabilization system consisting of three closely related subsystems (Fig. 1.1) [3] including:

- The spinal bones and joints or passive subsystem
- The muscles forming the active subsystem
- A central control unit, the CNS

1.1.1 Spinal Bones Joints and Ligaments

The passive subsystem plays a structural role, ensuring spinal stability, namely, within the elastic zone. It also has a transducer function carried out from a number of mechanoreceptors located within the joint capsules, discs and ligaments which send a continuous flow of proprioceptive inputs about the load status, spatial position and movement from each MS to CNS. On the basis of this information flow, CNS replays through an appropriate and coordinate muscle activity [4].

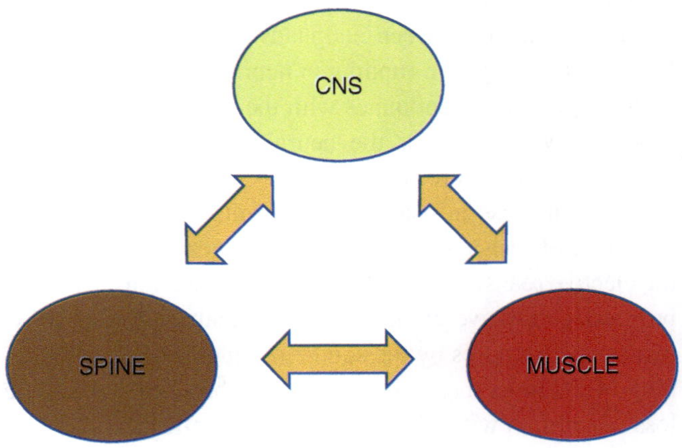

Fig. 1.1 Three strictly related subsystems control the stability of the spine: the spinal column, the muscles and the central nervous system. In case of damage to one subsystem, more compensatory work is played by the others in order to preserve stability

P. D'Aprile, A. Tarantino, *MRI of Degenerative Disease of the Spine*, https://doi.org/10.1007/978-3-030-73707-8_1

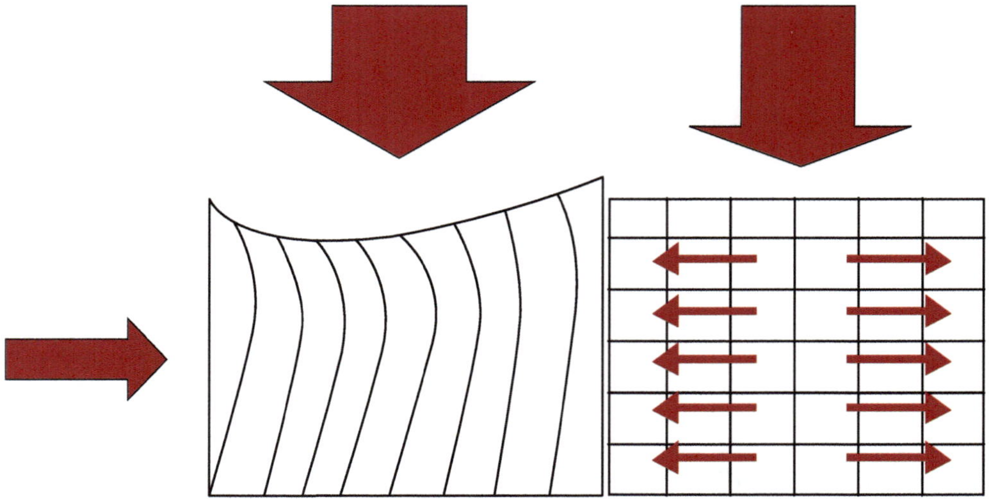

Figs. 1.2 and 1.3 The vertical compressive loads are first accepted by vertical trabecular columns which transmit forces between the endplates. The intrinsic tendency to bow of isolated vertical columns (first figure) is restrained by horizontal lamellae whose tension favours the radial dispersion of forces conferring resilience to the vertebral body (second figure)

The vertebral body is the key element of the load-bearing system. It mainly consists of spongy trabecular bone which plays a crucial role in determining the strength and resilience of the vertebral body. Compressive loads are first accepted by vertical trabecular struts joining directly the vertebral endplates. Vertical columns, if isolated, would tend to bow and lose their load-bearing capacity if these were not restrained and maintained right by tension of horizontal trabeculae (Figs. 1.2 and 1.3). It is this conversion of vertical loads in transverse tensions that confers weight-bearing resistance to vertebral body.

A solid bony block would be heavy and, like all crystalline structures, unable to bear dynamic loads which could fracture it, whereas, conversely, a box of cortical shell would easily collapse under compressive forces because of scarce resilience of cortical bone. Cancellous bone guarantees the best load/resistance ratio.

The resistance of vertebral spongiosa depends on either trabecular architecture or bone density.

The vertebral spongiosa of any vertebra contains four main trabecular systems having a quite constant orientation: a vertical system between endplates which transmits axial loads, a curved system running in neural arc and two curved systems joining the endplates with the articular and spinous processes which anchor the neural arc to vertebral body resisting shearing forces (Fig. 1.4).

The bone loss in osteoporosis results in an exponential reduction of resistance. During early stages of osteoporosis, the elective reabsorption of transverse connections leads to a progressive relative elongation of vertical columns, whose resistance decreases by the square of length. Later, the thinning of columns themselves also contributes to a quadratic loss of strength with a summation of both effects.

Out of any pathological change, vertebral endplates can fail by fracturing following repeated stresses.

When a vertebral body is compressed, a part of the energy applied to deform it will be lost and, when the load is removed, less energy is available for it to restore the initial shape, which is so not immediately regained. This mechanical phenomenon, defined as *hysteresis*, expresses the amount of energy lost during the deformation of any solid structure. By virtue of hysteresis, a structure regains its original shape at a rate and extent different to that at which it was deformed. If forces are applied with many repetitions and sufficient frequency, the vertebral body, like any material, is unable to recover and accumulate small weaknesses, losing gradually stiffness, and, finally, fails under a stress much less than that could damage it if applied a single time [5].

Failure fractures of the vertebral endplates may occur after as few as 30–80 applications of forces corresponding to 50–80% of ultimate compressive strength (normally between 3000 and 10,000 N). These forces are within the ranges occurring during normal daily activities [6].

Endplate fractures are now considered a possible cause of internal disc disruption and discogenic pain [7].

The annulus acts as the first ligament for restraining the complex 3D movements a vertebra can perform.

The oblique alternating arrangement of collagen fibres between adjacent lamellae (with a degree of 65–70° to endplate plane) and the degree of obliquity of fibres within each lamella both optimize the capacity to restrain movements in all directions. A steeper orientation of lamellar fibres would increase the resistance to distraction, but it would compromise that to sliding and twisting; a flatter inclination would enhance control of twisting, but it would lessen that of distraction and bending.

Adjacent to vertebral endplates, the disc acts as *shock absorber* of the forces transmitted to the head and brain during walking and jumping.

Both nucleus and inner annulus are involved in weight-bearing. The nucleus pulposus mainly works in the NZ bearing low axial loads, while the stiffer annulus fibrosus accepts a larger proportion of the highest loads. The densely packed lamellae confer compression stiffness to annulus, but, over

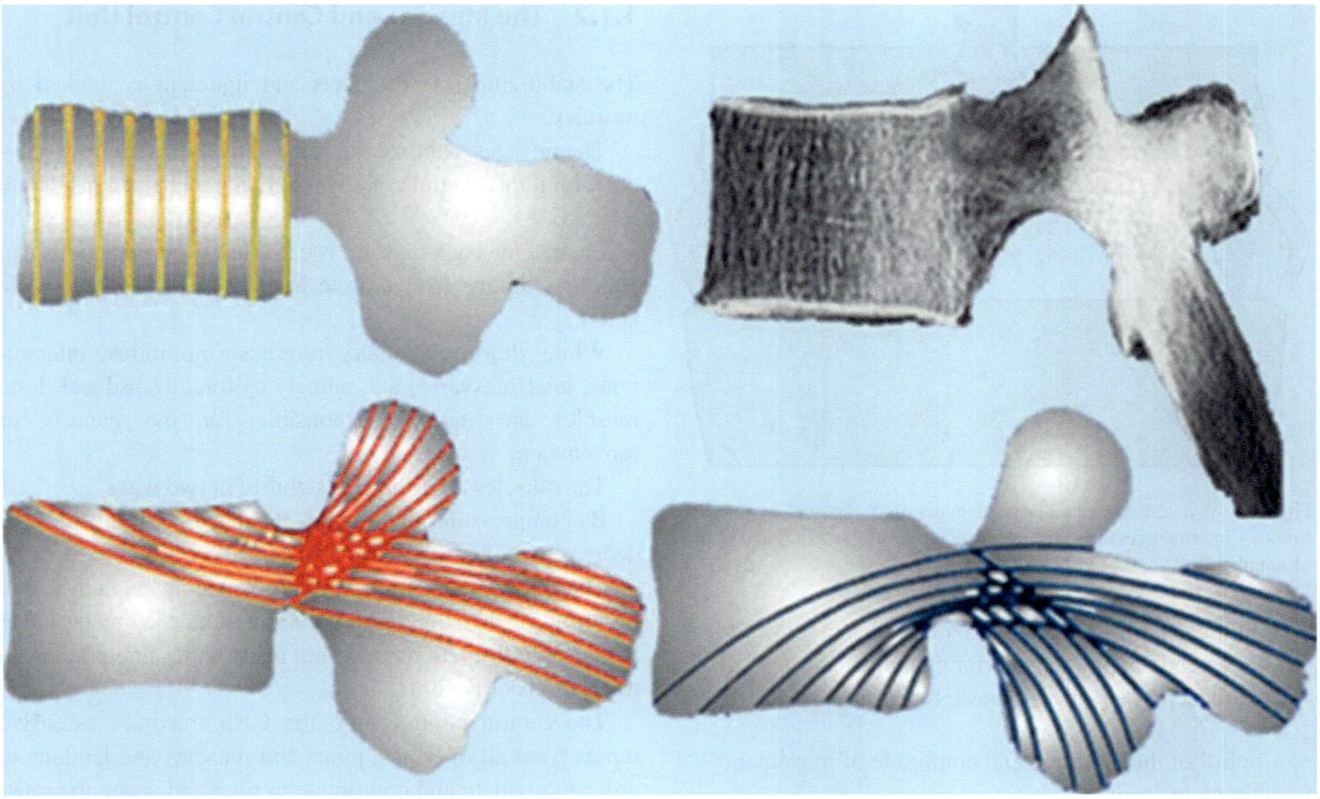

Fig. 1.4 The load-bearing capacity of the vertebral body depends on trabecular architecture. The vertebral spongiosa contains four main trabecular systems including a vertical system between endplates, a curved system running in neural arc and two curved oblique systems joining the endplates with the articular and spinous processes which anchor the neural arc to vertebral body resisting shearing forces

time, an isolated annulus under sustained loads tends to buckle and collapse.

The nucleus provides an internal bracing mechanism. Like a ball of fluid, the nucleus can be deformed but not compressed. Under axial compressive load, it expands radially stretching the annulus and pushing away the opposite endplates. The vertical pressure transmits part of load from one vertebra to the next, lessening the tension created in the annulus fibrosus. The radial pressure stretches and braces the annulus preserving the vertical orientation of lamellae, avoiding their buckling and increasing their capacity to transmit loads [8] (Fig. 1.5). The cooperative action of the nucleus and the annulus enhances the disc capacity of bearing higher and prolonged loads.

This mechanism is lost in case of degenerative depressurization of nucleus pulposus that leads to external and internal buckling of annular lamellae. Buckling accelerates and favours the further annulus disruption (Fig. 1.6).

In addition, under compression, a part of energy is used and stored to stretch the annulus and then released soon after the discharge of the spine. This momentary diversion of energy attenuates the speed of transmission of the force from a vertebra to another, preserving the adjacent endplates.

Under very high compressive loads, the first structure to fail is usually the endplate rather than the disc.

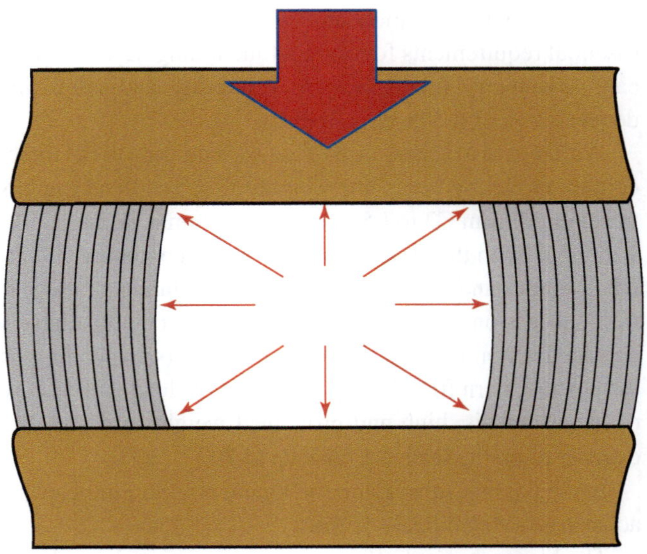

Fig. 1.5 A well-pressurized hydrated nucleus pulposus provides an internal bracing to annulus lamellae aiding annulus to contribute to weight-bearing. The cooperative action consents to disc to bear sustained and higher loads

The VB is exclusively designed to bear longitudinal loads and has no features that confer stability to intervertebral joints and limit movements within the horizontal plane [8].

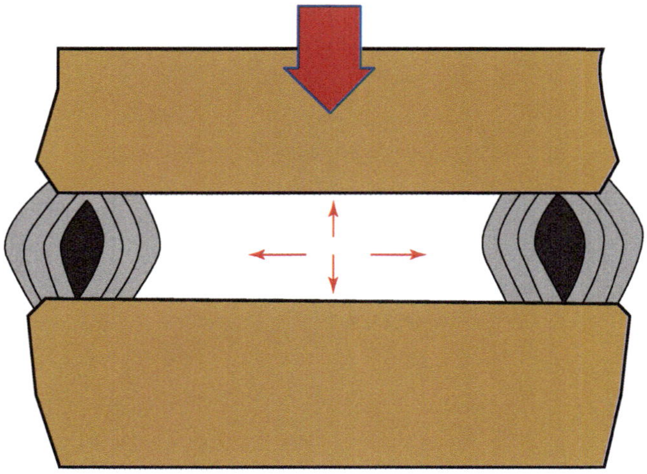

Fig. 1.6 As a consequence of disc degeneration, the nucleus pulposus loses its internal pressure favouring the collapse, buckling and tearing of annulus

For the stability in the horizontal plane, the VBs are totally dependent on the posterior elements.

The facet joints fulfil two basic functions:

- Control of the direction and amplitude of movement
- Sharing of loads

Facet joints resist sagittal translation and limit extension and axial rotation, protecting the discs from torsion injuries which normally occur over only 3° of rotation.

The spatial orientation and symmetry of the facets are essential requirements for correct functioning. Every significant asymmetry predisposes to instability and premature degeneration of the facets and discs.

With regard to acceptance of loads, according to the three-column model by Louis, the weight of the head and trunk is transmitted from C3 to L5 upon three columns arranged like a triangle, with the anterior column being composed of vertebral bodies and discs and the posterior columns of the vertical succession of the facet joints [9]. The columns have a balanced action for which the posterior facets, depending on the posture, born from 0% up to 33% of the load, but, in case of hyperlordosis, high and prolonged weight load and disc degeneration, the load can raise up to 70%.

In the passive subsystem, the ligaments and joint capsule act as passive stabilizers of MSs.

The biomechanical efficacy of any ligament depends not only on its intrinsic strength but also and more on the length of lever arm by which acts, the distance between the bony insertion and the instantaneous axis of rotation (IAR) of the vertebra which locates in the posterior part of vertebral body.

Specifically, the ISL and SSL, being located far apart from the IAR, work by a long lever arm and resist the spinal flexion more than the FL and PLL which function with shorter lever arms.

1.1.2 The Muscles and Central Control Unit

The stabilizing role of facets and ligament is flanked by muscles.

The muscles stabilize the spine actively and mainly operate within the neutral zone where ligaments and capsule are relaxed.

Each of the back muscles is capable of several actions. No action is unique to a muscle and no muscle has a single action.

While short segmentary muscles (multifidus, interspinous, intertransverse) act, namely as force transducer, long muscles are mainly responsible for the genesis of movements.

The muscles contribute to stability in two ways.

By compressing spinal segments, they limit joints motion, decreasing either the ROM or NZ [10].

The muscles also pull directly displacing segments, but, by virtue of their longitudinal orientation, they resist much better sagittal rotation but do not resist with same efficacy to translations or twisting.

The central control unit, the CNS, receives extensive inputs from all of bones, joints and muscles and tendons in order to regulate and coordinate in time and space the muscular posture and movement.

In case of damage to soft tissues and to mechanoreceptors after a single or repetitive trauma, corrupted transducer signals are sent to the CNS causing an inappropriate motor response with reduced temporal and spatial coordination.

The altered muscle response, in turn, increases the mechanical stress of bony and joint components and elicits an abnormal feedback response by FSUs and muscles themselves [11].

A vicious circle is finally created that leads to the development of inflammation, muscle fatigue and activation of nociceptors with onset and perpetuation of pain.

Patients with chronic low back pain have a delayed muscle response and offset in performing movements as well as a reduced postural control compared to asymptomatic subjects [12].

While the transverse abdominis and multifidus muscles stabilize the spine before initiating movement or accepting a load, in patients suffering from chronic spinal pain, such contractions are delayed [12].

1.2 Spine Instability

Spine instability is a frequent and often misdiagnosed cause of neck and back pain and disability.

Like stability, it also lacks a general universally accepted definition.

White and Panjabi defined instability as "the loss of the ability of the spine, under physiologic loads, to maintain its patterns of displacement so there is no initial or additional neurologic deficit, no major deformity, and no incapacitating pain" [13].

Pope and Panjabi qualified instability as a loss of stiffness, leading to abnormal and increased movement in the MS [14].

Even though the location and type of lesion in the MS determines the pattern of instability, as spinal movement is three-dimensional with coupled movements, tissue derangement tends to cause dysfunctional motions in more than one direction.

While the classical definitions of instability refer to a global increase of joint excursion, over the normal limits (terminal instability), abnormality can manifest not at the endpoints, but only during a step of range of motion, modifying the quality of motion.

In fact, the instability is not an all-or-nothing phenomenon, and a complete instability is rare. Each spinal component concurs to stability, and a number of studies have tested the contribution of every single structure.

In many clinical and experimental situations, instability consists of an enlarged neutral zone with excessive displacement early in range under minor loads (looseness), despite a normal ultimate joint strength.

In the light of relative importance of the NZ, Panjabi redefined instability as the reduced ability by the stabilizing systems of the spine to maintain the neutral zones of the MSs within physiological limits so that deformity, neurological deficit or disabling pain does not occur [3].

When an MS undergo a loss of stiffness, owing to a reduction of one of its restraints that resists a given movement, under an external force, it can have acceleration and a momentary lapse of control in early, middle or late range which is felt as instability [15].

Instability can stem from a mismatch between a pattern of motion programmed for a given usual movement and the proprioceptive feedback. The CNS relieves the mismatch and replays with a sudden muscle reflex experienced as a jerk or a catch [15].

1.2.1 Degenerative Instability

Degenerative instability is considered a common cause of acute and chronic spinal pain and disability as well as a frequent indication for surgery.

Degenerative instability has been defined as a change in vector forces relating the MSs generating abnormal, imbalanced and paradoxical movements.

A degenerative primum movens, involving generally the disc, primes disorders of movement which, in turn, increase the original bony, articular and biomechanical abnormalities, and extends them to other joints of the same and adjacent segments transforming a segmental into a regional pathology.

Because of degenerative disc collapse, the annulus and ligaments become lax and redundant favouring anterior, posterior and vertical subluxation of the vertebral bodies.

During the evolution of degenerative instability, Kirkaldy-Willis and Farfan distinguished three main biomechanical and clinical phases forming a so-called degenerative cascade: painful dysfunction, instability and restabilization [16].

During the instability phase, several radiological signs can be found including endplate oedema (Modic type 1 changes), peduncle and isthmus oedema, traction spurs [17], extended discal vacuum associated with mild disc space narrowing, joint effusion and facet joint gapping over 1 mm [18], synovial cysts, anterolisthesis and retrolisthesis [16].

All these signs of conventional imaging are indirect and their specificity and the clinical relevance for diagnosing instability are not consistent in the different reports and need to be established definitively.

Open MR systems allow positional-dynamic studies in either standing or seated positions to detect increased and abnormal intersegmental movements.

Positional-dynamic MRI studies may disclose dysfunctional movements which can worsen or uncover a central canal, lateral recesses and/or foraminal stenosis, disc protrusion or disc extrusion [19].

By comparing the results of traditional and functional MR in a small cohort of patients, Smith reported abnormal findings detected only by dynamic studies in 52% of patients with appropriate successful treatment in all cases of LBP and sciatica [20].

Axial-loaded CT (AL-CT) and MR (AL-MR) simulate the weight-bearing upright position and depict several findings including hypermobility, appearance of or increase in listhesis and the appearance or increase of canal and/or foraminal stenosis [21]. These findings can be observed alone (elementary modifications) or coexist in various patterns referred to as complex dynamic modifications [21].

Abnormal motion patterns in axial-loading imaging tend to evolve in a quite stereotyped way up to degenerative listhesis [21]. A basic drawback of axial-loading imaging is the impossibility to reflect postural changes related to muscle tone and physiological loads that are not uniform at different levels but increase in the caudal direction along the lumbar spine, so upright/positional MR is considered to outweigh axial-loaded MR and CT.

When spinal degeneration further progresses, in the final phase of "restabilization", the fibrosis of the joint capsules, the formation of osteophytes, the marked discal collapse and the remodelling of vertebral bodies increase stiffness and favour an overall reduction of mobility.

The final phase of restabilization is associated with significant disc collapse, radial remodelling of vertebral bodies, claw and "wrap around bumper" osteophytes [22], Modic type 3 changes, facet sclerosis and neoarthrosis between the spinous processes [21].

A spontaneous restabilization may occur even in case of spondylolisthesis whose presence does not always imply actual instability [16]. Disc collapse and osteophytes may block the progression of slippage, often with secondary improvement of pain. In effect, despite widespread opinion, spondylolisthesis is not always associated with increased motion.

A 10-year follow-up study found progression of slippage only in 30% of cases and 65% of patients who were initially neurologically normal did not worsen and could be treated conservatively [23].

The relation between instability and pain has been long debated and often is hard to be demonstrated. In a hypermobile segment, pain can be aggravated by the movement because of excessive engagement of irritated restraints, not necessarily by instability which can be present as an independent and parallel phenomenon.

According to Mulholland, abnormal movements detectable in a degenerative spine are not necessarily the cause of pain and instability is often a myth [24]. In many cases, spinal pain is due to an abnormal, irregular distribution of loads between joint surfaces. In fact, pain may persist after technically successful fixations or unexpectedly resolves also in cases of pseudarthrosis. Pain seems to be often elicited primarily from load stresses caused by the posture or powerful muscle contraction such as that of the erector muscles during lifting tasks rather than by movement itself.

As stressed by Bogduk, instability is a biomechanical term and a diagnosis too often abused.

The concept of enlarged neutral zone may contribute to justify the many cases of suspected but not ascertained instability.

Despite all efforts in this clinical topic, a definitive diagnosis remains often elusive.

Acknowledgement We would like to thank Dr. *Roberto Izzo* for his contribution in writing this chapter.

References

1. Kirkaldy-Willis WH (1985) Presidential symposium on instability of the lumbar spine. Introduction. Spine 10:254
2. White AA, Panjabi MM (1990) Clinical biomechanics of the spine, 2nd edn. JB Lippincott, Philadelphia, PA
3. Panjabi MM (1992) The stabilizing system of the spine. Part II. Neutral zone and instability hypothesis. J Spinal Disord 5:390–397
4. Panjabi MM (1992) The stabilizing system of the spine. Part I. Function, dysfunction, adaptation and enhancement. J Spinal Disord 5:383–389
5. Bogduk N (2012) Basic biomechanics. In: Bogduk N (ed) Clinical and radiological anatomy of the lumbar spine. Churchill-Livingstone Elsevier, Edinburgh, pp 61–72
6. Hansson TH, Kelelr TS, Spengler DM (1987) Mechanical behaviour of the human lumbar spine. II. Fatigue strength during dynamic compressive loading. J Orthop Res 5:479–487
7. Bogduk N (1992) Sources of low back pain. In: Jayson MIV (ed) The lumbar spine and back pain. Churchill-Livingstone, Edinburgh, pp 61–68
8. Bogduk N (2012) The interbody joint and the intervertebral discs. In: Bogduk N (ed) Clinical and radiological anatomy of the lumbar spine. Churchill Livingstone Elsevier, Edinburgh, pp 11–27
9. Louis R (1989) Chirurgia del rachide. Piccin ed, Padova, pp 67–69
10. Wilke HJ, Wolf S, Claes L et al (1995) Stability increase of the lumbar spine with different muscle groups: a biomechanical in vitro study. Spine 20:192–198
11. Panjabi MMA (2006) Hypothesis of chronic back pain: ligament subfailure injuries lead to muscle control dysfunction. Eur Spine J 15:668–676
12. Luoto S, Hurri H, Alaranta H (1995) Reaction times in patients chronic low-back pain. Eur J Phys Med Rehabil 5:47–50
13. White AA III, Panjabi MM (1978) The basic kinematics of the human spine. Spine 3(1):12–20
14. Pope MH, Panjabi M (1985) Biomechanical definitions of spinal instability. Spine 10:255–256
15. Bogduk N (2012) Instability. In: Bogduk N (ed) Clinical and radio-logical anatomy of the lumbar spine. Churchill Livingstone Elsevier, Edinburgh, pp 207–216
16. Kirkaldy-Willis WH, Farfan HF (1982) Instability of the lumbar spine. Clin Orthop Relat Res 165:110–123
17. Macnab I (1971) The traction spur: an indicator of segmental instability. J Bone Joint Surg Am 53:663–670
18. Chaput C, Padon D, Rush J et al (2007) The significance of increased fluid signal on magnetic resonance imaging in lumbar facets in relationship to degenerative spondylolisthesis. Spine 32(17):1883–1887
19. Alyas F, Connell D, Saifuddin A (2008) Upright positional MRI of the lumbar spine. Clin Radiol 63:1035–1048
20. Smith FW (2005) Positional upright imaging of the lumbar spine modifies the management of low back pain and sciatica. European Society of Skeletal Radiology, Oxford, p 2005
21. Cartolari R (1997) Functional evaluation of the lumbar spine with axial-loaded computer tomography and cine ALCT. Riv Neuroradiol 10:569–584
22. Fujiwara A, Lim TH, An HS et al (2000) The effect of disc degeneration and facet joint osteoarthritis on the segmental flexibility of the lumbar spine. Spine 25(23):3036–3044
23. Matsunaga S, Ijiri K, Hayashi K (2000) Nonsurgically managed patients with degenerative spondylolisthesis: a 10- to 18-year follow-up study. J Neurosurg 93:194–198
24. Mulholland RC (2008) The myth of lumbar instability: the importance of abnormal loading as a cause of low back pain. Eur Spine J 17:619–625

Suggested Readings

Hansen BB, Nordberg CL, Hansen P et al (2019) Weight-bearing MRI of the Lumbar Spine. Spinal Stenosis and Spondylolisthesis. Semin Musculoskelet Radiol 23(6):621–633

Harvey S, Hukins D, Smith F et al (2016) Measurement of lumbar spine intervertebral motion in the sagittal plane using videofluoroscopy. J Back Musculoskelet Rehabil 29(3):445–457

Lao LF, Zhong GB, Li QY et al (2014) Kinetic magnetic resonance imaging analysis of spinal degeneration: a systematic review. Orthop Surg 6(4):294–299

Michelini G, Corridore A, Torlone S et al (2018) Dynamic MRI in the evaluation of the spine: state of the art. Acta Biomed 89(1-S):89–101

Muto M, Giurazza F, Guarnieri G et al (2016) Neuroimaging of spinal instability. Magn Reson Imaging Clin N Am 24(3):485–494

Oichi T, Taniguchi Y, Oshima Y et al (2020) Pathomechanism of intervertebral disc degeneration. JOR Spine 3(1):e1076

Segebarth B, Kurd MF, Haug PH et al (2015) Routine upright imaging for evaluating degenerative lumbar stenosis: incidence of degenerative spondylolisthesis missed on supine MRI. J Spinal Disord Tech 28(10):394–397

Splendiani A, Perri M, Grattacaso G et al (2016) Magnetic resonance imaging (MRI) of the lumbar spine with dedicated G-scan machine in the upright position: a retrospective study and our experience in 10 years with 4305 patients. Radiol Med 121:38–44

Vincent SA, Anderson PA (2018) The unstable spine: a surgeon's perspective. Semin Ultrasound CT MR 39(6):618–629

Wang XD, Feng MS, Hu YC (2019) Establishment and finite element analysis of a three-dimensional dynamic model of upper cervical spine instability. Orthop Surg 11(3):500–509

2 MRI in Degenerative Disease of the Spine

Degenerative spinal pathology is one of the most common causes of pain in society. Degenerative disease of the spinal column is highly prevalent in the general population, and its incidence increases with age.

Pain is the main symptom among those individuals most commonly associated with this pathologic condition; others are neurologic disorders (i.e. sensory, motor, neurovegetative dysfunctions).

Different factors, both individually and concomitantly, can result in degenerative processes of the spine, such as mechanical (e.g. postural anomalies, heavy weight-bearing, sports), anatomic (e.g. malformations, dysplasias) and metabolic factors (e.g. diabetes).

The lumbar spine is most frequently involved; up to 70–80% of people have low back pain during their life-time [1].

It is understood that only a certain number of patients with back pain will be found to have a disc herniation, spinal stenosis or well-known causes of pain; in the other cases, it may be difficult to discover the source of pain. It is equally well understood that the syndrome may arise from the posterior elements/perispinal tissues of the lumbar spine, which are richly innervated [2–4].

The diagnostic techniques of computed tomography (CT) and magnetic resonance imaging (MRI) have made an important contribution to the study of degenerative diseases of the spinal column. In particular, MRI provides a very sensitive method for examining degenerative phenomena of the spine, even in the initial stages of the disease lifetime [1–3, 5–9].

However, traditional MRI of patients with low back pain does not always enable clear identification of pain aetiology. In our experience, T2-weighted sequences with fat saturation and, when indicated, T1-weighted sequences with fat saturation after intravenous administration of contrast medium provide a more sensitive picture of the degenerative changes of the spinal column and occasionally disclose pathologic conditions unsuspected during a "standard" MRI examination [1–3, 5].

All the patients in this series were examined with a 1.5 T MR system (Siemens Symphony TIM) by using the following basic study protocol:

- TSE/SE T1-weighted images on the sagittal plane (and axial plane on the lumbosacral spine)
- TSE T2-weighted images with fat saturation on the sagittal plane
- TSE T2-weighted images with fat saturation on the axial plane (eventually to be conducted on the pathologic area, for a better spatial characterization of the oedematous lesion)
- GE T2*-weighted images on the axial plane on the cervical spine
- TSE/SE T1-weighted images with FS on the sagittal and axial planes following administration of contrast medium (eventually to be conducted to identify the active inflammatory stage of the disease)

An efficient spinal imaging protocol must comprise T2-weighted sequences with fat suppression, in particular with fat saturation technique or STIR sequences, in order to clearly visualize hyperintensity corresponding to oedematous lesions, otherwise not easily identifiable with "standard" imaging sequences without fat suppression (Fig. 2.1).

In the same way, administration of contrast medium must be followed by T1 sequences with fat saturation, in order to clearly identify the active inflammation.

The indication for contrast medium administration was based on evidence of osteo-articular or muscular ligamentous oedema in T2-weighted images with fat saturation. In some selected cases, we administered contrast medium although the basic scan failed to disclose oedematous lesions on T2-weighted images (e.g. in cases of clinical-radiological discrepancy).

In this series, we administered intravenous paramagnetic contrast medium (Dotarem—Guerbet—0.5 mmol/mL, 0.2 mL/kg dose).

P. D'Aprile, A. Tarantino, *MRI of Degenerative Disease of the Spine*, https://doi.org/10.1007/978-3-030-73707-8_2

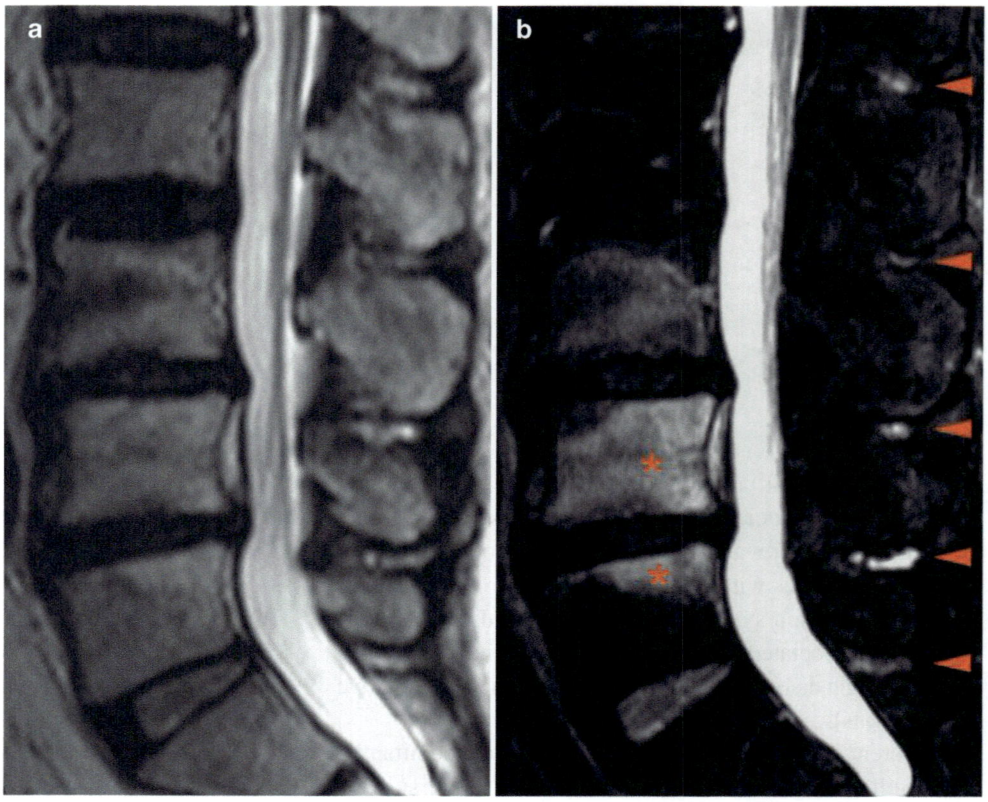

Fig. 2.1 (**a**, **b**) "Standard" sagittal TSE T2-weighted image without fat saturation (**a**) and sagittal TSE T2-weighted image with fat saturation (**b**). Hyperintense areas in fat-suppressed T2-weighted image in the L3-L4-L5 vertebral bodies, indicating oedema of the bone marrow (**b**, *asterisks*). Note that the sequence without fat saturation does not detect the same lesions in the same way (**a**). Note also hyperintense lesions of the interspinous ligaments in T2-weighted images with fat saturation (**b**, *arrowheads*). The same lesions cannot be defined in T2-weighted image without fat saturation (**a**)

The fat saturation technique consists of a spectral saturation of the fat, by adding a selective radiofrequency (RF) impulse on the fat frequency. To determine the fat frequency, the machine checks for the presence of approximately a 130-Hz peak, as compared with the resonance frequency of water, at which point it emits the RF impulse. The effect of the impulse is to excite the fat over 180°, whereby it will be unable to return the signal. Such a technique enables the saturation of the fat signal on almost all of the available sequences, from spin-echo to gradient-echo, using any type of MRI sequence (T1, T2, T2*).

We have to remember that fat signal can be suppressed also by using STIR sequences, but, in our experience, this technique has a long acquisition time, whereas FS technique substantially does not change the relative acquisition time.

Today, the correct diagnosis is important in effecting improved aeration outcomes: it will be reflected in an elevated benefit/cost ratio with regard to MRI and will enable more accurate therapy of the specific source of painful symptoms (e.g. microinvasive percutaneous treatment).

In this text-atlas, we deal with the following degenerative spinal changes, with particular attention on corresponding inflammatory aspects: disc degeneration, disc herniation, facet joint pathology (e.g. osteoarthritis, joint effusion, synovitis and synovial cysts), spondylolysis, canal stenosis, spinal/perispinal ligamentous degenerative inflammatory changes and perispinal muscular changes. Moreover, we show some unusual clinical cases.

2.1 Disc Degeneration

Discs are commonly the primary element of the spine that manifest degenerative alterations. As with every occurrence of arthrosis, such degenerative phenomena are largely due to genetics, long-term heavy weight-bearing and other complex factors.

From the morphological standpoint, disc degeneration results in loss of height, radial bulging, fissuring of the annulus fibrosus and disc herniation; moreover, degenerative disc alterations are typically accompanied by morpho-structural changes of the adjacent vertebral bodies (e.g. spondylosis and osteochondrosis).

These degenerative phenomena, and associated inflammatory component, are clinically important as they are associated with nonirradiating (discogenic) pain, caused by stimulation of the nerve terminals innervating the disc-vertebral body complex [4, 5] (Fig. 2.2).

MRI clearly depicts such degenerative phenomena to a superior degree than other imaging modalities. Among other findings, the degenerated disc demonstrates a reduction in signal intensity on T2-weighted images (principally due to dehydration processes and variations in proteoglycan composition) and a decrease in height; in the more advanced stages of degeneration, the disc collapses and may undergo cystic changes, gaseous degeneration and calcification.

Discal degenerative processes are usually accompanied by bone marrow changes in the supravertebral and subjacent

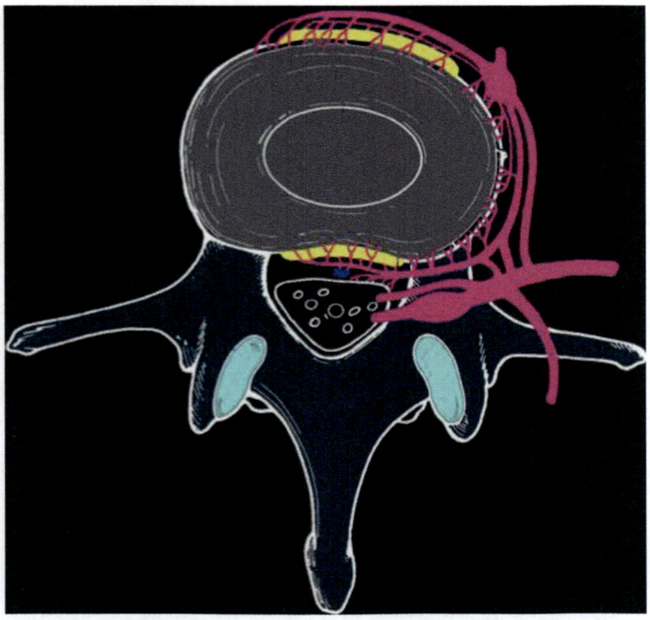

Fig. 2.2 Schematic figure depicting the rich innervation of the disc-vertebral body complex. (Modified from Jinkins)

vertebral bodies, which are currently classified as the following [10]:

Type I—fibrovascular replacement of the bone marrow
Type II—proliferation of the fatty marrow
Type III—osteosclerosis

In our experience, Type I alterations are more evident on T2-weighted images with fat saturation, since the suppression of the fat signal enhances the fibrovascular transforming phenomena and underlying bone marrow oedema. In addition, the use of T1-weighted sequences with fat saturation after administration of contrast medium frequently shows enhancement of this same bone marrow in parallel with the bone oedema (this event is normally marked in "traditional" T1-weighted sequences after contrast medium administration).

It is sometimes possible to detect contrast enhancement of the adjacent intervertebral disc, with or without associated disc changes; in our opinion, this finding can be named as "aseptic" or "sterile" discitis, of a degenerative nature [1, 5].

2.2 Disc Herniation

Disc herniation is one of the most common diseases, with very high social costs; it is the first cause for absenteeism from work and the main cause for surgery on the spine [11].

Herniated disc arises from the rupture of the annulus fibrosus and subsequent leakage of nucleus pulposus beyond the margins of the same annulus.

The aetiology of disc herniation includes degenerative disc disease, repeated trauma and genetic factors [9].

Symptoms of disc herniation originate from compression of nerve roots and/or spinal cord, depending on the level and position of the hernia.

In particular, radicular pain is caused by mechanical compression, inflammatory effects, vascular and biochemical modifications caused by the contact between the disc and nerve root [11].

Patients affected by herniated disc many times begin a diagnostic and therapeutic route involving neurosurgeons, orthopaedics, neurologists and physiatrists.

Diagnosis involves the collection of anamnestic data, physical examination, diagnostic imaging (MRI, CT) and electromyography.

MRI represents the gold standard diagnostic technique, exquisitely delineating disc herniation and the relationship to adjacent soft tissues.

It is important to describe the precise location of the herniated disc. The relationship of the disc material to surrounding structures should also be mentioned in describing a disc herniation.

The hallmark of a herniated disc is a focal contour abnormality along the disc margin, with a soft tissue mass displacing the epidural fat, thecal sac or nerve root. The herniated disc is usually contiguous with the corresponding disc by a narrow waist, which is the site of a radial tear in the annulus [9]. In some cases, a free disc fragment can develop, that is, no longer in continuity with the parent disc and can migrate inferior or superior to the parent disc level.

Unusual MR findings include atypical signal intensity or uncommon location. Some herniated discs present different signal intensity with respect to the disc parent, showing high signal intensity on T1- or T2-weighted images.

Unusual locations include extraforaminal or atypical migratory disc patterns. Sometimes disc herniation occurs completely outside the canal (e.g. the so-called far lateral herniation); rarely disc fragments are sequestered posterior to the thecal sac.

It is well known that contrast-enhanced MRI has a major role in the examination of the operated spine (i.e. diagnosis of recurrent hernia versus postoperative scar). Disc material usually does not enhance, showing peripheral contrast enhancement due to granulation tissue, whereas epidural scar demonstrates intense and homogeneous enhancement.

Contrast-enhanced MRI has a more limited use in the routine examination of the unoperated spine; however, a situation exists where the administration of contrast medium is valuable and should be considered. In particular, contrast-enhanced images are helpful in the following cases of differential diagnosis: foraminal herniated disc versus nerve sheath tumour, intense peridiscal inflammatory response that can mimic infections and in some situations of clinical-radiological discrepancy.

In all cases, an efficient imaging protocol must comprise fat-saturated T2-weighted sequences (in order to detect oedematous lesions) and, in selected cases, contrast-enhanced T1-weighted sequences with fat saturation (in order to detect inflammatory components of the lesions or clarify diagnostic doubts).

2.3 Canal Stenosis

Canal stenosis consists of narrowing of the central spinal canal, lateral recesses, neural foramina or a combination of these locations. This condition can be congenital or acquired or result from a combination of both factors.

Acquired (degenerative) causes are multiple: disc bulges or herniations, spondylosis, marginal osteophytes, facet joint arthrosis, calcification of the ligamenta flava and spondylolisthesis.

Stenosis is also documented after surgical procedures as a result of exuberant degeneration [11].

The lumbar and cervical regions are most commonly affected.

Symptoms of canal stenosis depend on the compression of the spinal cord or nerve roots, including pain, numbness, muscle weakness and problems with bladder or bowel function.

Typical symptoms of lumbar stenosis are neurogenic claudication, with inability of the patient to walk long distance and with sensation of heavy legs and progressive lack of strength [11].

CT and MRI with axial acquisitions allow to accurately measure the amplitude of the canal, both central and lateral.

2.4 Facet Joint Pathology (Joint Effusion, Synovitis, Synovial Cysts, Osteoarthritis)

Typical degenerative changes of the zygapophyseal joints include erosion of the articular cartilage associated with joint space narrowing, periarticular hyperostosis with osteophyte formation, subchondral bone changes (e.g. eburnation, erosion, cysts), joint subluxation (i.e. with consequent joint space widening and anterior/posterior degenerative spondylolisthesis) and soft tissue changes (e.g. joint effusion, thickening/calcification of the ligamenta flava, facet joint synovial cyst formation) [2, 8, 9].

We underline that these posterior spinal structures are richly innervated primarily, although not solely, from the dorsal rami of the spinal nerves (Fig. 2.3) [4], so justifying the painful symptomatology.

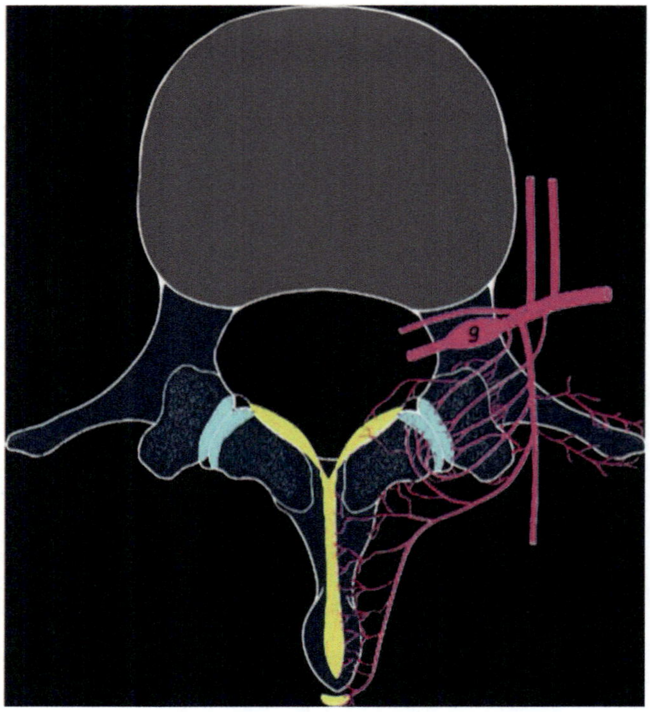

Fig. 2.3 Schematic figure depicting the rich innervation of the posterior vertebral compartment, arising from the dorsal branch of the spinal nerve (g = spinal ganglion). (Modified from Jinkins)

Facet joint changes are easily recognized with standard MRI sequences. However, by using T2-weighted sequences with fat saturation and, when indicated intravenous contrast medium administration, it is possible to uncover additional otherwise occult potentially clinically pertinent findings. For example, T2-weighted sequences enable the clear, unambiguous visualization of joint effusions, subchondral bony changes (e.g. marrow oedema) and periapophyseal soft tissue changes (e.g. oedema/sterile inflammation). Contrast media administration further confirms the presence and extent of such inflammatory-degenerative phenomena. Isolated contrast enhancement of the synovial surfaces may be termed synovitis; contrast enhancement of the subchondral bone in association with the typical osteoarthritic degenerative alterations may be termed osteoarthritis; periapophyseal contrast enhancement may be defined as periapophyseal soft tissue degenerative inflammatory reaction [2].

With regard to posterior spinal facet joint synovial cysts, such degenerative alterations may extend into the spinal canal or alternatively may have a posterior perispinal/extraspinal soft tissue location [2, 6–8]. Intraspinal synovial cysts can extend into the central spinal canal and/or into the spinal neural foramen, where they may respectively encroach on the thecal sac/cauda equina or upon the exiting spinal nerve and therefore can be the source of radicular pain or spinal claudication.

Extraspinal synovial cysts develop postero-inferiorly to the corresponding posterior spinal facet joint. Their clinical manifestation is controversial; logically, the symptomatology probably arises from degenerative changes of the corresponding facet joint, including the neurologically competent synovium; these posterior perispinal/extraspinal soft tissue synovial cysts obviously will not impinge upon major neurologic structures [2].

Such synovial cysts may not be detectable if T2 sequences with fat saturation are not acquired. Synovial cysts may or may not reveal a thin rim of enhancement after the intravenous injection of gadolinium, enhancement perhaps indicating the presence of an inflammatory component.

The pathogenesis of synovial cysts is linked to degenerative joint disease likely associated with joint effusion and elevation of intra-articular pressure; combined with kinetic weight-bearing manoeuvres, the joint fluid theoretically creates a sudden or chronic progressive expansion of the synovial surface into the form of an aneurismal sac. Naturally, most or all of these synovial cysts communicate with the adjacent facet joint. Histologically, these cysts may be lined by synovial tissue (i.e. true synovial cysts) or not lined with synovium (i.e. neocysts or pseudocysts lined by fibrous tissue) [2, 6, 7].

2.5 Spondylolysis

Spondylolysis is a fracture of the pars interarticularis. The pathogenesis of this alteration is believed to involve repeated microfractures of the pars, eventually resulting in a permanent defect. The pars lesion becomes bridged by a fibrocartilaginous bar and may develop into a pseudarthrosis; occasionally, bony union of a pars defect occurs [12].

In some cases, especially those without spondylolisthesis, visualization of the pars defect may be difficult to detect on T2-weighted imaging without fat saturation, and intravenous contrast medium-enhanced images permit clear recognition of these "hidden" fractures [2]. In particular, in the acute-inflammatory phase, areas of T2 hyperintensity and contrast enhancement appear in the region of the pars interarticularis defect, pedicle and occasionally within the immediately adjacent soft tissues. These changes persist for months to years and are presumably a reaction of the bone marrow and soft tissues to increased local mechanical stresses.

2.6 Spinal/Perispinal Ligamentous Degenerative Inflammatory Changes

The ligaments of posterior vertebral compartment, and in particular the interspinous ligaments together with the related adjacent spinous processes and perispinous soft tissues, are thought to be a possible source of low back pain [2, 13–15]. These osseous and ligamentous tissues may undergo extensive degenerative inflammatory alteration. Sudden trauma may induce an acute interspinous ligament sprain, with minor or major/complete tears of the ligamentous fibres; chronic repetitive microtrauma occurring during normal daily activities results in progressive degenerative changes of these structures [16].

According to the published literature, the fundamental factors responsible for chronic progressive interspinous injury include the following: variable but normal hyperlordosis of the spinal segments at and suprajacent to the lumbosacral junction, with consequent bony collision of the opposed vertebral spinous processes (i.e. Baastrup's phenomenon) and injury of the intervening interspinous ligament [6, 7, 13, 14], and collapse of the intervertebral disc, with resultant narrowing of the respective interspinous space, collision of the spinous processes and injury of the interposed interspinous ligament [6, 7]. Such ligamentous degenerative changes may occur before, simultaneously with or following iso-segment intervertebral disc degeneration; furthermore, this may occur with only minor hyperlordosis.

Degenerative phenomena of the spinal ligaments has been evaluated histologically, biochemically and by MRI [15, 17–21]. Histologic examination may show varied degenerative changes in the interspinous ligaments: fragmentation and necrosis of the fibre bundle, proliferation of cells and vessels, fibrous inflammatory exudates, formation of pseudocystic cavities (i.e. formation of interspinous bursae), cartilaginous metaplasia and synovial metaplasia. These changes explain the variability of MRI signal in the region of the interspinous ligaments that may be either iso- or hyperintense on T1- and T2-weighted images and which frequently demonstrate contrast enhancement. In some cases, these ligamentous changes are not detectable on T2-weighted imaging using fat saturation, but only after the administration of intravenous contrast medium coupled with fat-saturated T1-weighted acquisitions [2].

Based upon published reports, there seems to be no specific terminology for these MRI/pathologic changes of the interspinous ligaments. Some authors use the definition of "interspinous bursitis" [8]. We think that the term bursitis should be applied only in the presence of an interspinous *pseudo-bursae* or pseudocysts (i.e. lined by fibrous tissue), which are related to interspinous pseudarthrosis and which demonstrate rim enhancement after the administration of intravenous contrast medium within the fibrous walls of the pseudocyst cavity. Actually, it is possible to find bursae that do not show contrast enhancement and ligaments without bursae that show contrast enhancement, so we prefer to distinguish between degenerative (i.e. no enhancement) and degenerative inflammatory (i.e. enhancement) changes of the spinal ligaments [2].

These ligamentous changes may present clinically with focal midline lumbar tenderness and pain on palpation as well as upon extension or flexion manoeuvres; such pain typically can be relieved by local anaesthetic/steroid injections. However, although low back pain has been attributed to these interspinous alterations, clinical significance of the above-mentioned findings is controversial, as similar changes may be observed in asymptomatic individuals. In our experience, contrast enhancement of the ligaments corresponds generally to local painful symptomatology. Upright, weight-bearing and dynamic kinetic MRI of the spine may also be helpful in the clinical-radiological correlation of such ligamentous pathology [22].

Chronic degenerative inflammatory changes may involve not only the interspinous ligaments but also the supraspinous ligaments and the ligamenta flava; in many instances, several or all of these structures are involved, at one level or at multiple levels.

2.7 Muscular Changes

Occasionally, in patients with low back pain, MRI detects alterations of the intrinsic posterior perispinal lumbosacral muscles (e.g. interspinalis, multifidus muscles).

It is possible to postulate that three-dimensional lumbar intersegmental hypermobile instability, exceeding the normal range of motion, may predispose and precipitate various pathologic degenerative muscular alterations, including spasm, sprain, inflammation and acute-subacute degeneration [2]. These changes can be caused by either one or both of two mechanisms related to neuromuscular autotrauma: rupture-avulsion of the intrinsic spinal muscles or traumatic denervation of the nerves supplying the intrinsic spinal muscles (i.e. rupture-avulsion of the medial branch of the dorsal ramus of the spinal nerve) [16, 23].

MRI clearly visualizes the above-mentioned muscular alterations. In particular, T2-weighted images with fat saturation show hyperintensity of the perispinal muscular tissue, otherwise not identifiable with standard imaging sequences without fat suppression; typically, these same muscle fibres showed enhancement after the intravenous administration of contrast medium.

Such muscular changes may be directly (e.g. intrinsic spinal muscle sprain/rupture) or indirectly (e.g. intrinsic spinal muscle spasm) involved in the pathogenesis of low back pain. It is possible to find a close clinical-radiological correlation between the anatomic distribution of pain and the perispinal muscle alterations as visualized by MRI. In some patients with low back pain, these changes may be the only abnormal finding on MRI.

References

1. D'Aprile P, Tarantino A, Strada A et al (2002) Potenzialità delle sequenze Fat Suppression e del Gadolinio nello studio RM della patologia degenerativa lombare. Riv Neuroradiol 15:679–697
2. D'Aprile P, Tarantino A, Jinkins JR et al (2007) The value of fat saturation sequences and contrast medium administration in MRI of degenerative disease of posterior/perispinal elements of the lumbosacral spine. Eur Radiol 17:523–531
3. Tarantino A, D'Aprile P et al (2003) Syndrome da low back pain. Sequenze RM Fat Saturation e Gadolinio nello studio del compartimento posteriore del rachide lombare. Riv Neuroradiol 16(Suppl 1):265–266
4. Jinkins JR (2004) The anatomic and physiologic basis of local, referred and radiating lumbosacral pain syndromes related to disease of the spine. J Neuroradiol (Paris) 31:163–180
5. D'Aprile P, Tarantino A, Lorusso V et al (2006) Fat saturation technique and gadolinium in MRI of lumbar spinal degenerative disease. Neuroradiol J 19:654–671
6. Jinkins JR (2002) Acquired degenerative changes of the intervertebral segments at and supradjacent to the lumbosacral junction. Riv Neuroradiol 15:359–392
7. Jinkins JR (2004) Acquired degenerative changes of the intervertebral segments at and supradjacent to the lumbosacral junction: a radioanatomic analysis of the nondiscal structures of the spinal column and perispinal soft tissues. Eur J Radiol 50:134–158
8. Wybier M (2001) Imaging of lumbar degenerative changes involving structures other than disk space. Radiol Clin N Am 39(1):101–114
9. Czervionke LF, Haughton VM (2002) Degenerative disease of the spine. In: Atlas SW (ed) Magnetic resonance imaging of the brain and spine, vol II, 3rd edn. Lippincott, Philadelphia, PA, pp 1633–1713
10. Modic MT, Steinberg PM, Ross JS et al (1988) Degenerative disk disease: assessment of change in vertebral body marrow with MRI. Radiology 166:193–199
11. Scarabino T, Pollice S (2014) Imaging spine after treatment. A case-based atlas. Springer, Milan
12. Ulmer JL, Elster AD, Mathews VP, Allen AM (1995) Lumbar spondylolysis: reactive marrow changes seen in adjacent pedicles on MR images. AJR Am J Roentgenol 164:429–433
13. Baastrup CI (1933) On the spinous processes of the lumbar vertebrae and the soft tissue between them and on pathological changes in that region. Acta Radiol 14:52–54
14. Baastrup CI (1936) Le 'lumbalgo' et les affections radiologiques des apophyses épineuses des vertèbres lombaires, de la 1 re vertèbre sacrèe et des parties interepinéuses. J Radiol Electrol 20:78–93
15. Fujiwara A, Tamai K, An HS et al (2000) The interspinous ligament of the lumbar spine. Magnetic resonance images and their clinical significance. Spine 25(3):358–363
16. Jinkins JR (2002) Lumbosacral interspinous ligament rupture associated with acute intrinsic spinal muscle degeneration. Eur Radiol 12:2370–2376
17. Rissanen PM (1962) "Kissing-spine" syndrome in the light of autopsy findings. Acta Orthop Scand 32:132–139
18. Bywaters EGL (1979) Lesions of bursae, tendons and tendon sheaths. Clin Rheum Dis 5:883–925
19. Goobar JE, Sartorius DJ, Hajeck PC et al (1987) Magnetic resonance imaging of the lumbar spinous processes and adjacent soft tissues: normal and pathologic appearances. J Rheumatol 14:788–797
20. Sartoris DJ, Resnick D, Tyson R, Haghighi P (1985) Age-related alterations in the vertebral spinous processes and intervening soft tissues: radiologic-pathologic correlation. AJR Am J Roentgenol 145:1025–1030
21. Yahia H, Drouin G, Maurais G et al (1989) Degeneration of the human lumbar spine ligaments: an ultrastructural study. Pathol Res Pract 184:369–375
22. Jinkins JR, Dworkin JS, Damadian RV (2005) Upright, weight-bearing, dynamic-kinetic MRI of the spine: initial results. Eur Radiol 15(9):1815–1825
23. Fleckenstein JL, Chason DP (1999) Skeletal muscles. In: Stark DD, Bradley WG (eds) Magnetic resonance imaging. Mosby, St. Louis, MO, pp 1057–1077

Suggested Readings

Clarençon F, Law-Ye B, Bienvenot P et al (2016) The degenerative spine. Magn Reson Imaging Clin N Am 24(3):495–513

Gallucci M, Limbucci N, Paonessa A et al (2007) Degenerative disease of the spine. Neuroimaging Clin N Am 17(1):87–103

Hansen BB, Nordberg CL, Hansen P et al (2019) Weight-bearing MRI of the Lumbar Spine. Spinal Stenosis and Spondylolisthesis. Semin Musculoskelet Radiol 23(6):621–633

Khalatbari K, Ansari H (2008) MRI of degenerative cysts of the lumbar spine. Clin Radiol 63(3):322–328

Mann E, Peterson CK, Jürg Hodler J et al (2014) The evolution of degenerative marrow (Modic) changes in the cervical spine in neck pain patients. Eur Spine J 23(3):584–589

Parizel PM, Van Hoyweghen AJL, Bali A et al (2016) The degenerative spine: pattern recognition and guidelines to image interpretation. Handb Clin Neurol 136:787–808

Sheng-yun L, Letu S, Jian C et al (2014) Comparison of modic changes in the lumbar and cervical spine, in 3167 patients with and without spinal pain. PLoS One 9(12):e114993

Splendiani A, Bruno F, Marsecano C et al (2019) Modic I changes size increase from supine to standing MRI correlates with increase in pain intensity in standing position: uncovering the "biomechanical stress" and "active discopathy" theories in low back pain. Eur Spine J 28(5):983–992

MRI in Postoperative Spine

3

3.1 Surgery

Surgery in degenerative disease of the spine is used when conservative management fails. Main indications to surgery are the following: discal hernia, spinal canal stenosis, spondylolisthesis, post-discectomy syndromes. It is important to point out that surgery should be done only in case of real indication, with minimal invasiveness.

The two most common surgical approach in spine degenerative pathology are: decompression for the treatment of herniated disc and stabilization/fusion.

Decompression surgery consists of removing part of the bone and disc material over the suffering nerve root. Traditional techniques are microdiscectomy and discectomy, both carried out in order to solve the compression and delete the discal material that triggers the inflammatory process responsible for the pain.

Microdiscectomy consists of full or partial removal of the nucleus pulposus with the aid of the surgical microscope. Standard discectomy instead involves open air full or partial removal of the herniated nucleus pulposus.

Decompressive surgery is performed by the following three main techniques: laminotomy (bone resection limited to small segments of the adjacent laminae), laminectomy (resection of the entire lamina), facetectomy (resection of part or full facet joint).

Laminectomy may be either unilateral or bilateral; in the latter case, it involves excision of both laminae and the spinous process. Laminectomy is generally performed in cases when removal of larger disc material is necessary or to treat central canal or lateral recess stenosis. The addition of complete or partial facetectomy to a laminectomy is primarily done when there is nerve root compression necessitating access to the neural foramen; however, overexcision of the facet joint can lead to instability and spondylolisthesis, so it is paramount to leave as much of the facet joint as possible [1–3].

Surgical approaches for decompressive procedures vary widely and are categorized depending on the direction from which the spine is approached (posterior, anterior, lateral). The posterior approach is most often used, due to an optimal access to the posterior vertebral elements, spinal canal and intervertebral disc.

The second most common surgical approach in spine degenerative pathology is represented by stabilization/fusion. Spinal stabilization and fusion procedures are used to stabilize the spine, maintain or improve alignment or replace removed osseous or soft tissue structures of the spine. This can be done for a variety of reasons, including recurrent disc disease, spondylolisthesis, stenosis [3].

These procedures can be performed with traditional approach (known as fusion surgery) or with more recent dynamic stabilization (non-fusion surgery) [4–6].

Spinal fusion consists of fusion of two or more adjacent vertebral bodies after removal of the intervertebral disc, in order to stop the motion at a painful vertebral segment, stabilizing the spine and maintaining anatomic alignment.

Spinal fusion involves the insertion of a bone graft of bone graft substitute between two adjacent vertebral bodies, with or without any material in the space left by disc removal. Bone graft stimulates growing of new bone to fuse the opposing vertebral bodies. Bone fusion occurs within 4–5 months after surgery. Before fusion, some devices are used to provide stability of that spine segment. Devices commonly used are rods and plates, cross bars, translaminar or facet screws, transpedicular screws, interbody and interspinous spacers [6, 7].

The most common hardware used in posterior spinal fusion are rods in combination with either lateral mass screws in the cervical spine or transpedicular screws in the thoracic and lumbar spine. The screws traverse the lateral mass or pedicle, entering the lateral aspect of the vertebral body anteriorly. The screws should not extend into the spinal canal or neural foramen, and they should not protrude anterior to the ventral aspect of the vertebral body cortex.

Interbody spacers are solid or open structures placed in the intervertebral disc space after discectomy to promote fusion, maintain alignment and provide spinal column

P. D'Aprile, A. Tarantino, *MRI of Degenerative Disease of the Spine*, https://doi.org/10.1007/978-3-030-73707-8_3

support. Spacers can be composed of titanium, carbon fibre, polyetheretherketone and are often filled with bone graft material to further promote osseous fusion between vertebral bodies. Most spacers contain radiopaque markers for better evaluation of their position on imaging. Although placement of the spacer may be different depending on the patient and product, a general rule is that a posterior marker located approximately 2 mm anterior to the posterior cortex of the adjacent vertebral body indicated good position [1, 3–5].

Disc arthroplasty consists of removal of the intervertebral disc and replacement with an artificial disc that contains core material, such as polyethylene between two metal plates that are attached to the adjacent vertebral bodies. Disc arthroplasty is designed to allow motion and provide cushioning similar to a healthy disc [3, 5, 8].

Interspinous devices, also known as "interspinous spacers" or "dumping devices", are used for the treatment of low back pain and sciatic pain originated from degenerative disc disease, facet joints disease, segmental instability, central spinal canal stenosis and foraminal stenosis. Interspinous devices mainly used are X-stop, DIAM, Wallis, Viking, Coflex, Ellipse, In Space [5–7].

Rational use of interspinous devices, positioned between the spinous processes, is based on reduction of load on disc and facet joints, increasing disc space height and foraminal height, widening of the central spinal canal, thereby decreasing epidural pressure and nerve root compression (Figs. 3.1 and 3.2).

Implantation of interspinous devices is less invasive than disk arthroplasty or conventional fusion. The procedure leaves both anterior and posterior longitudinal ligaments intact and, in some cases, also part of interspinous and supraspinous ligaments remains intact. This surgery substantially does not have any risk. Specific complications are fracture of spinous processes, implant migration, infection and dural injury.

In case of symptomatic cervical degenerative disc disease and herniation, the most common surgical treatment is the anterior cervical discectomy with intervertebral fusion. In this case, the removal of cervical disc herniation is done through an anterior approach, followed by disc removal, canal decompression, anterior vertebral fusion with insertion of bone graft into the evacuated disc space [6, 9, 10].

This approach has several advantages for both the surgeon (good access to the spine through an uncomplicated pathway) and the patient (less incisional pain). Moreover, chance of recurrent hernia is little because most of the disc is removed [6].

Surgical complications can be infections and nerve root/spinal cord damage.

There may be a recurrence or a fibrous scar that can compress and irritate the affected nerve root and require a second operation (the risk of reoperation is around 3–15%) [6]. Moreover, with the lack of disc, the supradjacent and subadjacent discs work harder, increasing risk of other hernias.

3.2 Imaging

Failed Back Surgery Syndrome (FBSS) is a generalized term used to describe varied spinal symptoms of patients who have had unsuccessful results after spinal surgery. FBSS is a fairly common problem encountered in neurosurgical practice. This syndrome is characterized by recurrent or residual back pain after spinal surgery and has a reported incidence of 5–40% [1, 11].

FBSS has a wide spectrum of causes. The common causes include residual/recurrent disc herniation, epidural fibrosis or postoperative scarring, infection, arachnoiditis, mechanical instability following surgery, spinal stenosis and surgery at the wrong level.

Imaging plays a crucial role in postoperative spine, allowing a precise identification of causes and guiding the appropriate therapy.

Plain radiographs can be used to assess the alignment of the spine, positioning of devices, implant fractures, changes in the bone implant, so they have a role both in immediate postoperative period and in follow-up (Fig. 3.3). X-rays must be executed in antero-posterior and lateral-lateral views, eventually in oblique position. Dynamic radiographs in flexion and extension provide information about instability. Obviously, X-rays are not helpful to evaluate soft tissues and discs.

CT with multiplanar and 3D reconstructions can accurately show bony details, vertebral alignment, instrumentation and implant alignment (Fig. 3.4). CT cannot reliably differentiate residual disc from scar tissue. Moreover, beam-hardening artifacts caused by metallic devices limit evaluation of adjacent soft tissues. The radiation dose should also be taken into account. With these considerations, CT should be used only for targeted examination and specific indications [3].

Currently, MR is the imaging modality of choice in postoperative spine, in the evaluation of patients with persisting or recurrence of pain with characteristics similar or different than previous surgery. MR allows, by virtue of its known peculiarities (high sensitivity, multi-parametric, high contrast spatial resolution, simultaneous display of containing and contained), a correct diagnosis and therefore precise therapeutic indications. The treatment of FBSS is challenging and varies from conservative management to reoperation.

MRI is ideal for soft tissue sensitivity, but it is known that metal devices cause magnetic field disturbances, leading to artifacts which complicate image interpretation. Metal artifacts reduce image quality by causing anatomical distortion,

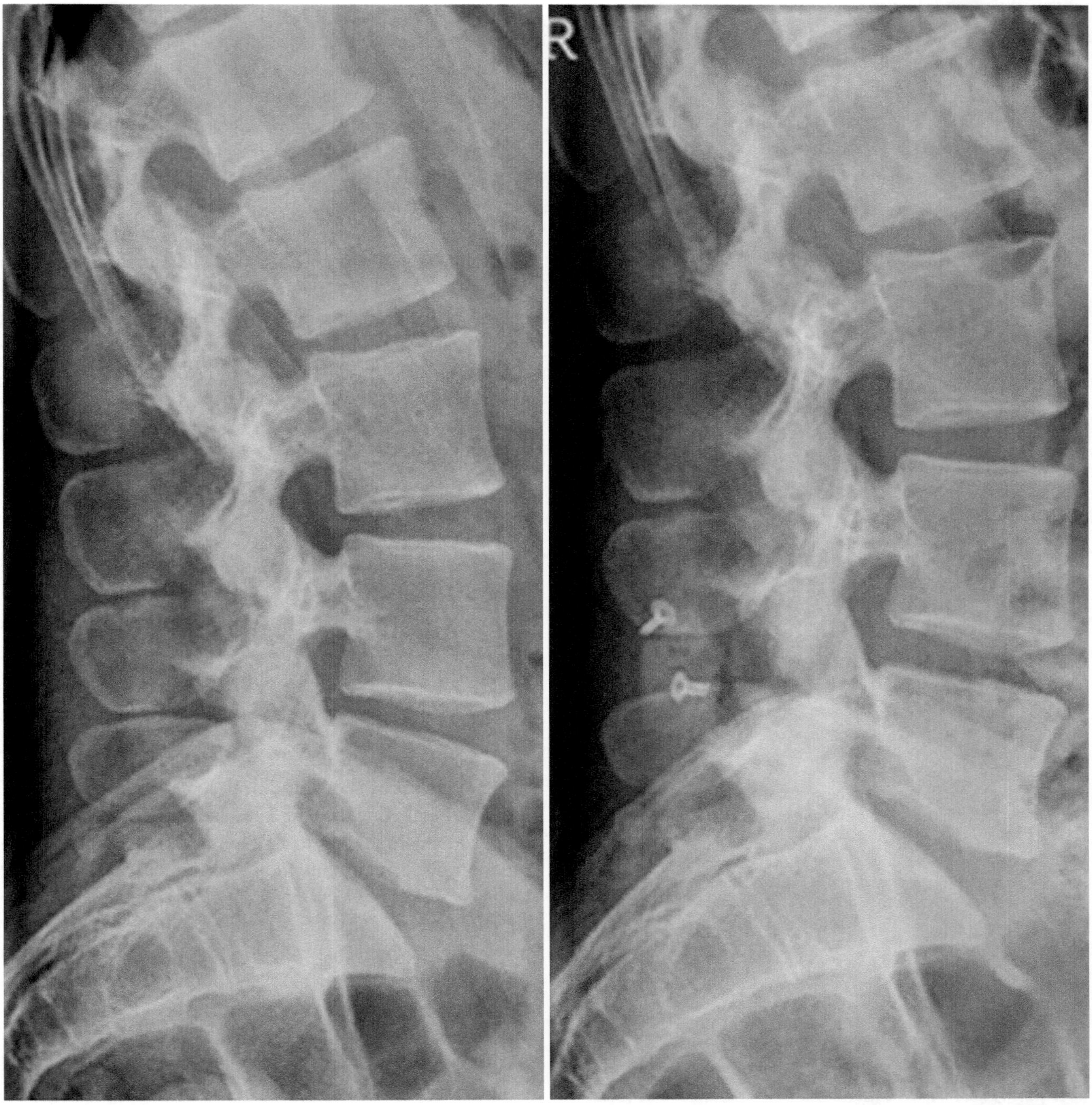

Figs. 3.1 and 3.2 Lateral radiograph of the lumbar spine before and after positioning of interspinous device at L4/L5. Postoperative RX shows widening of the same interspinous space

signal loss and inhomogeneous fat suppression. These artifacts present as signal voids surrounded by a peripheral rim of high signal intensity, following the shape of a device.

Artifacts by ferromagnetic material, in the past often present and able to affect imaging quality, are currently less evident thanks to new synthesis material (titanium display relatively mild artifacts, while stainless steel displays severe artifacts) and to the use of particular MR sequences less sensitive to magnetic susceptibility (e.g. Fast SE, Turbo SE). Therefore, they no longer represent an obstacle or a contraindication to MRI examination [6, 12–16].

Post-surgery MR examination does not differ significantly from a basic study including conventional sagittal and axial T1- and T2-weighted images (e.g. TSE, FSE) shortly affected by artifacts caused by metal or any other surgical material used [6].

In case of metallic devices (clips, stabilizers, prostheses), SE and GE sequences should be avoided because particularly

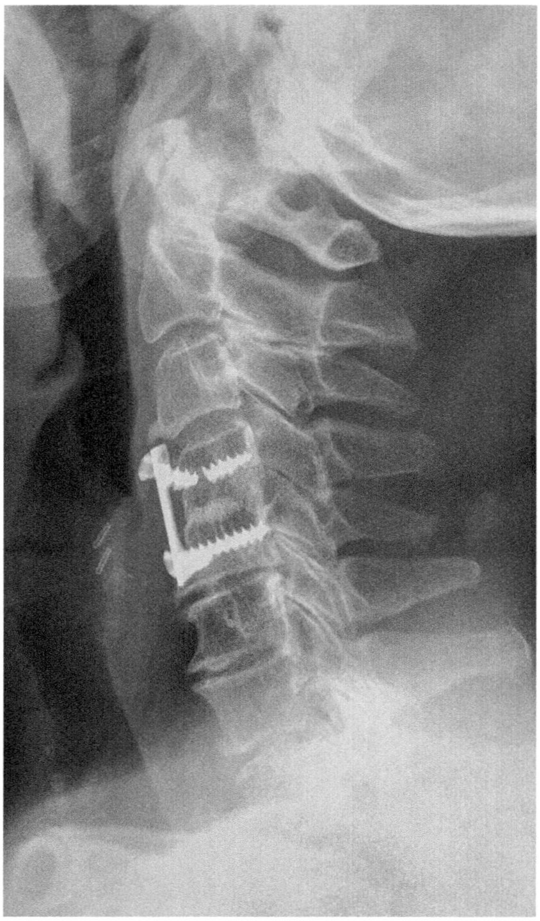

Fig. 3.3 Lateral radiograph of the cervical spine. Fusion and stabilization at C4/C5, with breakage of the upper screw

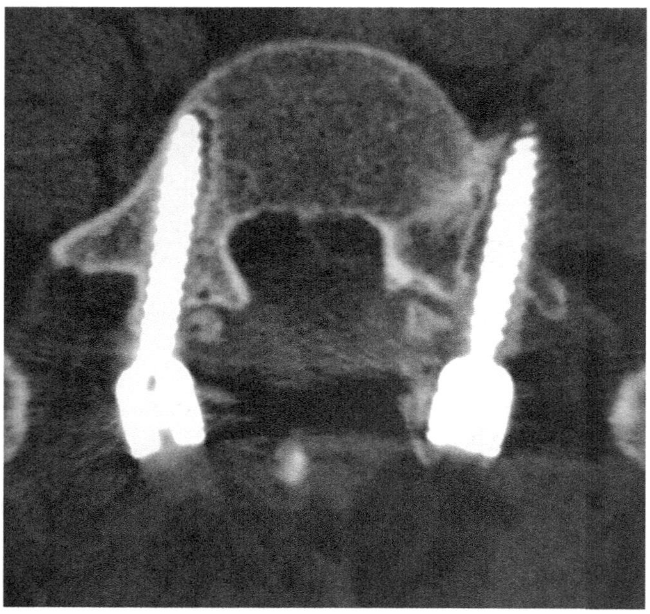

Fig. 3.4 Lumbar axial TC image. Laminectomy and stabilization with pedicle screws at L5. The left screw protrudes beyond the lateral margin of the vertebra. There is also bilateral periprosthetic osteolysis

sensitive to magnetic susceptibility [6, 17] (Figs. 3.5, 3.6, and 3.7).

An efficient MR study protocol must comprise fat-suppressed T2-weighted sequences, in particular with fat saturation technique or STIR sequences, in order to clearly visualize hyperintensity corresponding to oedematous lesions, otherwise not easily identifiable with "standard" imaging sequences without fat suppression.

In case of post-surgery MR examination, there is indication to the administration of contrast medium, in order both to identify the active inflammation and make differential diagnosis between herniated disk recurrence and scarring phenomena. Also in this case, contrast medium administration must be followed by T1-weighted sequences with fat saturation, to best emphasize pathology within spinal or epidural adipose tissue.

We have to underline that fat saturation technique is sensitive to magnetic field inhomogeneity and vulnerable to susceptibility and metallic artifacts.

Imaging of the spine in the early postoperative period should be done with particular attention. First of all, there are some "normal" changes of MR signal after uncomplicated discectomy. In the early postoperative period, there is normal contrast enhancement of the post discectomy disc space, vertebral endplates, perispinal muscles, facet joints and the nerve roots.

In particular, intervertebral disc can appear hypointense in T1 and hyperintense in T2 with associated disruption of the annulus fibrosus. A thin linear contrast enhancement of the disc, paralleling the endplates and converging within the posterior annulus at the site of curettage, is an expected finding after discectomy: this finding is named "mechanical or chemical discitis". Occasionally, after discectomy, moderate signal changes of the adjacent subchondral spongiosa may occur, with hypointensity in T1, hyperintensity in T2 and mild contrast enhancement, in relation to oedema: this finding is named aseptic spondylodiscitis.

All these findings, not associated with increase of inflammatory markers, do not have pathological significance and gradually resolve over a period of 4–5 weeks and in any case no later than 6 months [1, 3, 17–19].

In early postoperative period, another possibility to consider is that mass effect from postsurgical oedema and haemorrhage may efface the thecal sac, simulating disc herniation.

As above mentioned, in the 2 months after discectomy, persistence of symptoms arising from compression on roots and dural sac can be related to residual or recurrent hernia and/or exuberant scar, so this is generally the most frequent differential diagnosis.

Studies indicate that disc herniation is responsible for 7–37% of cases of FBSS [11, 20, 21]. Usually, discal hernia causes mass effect, nodularity, impression on the dural sack

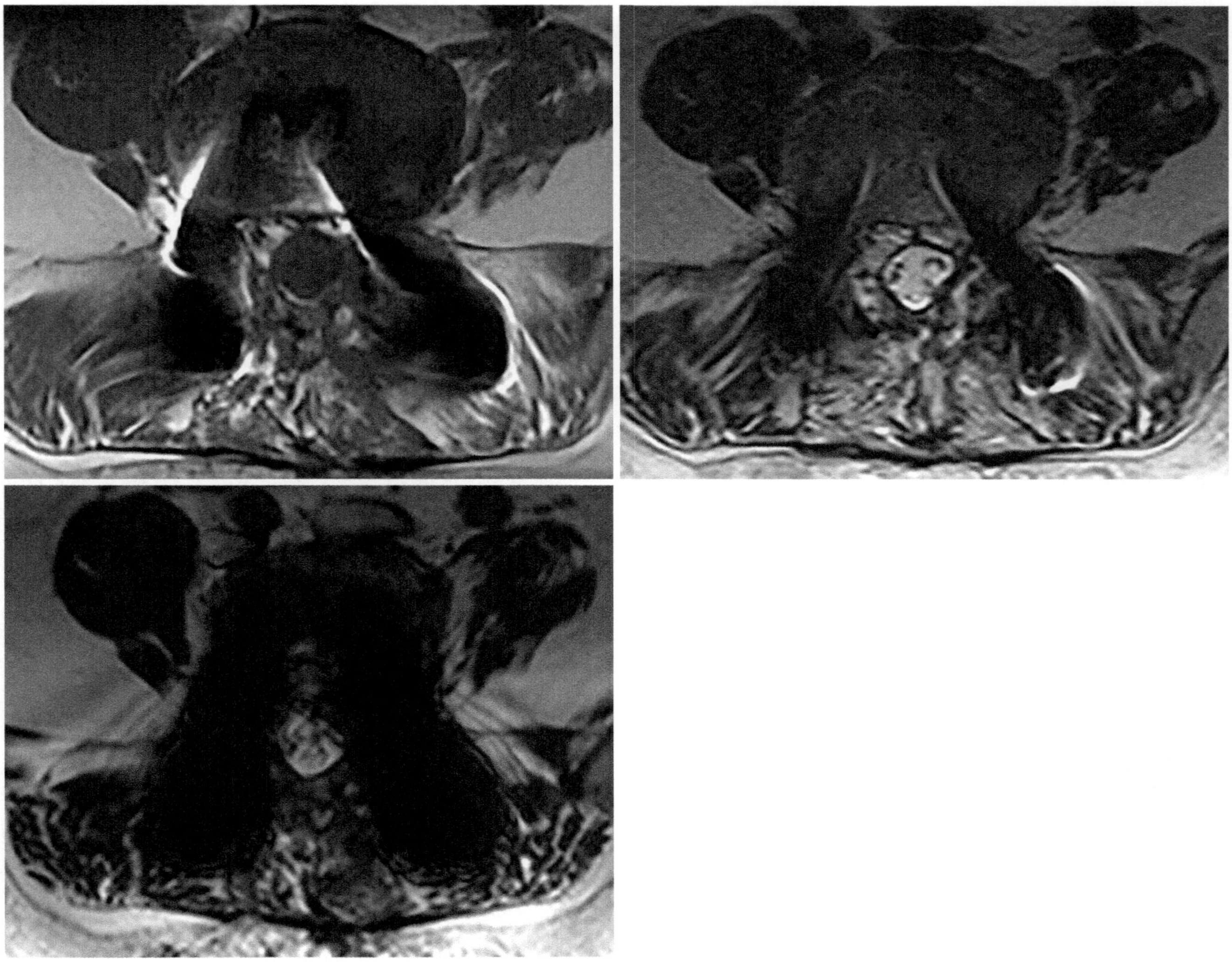

Figs. 3.5–3.7 Axial TSE T1-weighted image, axial TSE T2-weighted image, axial GE T2*-weighted image. Laminectomy, interbody spacer and pedicle screws. Note artifacts due to metallic devices that are more marked in GE T2*-weighted image than in TSE images

without dural traction, generally in continuity with the corresponding disc. There is no early contrast enhancement for lack of vascularization; sometimes, early peripheral contrast enhancement with delayed central diffusion due to the presence of granulation tissue can be found; in later phase (1 month), contrast enhancement can occur for a diffusion mechanism.

Conversely, surgical scar more often lacks mass effect, has linear configuration, there is dural traction and contiguity with the disc. However, exuberant scar tissue can surround the dural sac with possible compression mechanism. Contrast enhancement is early, intense and diffused thanks to neoangiogenesis; the trend is to significantly disappear at least after 1 year [6, 22, 23]. Therefore, contrast-enhanced MR images acquired within 7–10 min are important for differential diagnosis. However, some degree of epidural scarring occurs after all laminectomies and discectomies.

Complications of surgery are spondylodiscitis, radiculitis, arachnoiditis, CSF fistula, haematoma, seroma, meningoceles.

Postoperative spondylodiscitis has been reported in up to 3% of patients in various series [1, 11, 24]. More rarely isolated discitis or spondylitis may occur.

Generally, these infectious complications present at short time after surgery with recurrence of pain, fever, increase of inflammatory markers.

MR examination shows signal changes in the disc and subchondral bone (T1 hypointensity, T2 hyperintensity and contrast enhancement), with possible involvement of the spinal canal and perivertebral soft tissues.

Abscess may develop, alone or associated with spondylodiscitis. It is constituted by a fluid collection in the epidural space or perivertebral soft tissues. Typically, abscess is characterized by T2-hyperintensity and delineated by peripheral contrast enhancement. Diffusion-weighted imaging can also be helpful, demonstrating reduced diffusion.

Radiculitis can be a cause of residual or recurrent symptoms after lumbar surgery. It is characterized by abnormal contrast enhancement of nerve roots on MR imaging, secondary to temporary damage of the blood–nerve barrier caused by surgery or chronic compression before surgery. Nerve root enhancement in the immediate postoperative period may be a normal finding. Enhancement of 6 months after surgery is considered pathologic [25].

Arachnoiditis consists of inflammation of the arachnoid meninges and subarachnoid space. Although arachnoiditis may develop throughout the subarachnoid space, it is generally seen in the lumbar region where the cauda equina floats in ample CSF, thus justifying the well-known denomination of spinal/lumbar adhesive arachnoiditis.

As a result of inflammation, the nerve roots become adherent to each other and to the thecal sac. Three resultant morphological patterns have been described on the basis of imaging [26]:

- Type I: nerve roots are clumped together and distorted.
- Type II: nerve roots are adherent to the theca resulting in an empty thecal sac sign.
- Type III: nerve roots and theca are clumped together into a single soft tissue mass centrally within the spinal canal.

Lumbar spine arachnoiditis can result in leg pain, sensory changes and motor weakness.

Epidural hematoma may be a result of excessive intraoperative bleeding. A neurological deterioration may occur for compression mechanism, thus requiring decompression [27]. MR signal is variable in relation to the various stages of haemoglobin degradation.

Seromas are sterile cyst paraspinal collections, typically with CSF-like MR signal. Sterile fluid collections evolve slowly over time and usually resolve by 6 weeks; however, their appearance can be mistaken for infection because peripheral enhancement can occur [3]. Diffusion-weighted imaging can be helpful because seromas do not present restricted diffusion.

Meningoceles are CSF collections communicating with the subarachnoid space caused by arachnoid herniation through the surgical dural breach. Pseudomeningocele is an extrameningeal collection communicating with the subarachnoid space through a fistula. Both meningocele and pseudomeningocele may extend outside and inside the vertebral canal.

References

1. Van Goethem JW, Parizel PM, Jinkins JR (2002) MRI of the postoperative lumbar spine. Neuroradiology 44:723–739
2. Eliyas JK, Karahalios D (2011) Surgery for degenerative lumbar spine disease. Dis Mon 57(10):592–606
3. Eisenmenger L, Clark AJ, Shah VN (2019) Postoperative spine. What the surgeon wants to know. Radiol Clin N Am 57: 415–438
4. Murtagh RD, Quencer RM, Castellvi AE et al (2011) New techniques in lumbar spinal instrumentation: what the radiologist needs to know. Radiology 260(2):317–330
5. Rutherford EE, Tarplett LJ, Davies EM et al (2007) Lumbar spine fusion and stabilization: hardware, techniques and imaging appearances. Radiographics 27(6):1737–1749
6. Scarabino T, Pollice S (2014) Imaging spine after treatment. A case based atlas. Springer, Milan
7. Hunter TB, Yoshino MT, Dzioba RB et al (2004) Medical devices of the head, neck and spine. Radiographics 24:257–285
8. Thakkar RS, Malloy JP, Thakkar SC et al (2012) Imaging the postoperative spine. Radiol Clin N Am 50(4):731–747
9. Hernandez R, Neroni M, Fiore C et al (2001) Cervical arthrodesis with interbody fusion titanium cages for cervical degenerative disease. Acta Medica Romana 39:383–394
10. Kim K, Isu T, Morimoto D et al (2012) Cervical anterior fusion with the Williams-Isu method: clinical review. J Nippon Med Sch 79:37–45
11. Dhagat PK, Jain M, Sing SN et al (2017) Failed back surgery syndrome: evaluation with magnetic resonance imaging. J Clin Diagn Res 11(5):TC06–TC09
12. Lee MJ, Kim S, Lee S et al (2007) Overcoming artifacts from metallic orthopedic implants at high-field-strength MR imaging and multi-detector CT. Radiographics 27(3):791–803
13. Petersilge CA, Lewin JS, Duerk JL et al (1996) Optimizing imaging parameters for MR evaluation of the spine with titanium pedicle screws. AJR 166:1213–1218
14. Rudish A, Kremser C, Peer S et al (1998) Metallic artifacts in MR imaging of patients with spinal fusion. A comparison of implants materials and imaging sequences. Spine 23:629–639
15. Viano AM, Gronemeyer SA, Haliloglu M et al (2000) Improved MR imaging for patients with metallic implants. Magn Reson Imaging 18:287–295
16. Tartaglino LS, Flanders AE, Vinitski S et al (1994) Metallic artifacts on MR images of the postoperative spine: reduction with fast spin echo techniques. Radiology 190:565–569
17. Splendiani A, D'Orazio F, Patriarca L et al (2017) Imaging of postoperative spine in intervertebral disc pathology. Musculoskelet Surg 101(suppl 1):S75–S84
18. Sahin N, Sargin S, Atik A (2015) Failed back surgery: a clinical review. Int J Orthop 2(5):399–404
19. Katayama Y, Matsuyama Y, Yoshihara H et al (2006) Comparison of surgical outcomes between macrodiscectomy and microdiscectomy for lumbar disc herniation: a prospective randomized study with surgery performed by the same spine surgeon. J Spinal Disord Tech 19:344–347
20. Slipman CW, Shin CH, Patel RK et al (2002) Etiologies of failed back surgery syndrome. Pain Med 3:200–214
21. Waguespack A, Schofferman J, Slosar P, Reynolds J (2002) Etiology of long-term failures of lumbar spine surgery. Pain Med 3:18–22
22. Gallucci M, Caulo M, Masciocchi C (2001) Il rachide operato. In: Dal Pozzo G (ed) Compendio di Risonanza Magnetica. Utet Ed, Torino, pp 1047–1071
23. Ross JS, Obuchowski N, Zepp R (1998) The postoperative lumbar spine: evaluation of epidural scar over a 1year period. AJNR 19:183–186
24. Hayashi D, Roemer FW, Mian A et al (2012) Imaging features of postoperative complications after spinal surgery and instrumentation. AJR 199:123–129

25. Lee YS, Choi ES, Song CJ (2009) Symptomatic Nerve Root Changes on Contrast-Enhanced MR Imaging after Surgery for Lumbar Disk Herniation. AJNR 30(5):1062–1067
26. Kunam VK, Velayudhan V, Chaudhry ZA et al (2018) Incomplete cord syndromes: clinical and imaging review. Radiographics 38(4):1201–1222
27. Leonardi MA, Zanetti M, Saupe N et al (2010) Early postoperative MRI in detecting hematoma and dural compression after lumbar spinal decompression: prospective study of asymptomatic patients in comparison to patients requiring surgical revision. Spine J 19:2216–2222

Part II

Clinical Cases

4 Osteochondrosis, Osteochondritis

Case 1: Osteochondrosis

- A 44-year-old man
- Persistent low back pain
- Limitation of motion of the spine

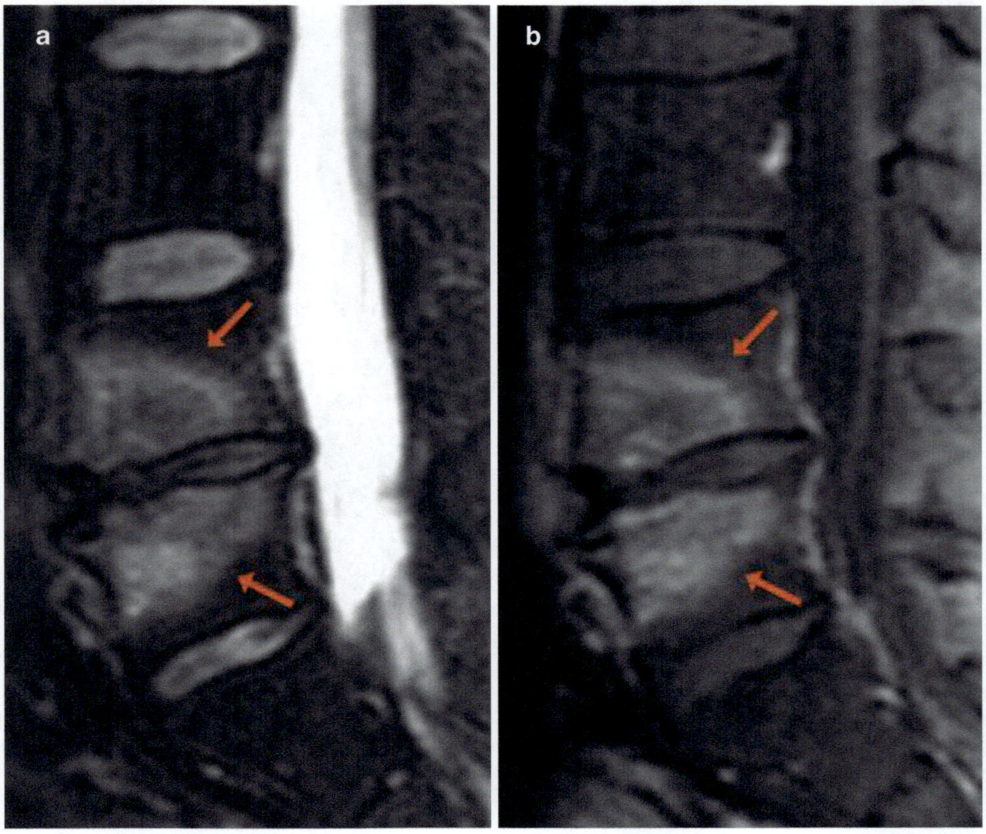

Fig. 1 (**a**, **b**) Sagittal TSE T2-weighted image with fat saturation (**a**) and sagittal SE T1-weighted image with fat saturation following administration of contrast medium (**b**). The opposing L4 and L5 vertebral bodies present hyperintense areas on T2-weighted imaging (**a** *arrows*), with enhancement after contrast medium administration (**b** *arrows*). Reduction in height of the corresponding L4/L5 intervertebral disc. Diagnosis: osteochondrosic degeneration in active inflammatory phase, with fibrovascular transformation of the bone marrow (Modic Type I)

P. D'Aprile, A. Tarantino, *MRI of Degenerative Disease of the Spine*, https://doi.org/10.1007/978-3-030-73707-8_4

Case 2: Osteochondrosis

- A 73-year-old woman
- Patient with persistent back pain that worsens in upright position and with movements

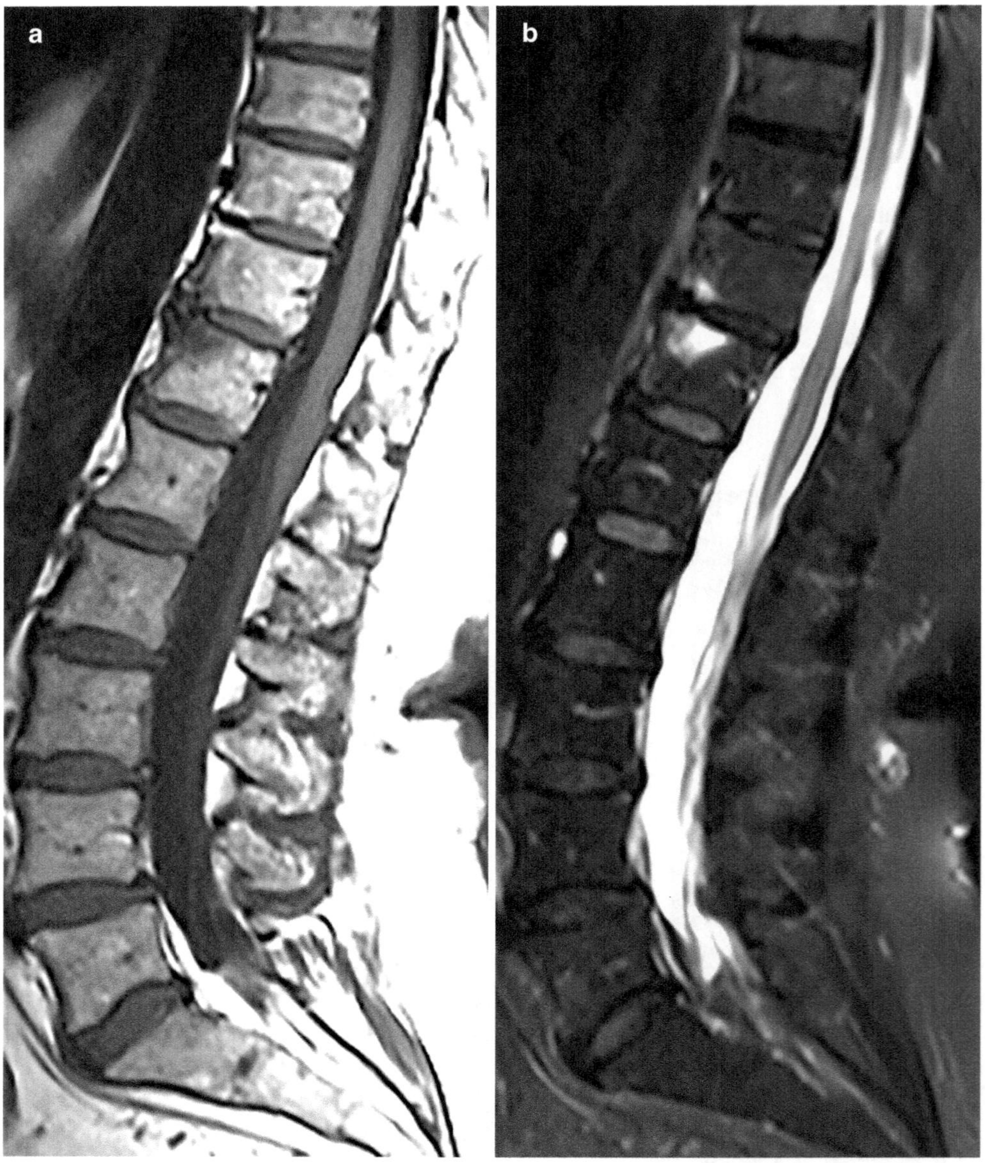

Fig. 2 (**a**, **b**) Sagittal TSE T1-weighted image (**a**), sagittal TSE T2-weighted image with fat saturation (**b**). Areas of hypointensity in T1 and hyperintensity in T2 in the opposite anterior corners of the vertebral bodies D11/D12. These alterations develop at the point of maximum load of the dorsal-lumbar spine, suggesting a degenerative mechanical pathogenesis. Diagnosis: osteochondrosis in active inflammatory phase

Case 3: Osteochondrosis

- A 44-year-old woman
- Patient with persistent back pain, more marked during prolonged upright position

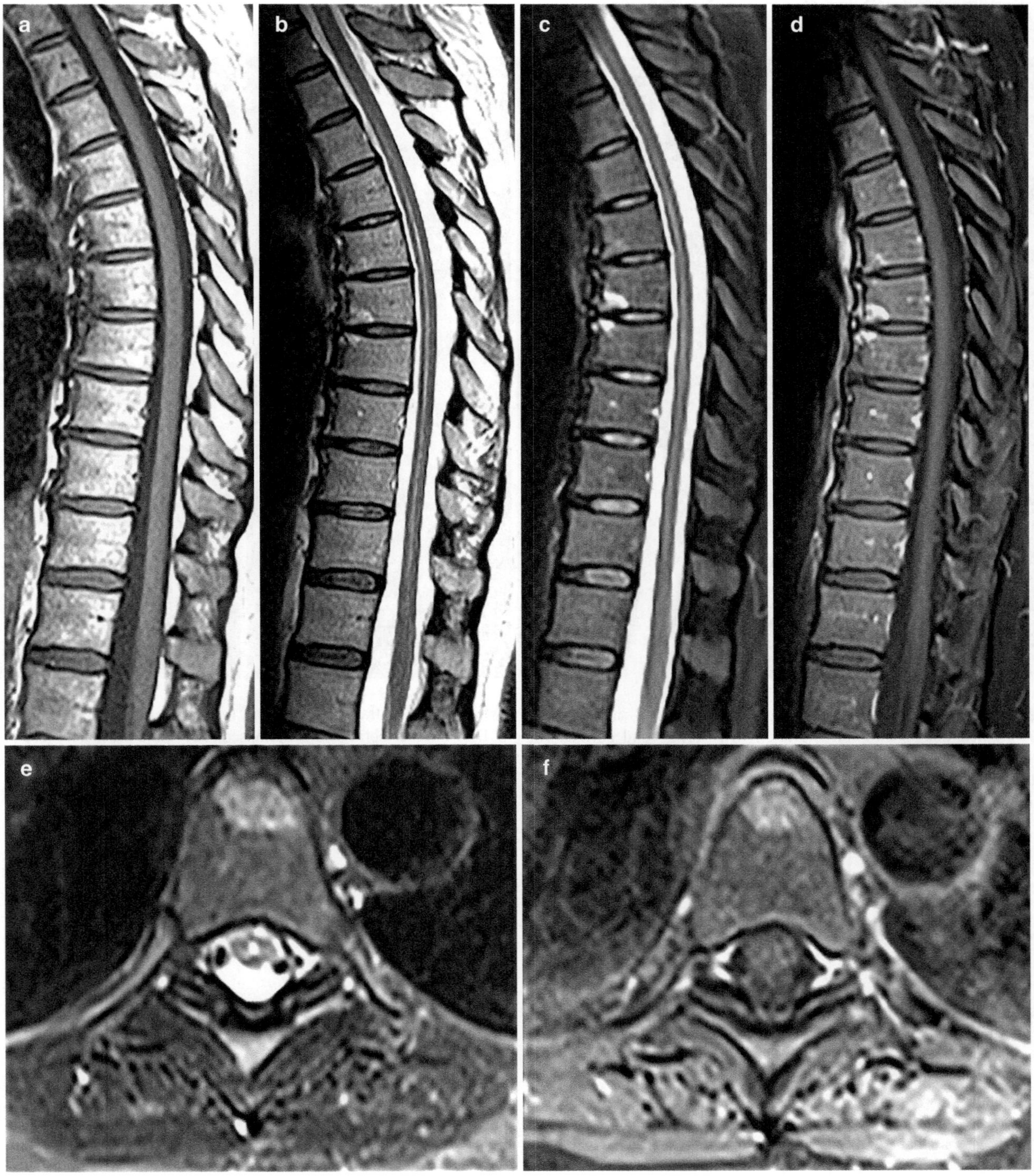

Fig. 3 (**a**–**f**) Sagittal TSE T1-weighted image (**a**), sagittal TSE T2-weighted image (**b**), sagittal and axial TSE T2-weighted images with fat saturation (**c**, **e**), sagittal and axial TSE T1-weighted images with fat saturation after administration of contrast medium (**d**, **f**). The opposite anterior corners D7/D8 show hyposignal in T1 (**a**), hypersignal in T2 (**b**, **c**, **e**), with contrast enhancement (**d**, **f**). Diagnosis: osteochondrosis in inflammatory phase. Note that these alterations develop at the apex of kyphosis, that is the point of maximum load of the patient, supporting the degenerative pathogenesis of the lesions

Case 4: Osteochondrosis

- A 32-year-old woman
- Chronic low back pain
- Limitation of motion of the spine in the frontal and lateral planes

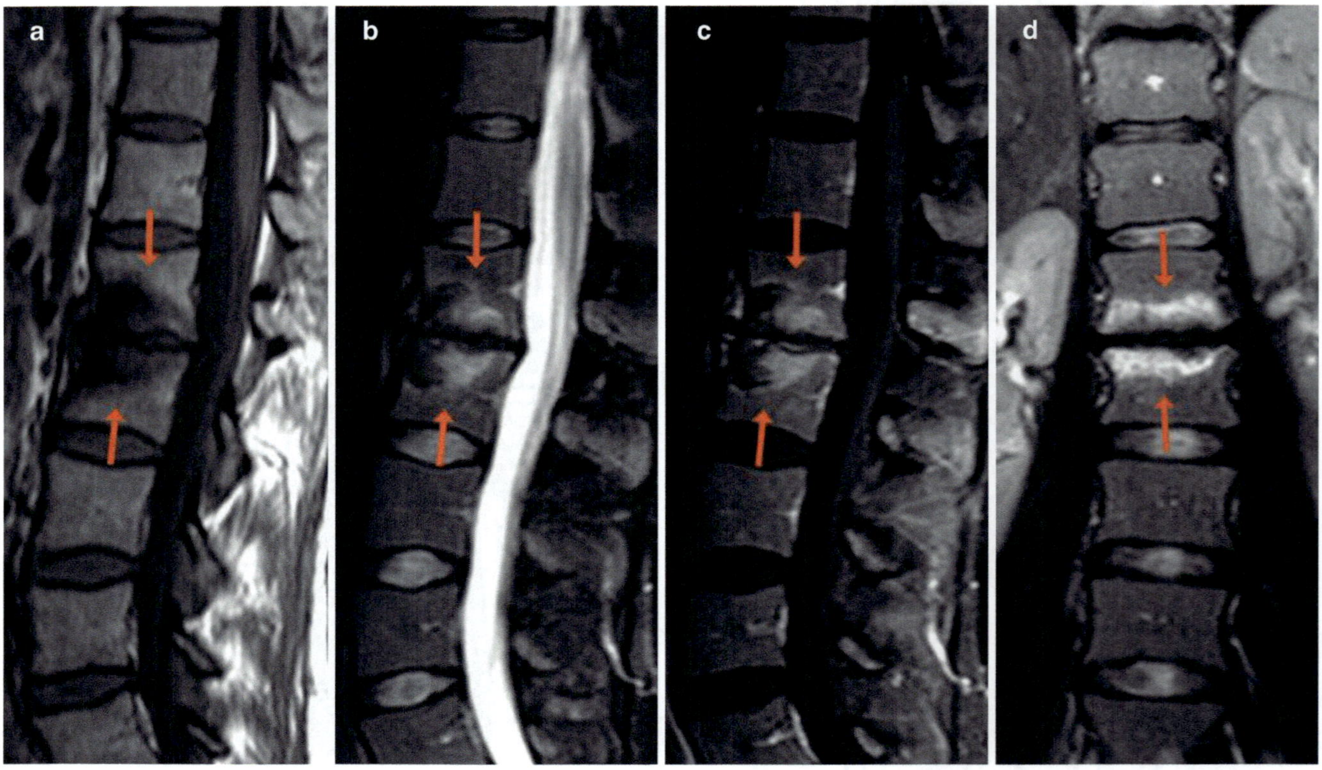

Fig. 4 (**a–d**) Sagittal SE T1-weighted image (**a**), sagittal TSE T2-weighted image with fat saturation (**b**), sagittal and coronal SE T1-weighted images with fat saturation after contrast medium administration (**c**, **d**). The opposing L1/L2 vertebral bodies show hypointense signal in T1 (**a**, *arrows*) and hyposignal/hypersignal in T2 (**b**, *arrows*), with partial contrast enhancement (**c**, **d**, *arrows*). The corresponding L1/L2 intervertebral disc is collapsed. The spine presents a loss of the physiological curve at the same level. Diagnosis: osteochondrosis in active inflammatory phase

Fig. 5 (**a–h**) Coronal TSE T2-weighted image (**a**), coronal, sagittal and axial TSE T2-weighted image with fat saturation (**b–d**, **g**, **h**), sagittal TSE T1-weighted images (**e**, **f**). Lumbar scoliosis, convex to the right (**a**, **b**). Osteochondrosic degeneration at L2/L3 on the left side and L4/L5 on the right side, in active inflammatory phase (**a–h**)

Case 5: Osteochondrosis

- A 56-year-old man
- Patient with chronic low back pain

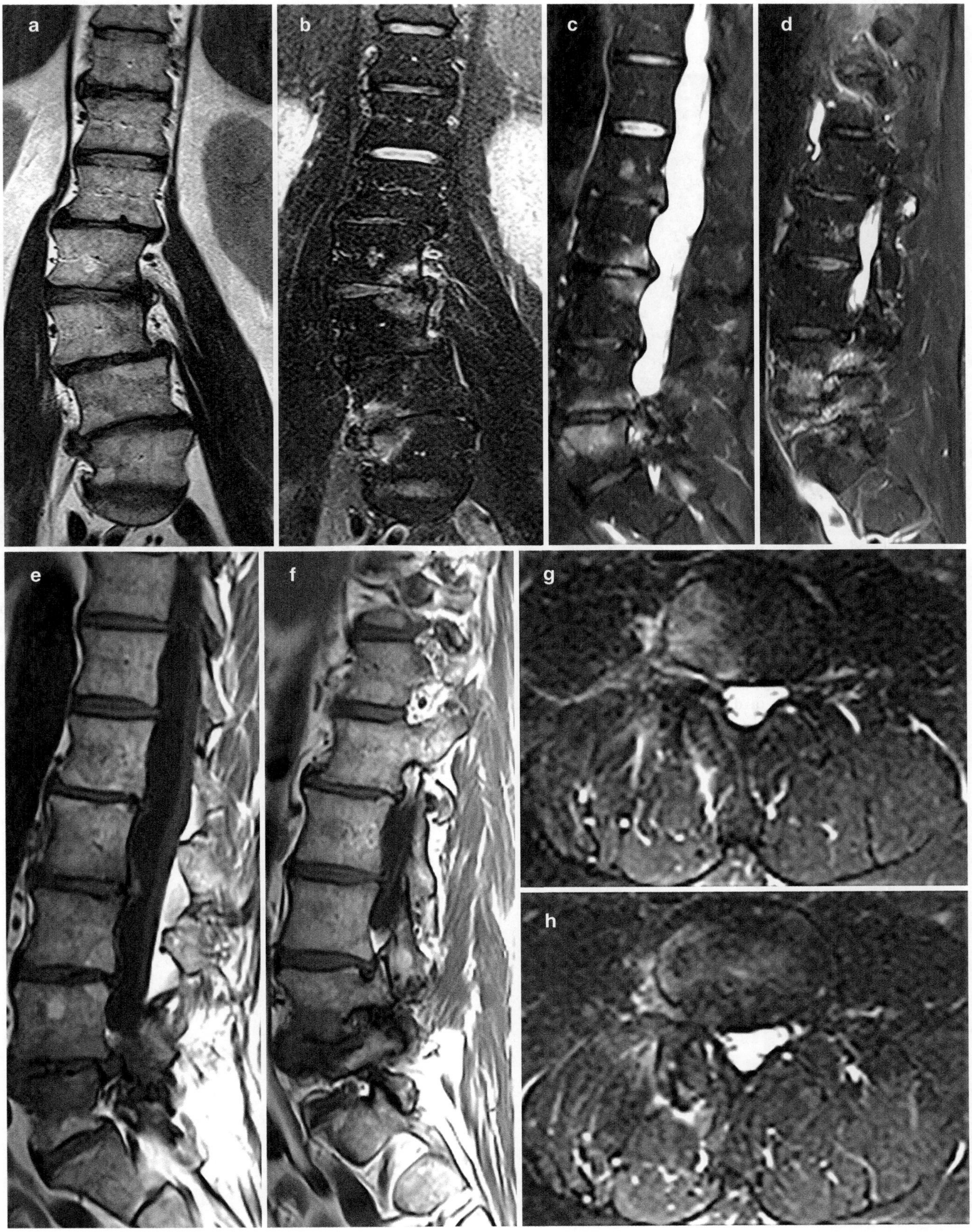

Case 6: Osteochondritis

- A 51-year-old woman
- Chronic low back pain

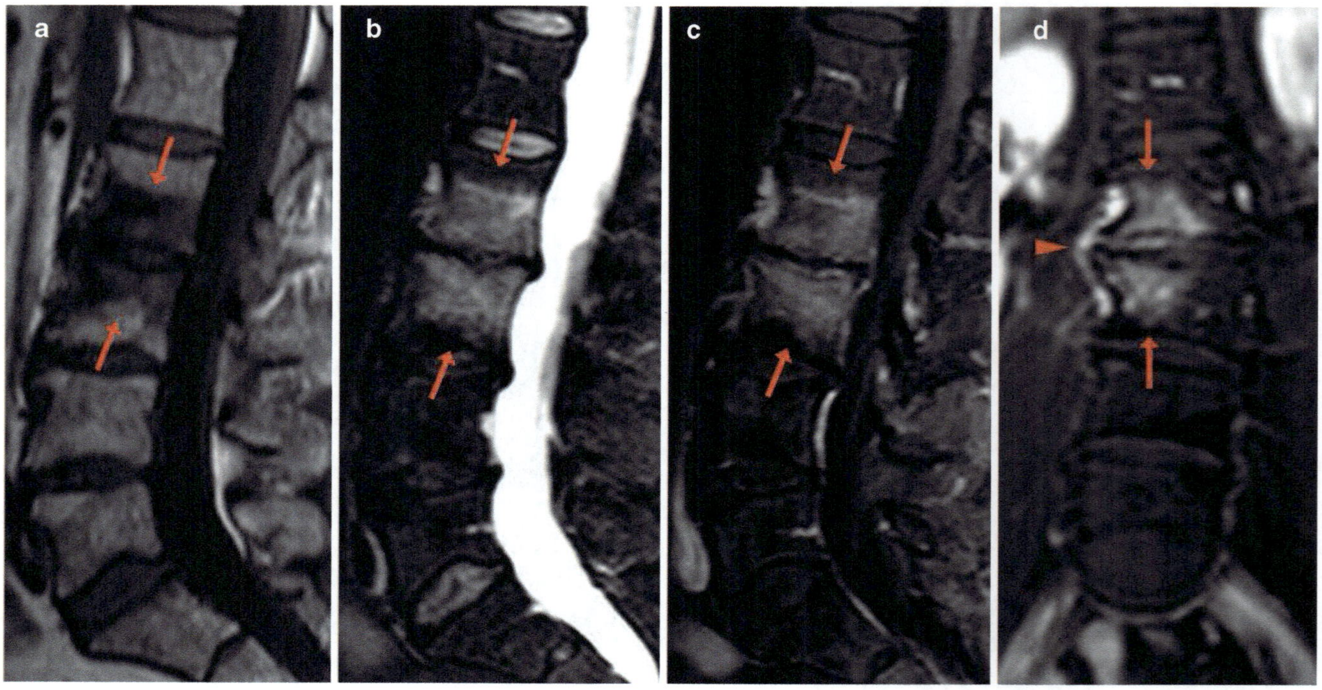

Fig. 6 (**a–d**) Sagittal SE T1-weighted image (**a**), sagittal TSE T2-weighted image with fat saturation (**b**), sagittal and coronal SE T1-weighted images with fat saturation after administration of contrast medium (**c**, **d**). Typical osteochondritis at L2/L3, with oedematous pattern of the subchondral bone, and contrast enhancement of the same areas and articular surfaces (**a–d**, *arrows*). Left-convex scoliosis (**d**). Note that signal changes develop on the right side of the intervertebral joint, corresponding to the point of greatest joint load in the scoliotic spine. Note also periarticular contrast enhancement on the right side at L2/L3 (**d**, *arrowhead*), indicating an aseptic reactive inflammation of the periarticular soft tissues

Case 7: Osteochondritis

- A 48-year-old woman
- Chronic low back pain
- Improvement with rest

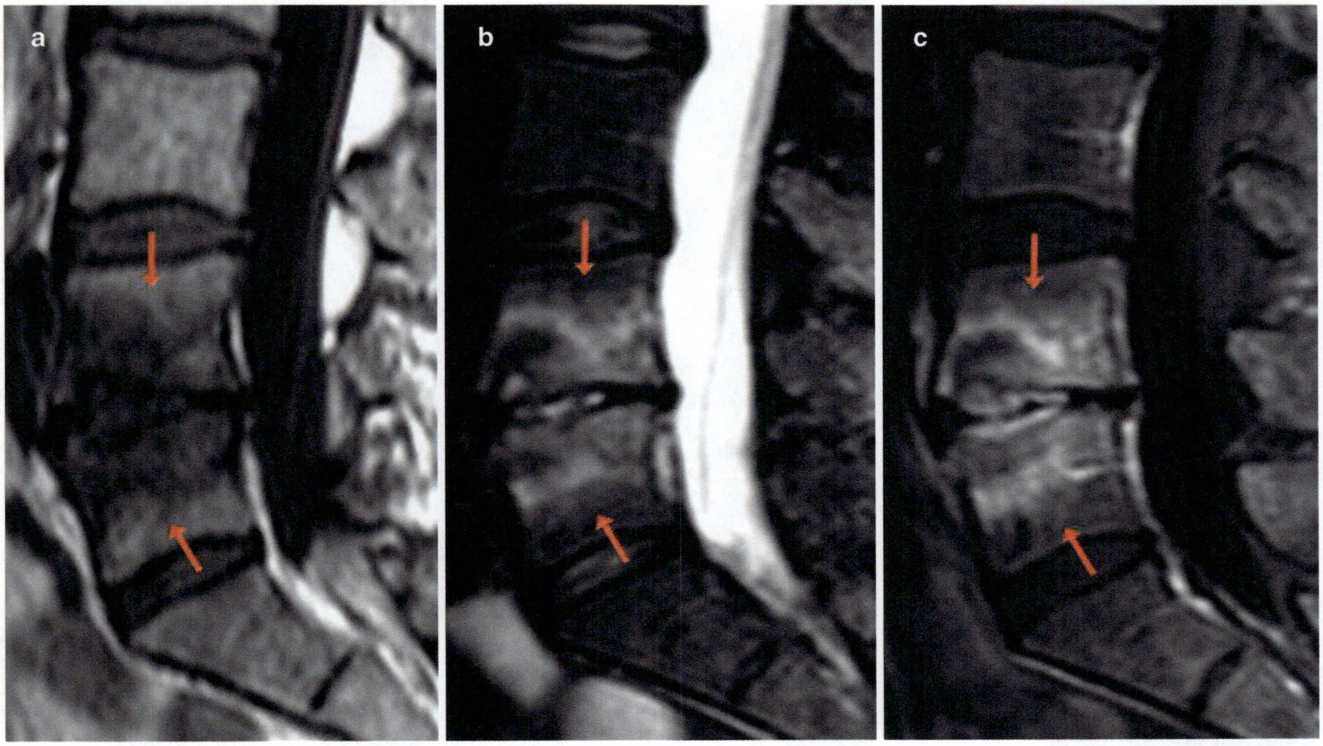

Fig. 7 (**a–c**) Sagittal SE T1-weighted image (**a**), sagittal TSE T2-weighted image with fat saturation (**b**), sagittal SE T1-weighted image with fat saturation following administration of contrast medium (**c**). The opposing L4 and L5 vertebral bodies present a hypointense band in T1 (**a**, *arrows*), with hyperintense signal in T2 (**b**, *arrows*) and contrast enhancement (**c**, *arrows*). The L4/L5 intervertebral disc is collapsed. The same disc shows hyperintense signal in T2 (**b**) and marginal contrast enhancement (**c**), due to sterile inflammation. Diagnosis: osteochondrosis in active inflammatory phase (i.e. osteochondritis)

Case 8: Osteochondritis. Aseptic Discitis

- A 50-year-old woman
- Chronic low back pain

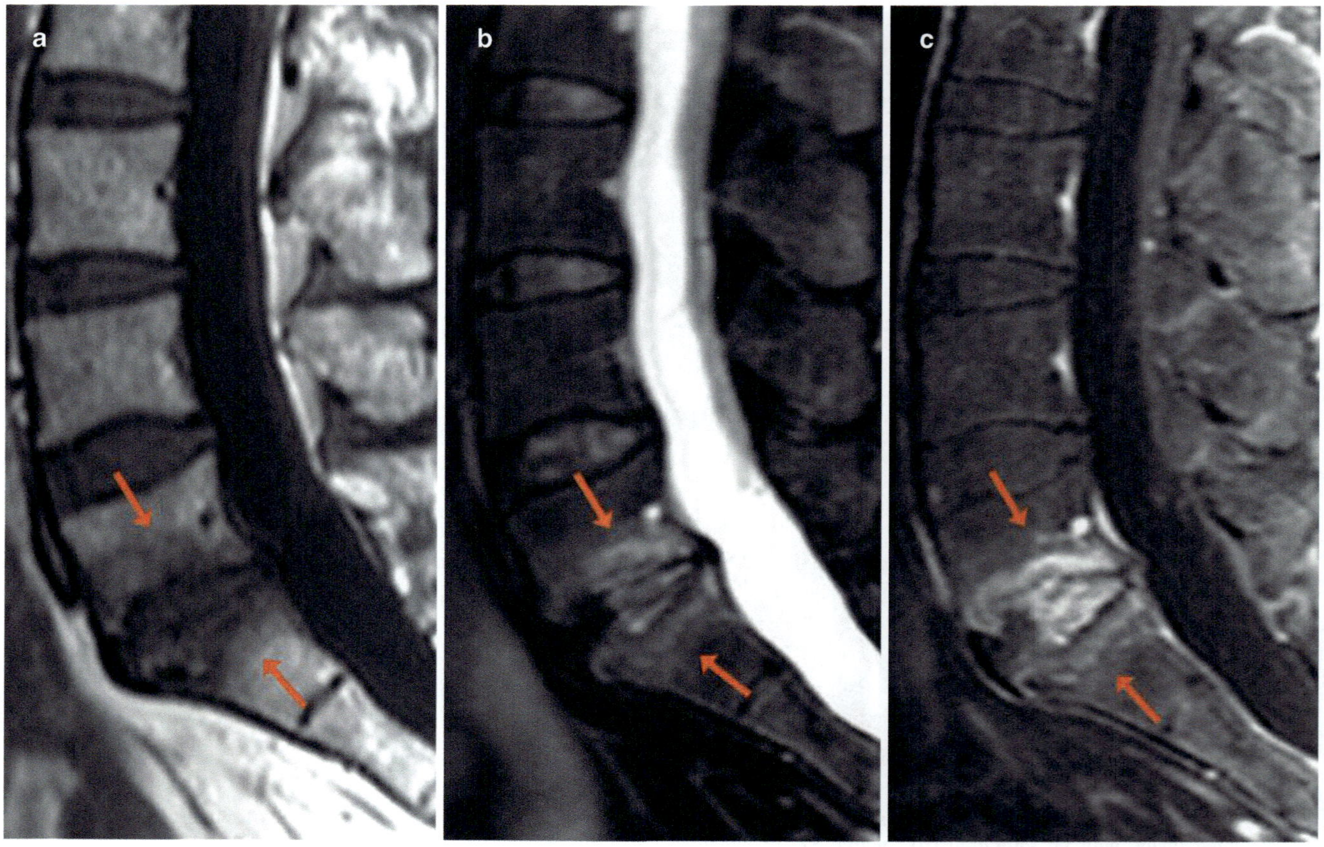

Fig. 8 (**a**–**c**) Sagittal SE T1-weighted image (**a**), sagittal TSE T2-weighted image with fat saturation (**b**), sagittal SE T1-weighted image with fat saturation following administration of contrast medium (**c**). Signal changes (hypointense in T1 and hyperintense in T2) and marked contrast enhancement of the subchondral cancellous bone, chondral surfaces and disc at L5/S1 (**a**–**c**, *arrows*). Erosion of the articular surfaces. Typical osteochondritis and aseptic discitis in active inflammatory phase

Case 9: Osteochondritis

- A 35-year-old woman
- Chronic low back pain
- Improvement with rest

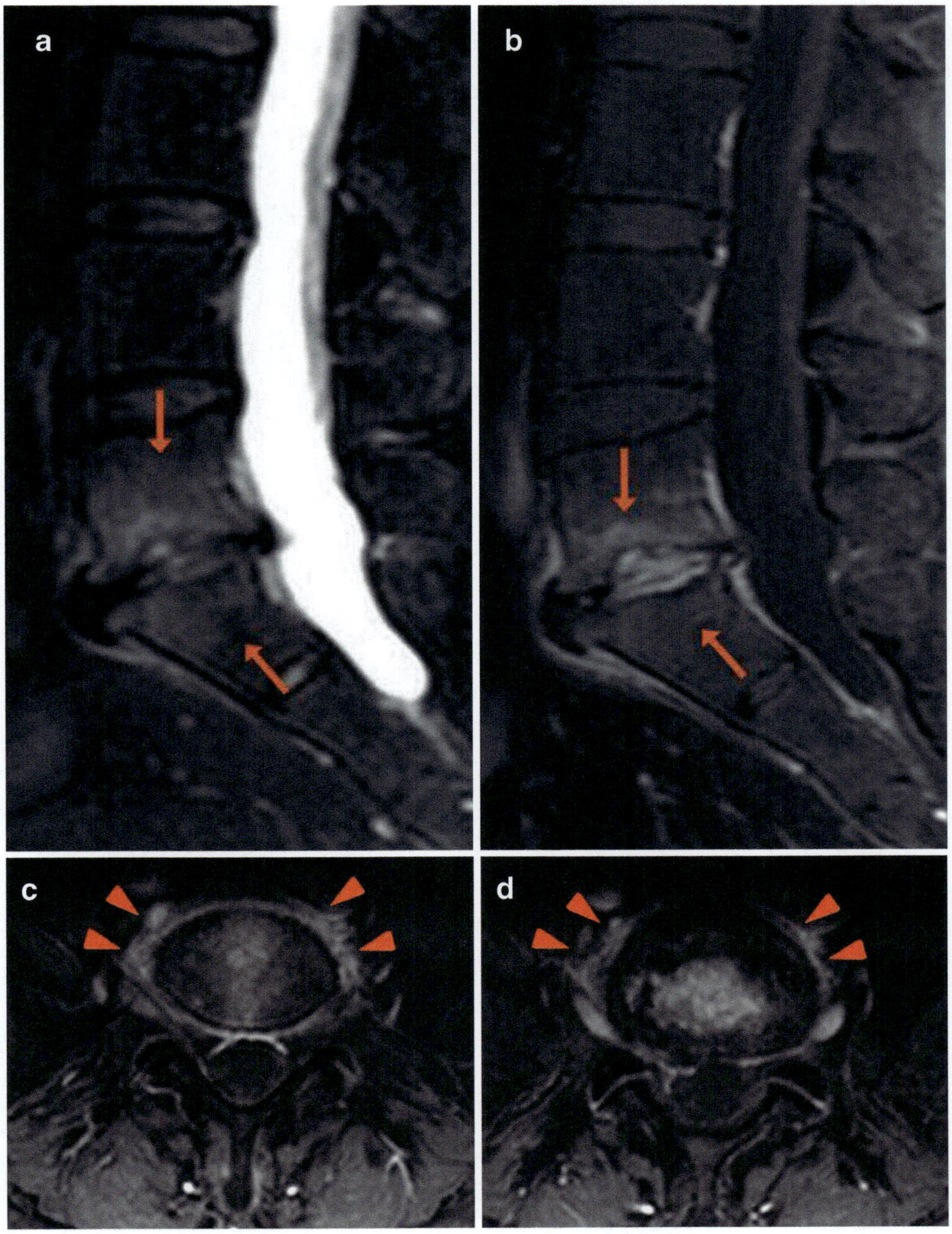

Fig. 9 (**a–d**) Sagittal TSE T2-weighted image with fat saturation (**a**), sagittal and axial SE T1-weighted images with fat saturation after administration of contrast medium (**b–d**). T2 hyperintensity (**a**) and contrast enhancement (**b**) of the subchondral cancellous bone, chondral surfaces and intervertebral disc at L5/S1, indicating osteochondritis in inflammatory phase, with reduction in height of the same disc (**a**, **b**, *arrows*). Note also peridiscal contrast enhancement, indicating inflammation of the peridiscal soft tissue (**c**, **d** *arrowheads*)

Case 10: Osteochondritis

- A 42-year-old man
- Back pain
- Limitation of motion of the thoracolumbar spine in the sagittal plane

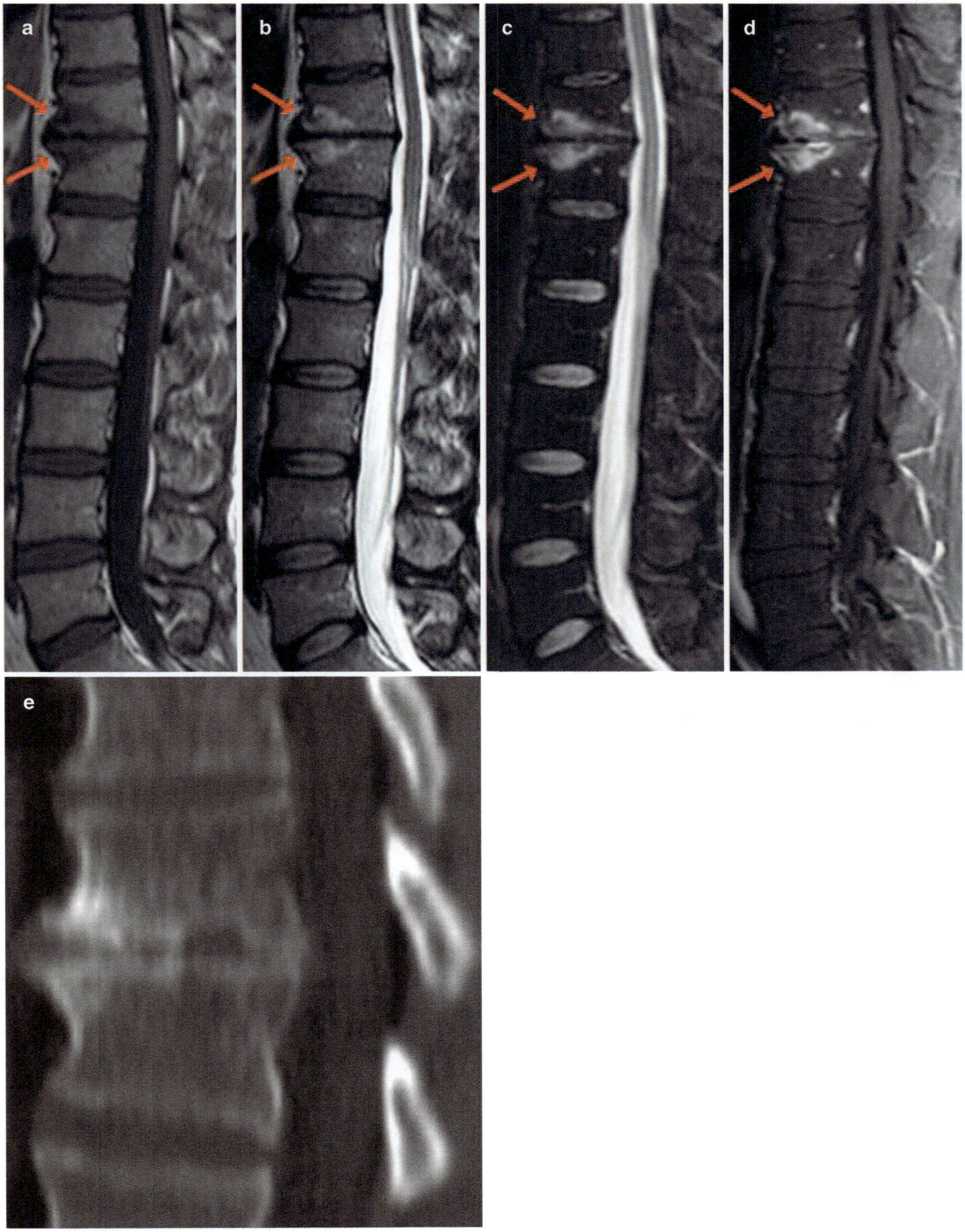

Fig. 10 (**a–e**) Sagittal SE T1-weighted image (**a**), sagittal TSE T2-weighted image (**b**), sagittal TSE T2-weighted image with fat saturation (**c**), sagittal SE T1-weighted image with fat saturation after contrast medium administration (**d**), sagittal CT image—MPR (**e**). T1 hypointensity (**a**) and T2 hyperintensity (**b, c**) of the subchondral cancellous bone at T11/T12, indicating fibrovascular transformation of the bone marrow and oedema (**a–c**, *arrows*). The signal change is more diffuse in the anterior corners of the vertebral bodies. Note that oedematous changes are more evident in T2-weighted images with fat saturation (**c**) than in T2 images without fat saturation (**b**). The intervertebral disc is reduced in height. Marked contrast enhancement of the same areas and chondral surfaces (**d**, *arrows*), indicating osteochondritis in active-inflammatory phase. CT image showing osteosclerosis of the anterior edges of the same vertebral bodies, erosions of the articular surfaces and osteophytosis (**e**)

Case 11: Osteochondritis

- A 58-year-old woman
- Patient with persistent back pain radiating anteriorly

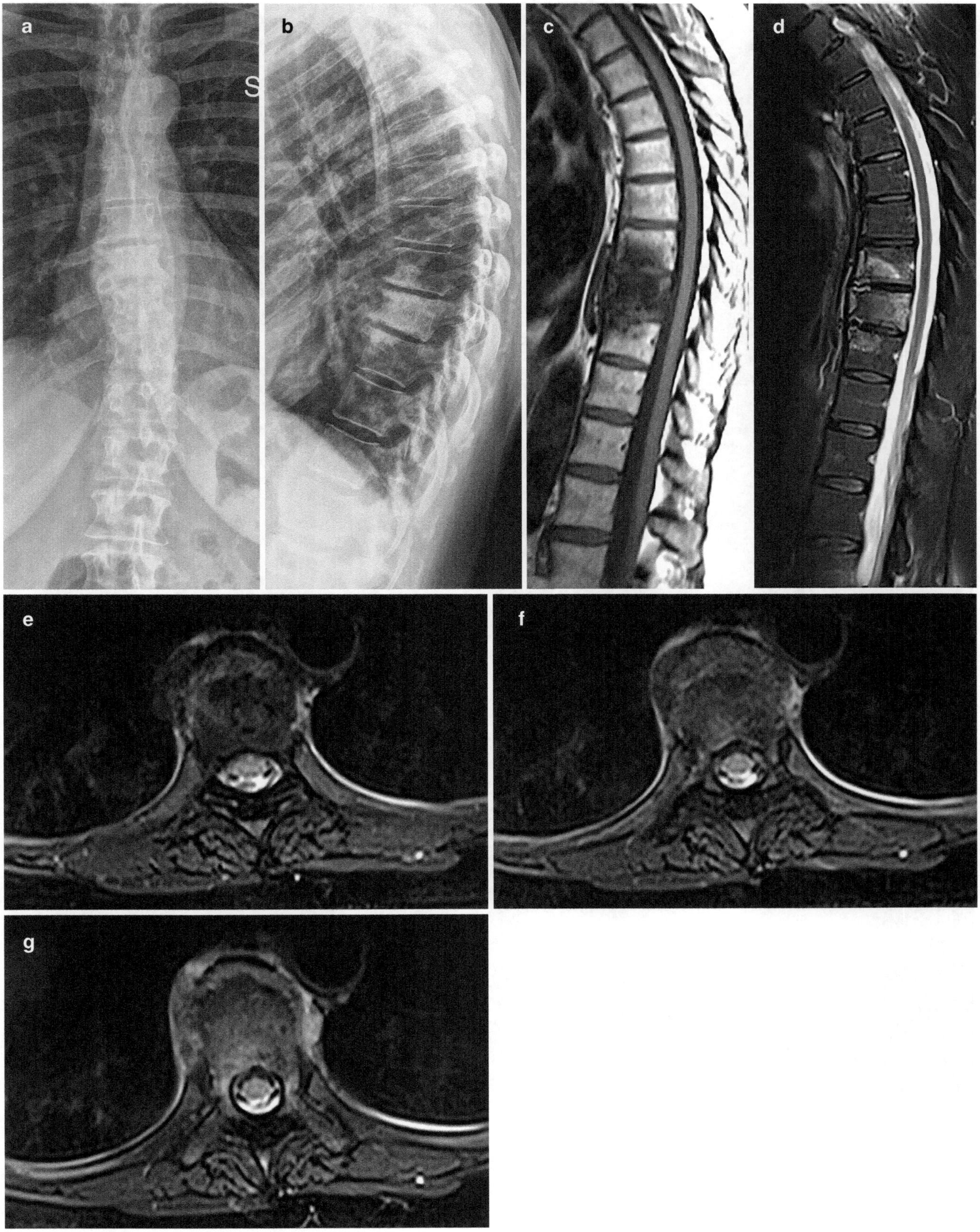

Fig. 11 (**a–o**) X-ray of the dorsal spine (**a, b**), sagittal TSE T1-weighted image (**c**), sagittal and axial TSE T2-weighted images with fat saturation (**d–g**), sagittal, axial and coronal TSE T1-weighted images with fat saturation after administration of contrast medium (**h–o**). Signal alteration, hypointense in T1 (**c**) and hyperintense in T2 (**d–g**), of the vertebral bodies D8-D9-D10, with contrast enhancement of the same vertebral bodies and part of the interposed chondral surfaces (**h–o**), indicating marked osteochondritis (**h–o**). There is also contrast enhancement of the perivertebral soft tissues at the same levels, due to reactive inflammation (**h–o**). Note: osteophytes, typically directed horizontally, and surrounding reactive inflammation (**b–o**)

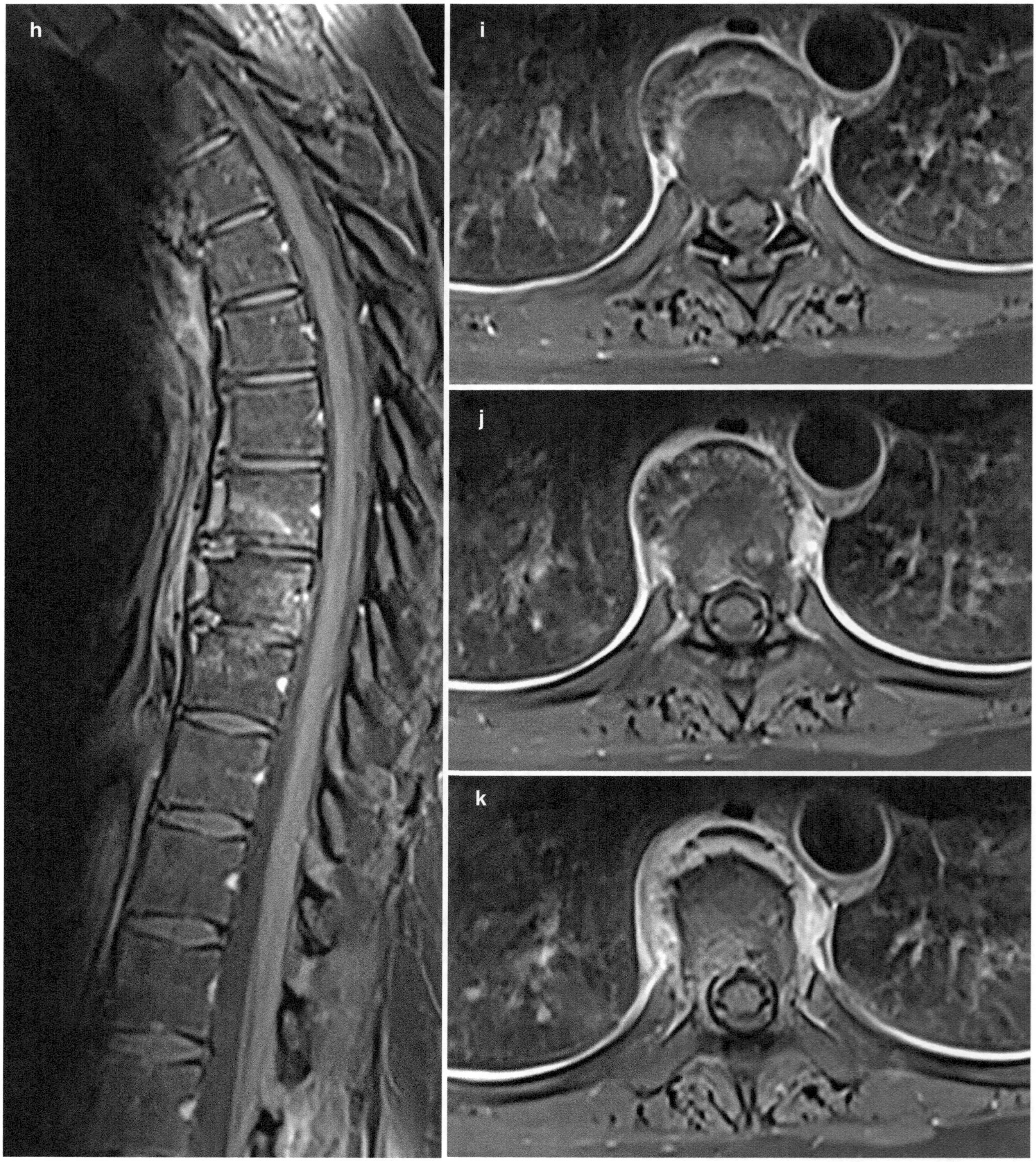

Fig. 11 (continued)

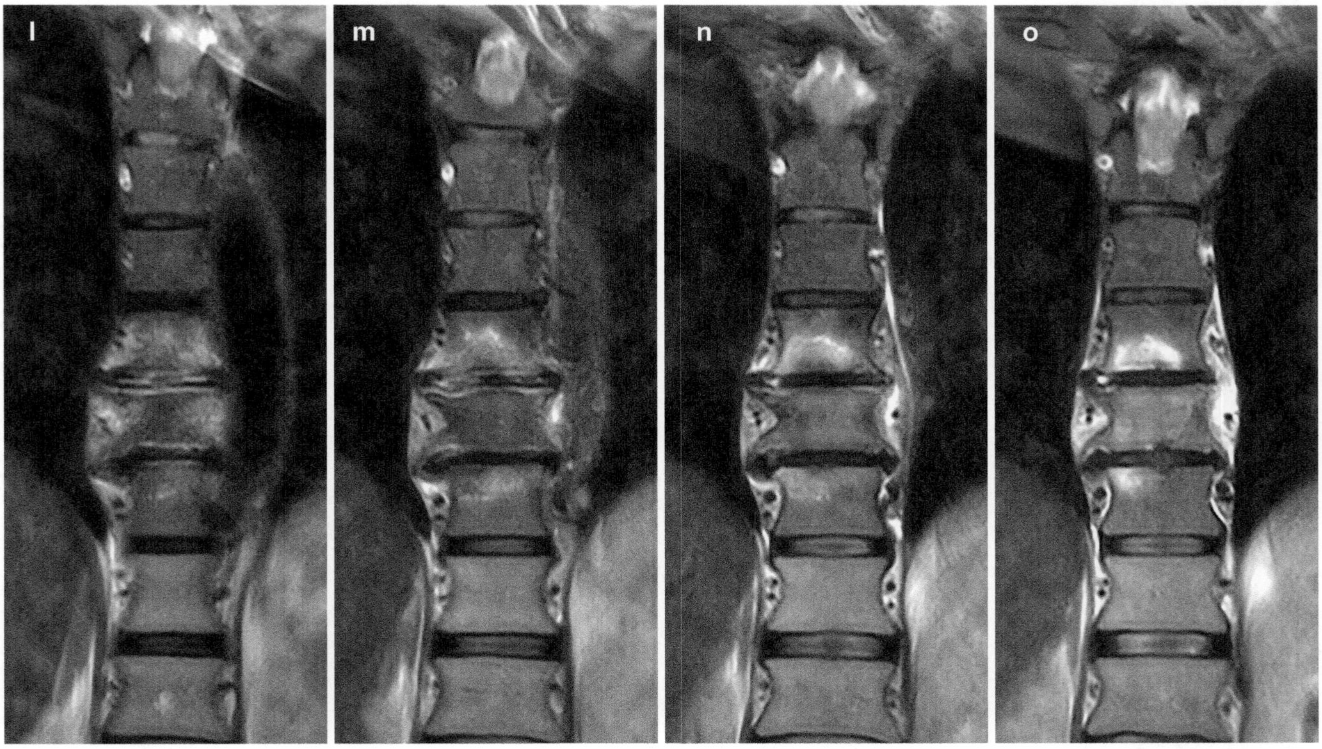

Fig. 11 (continued)

Facet Joint Pathology

5

Case 12: Facet Joint Effusion

- A 46-year-old woman
- Patient with chronic back pain, exacerbated by flexion and extension

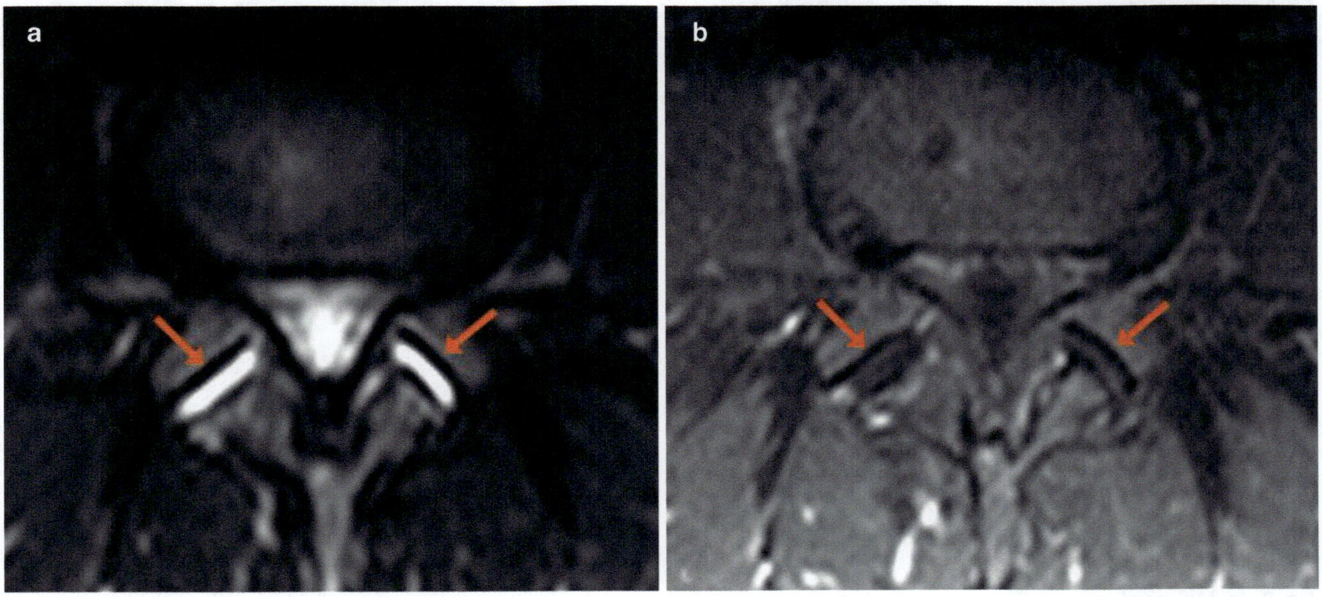

Fig. 1 (**a**, **b**) Axial TSE T2-weighted image with fat saturation (**a**), axial SE T1-weighted image with fat saturation following administration of contrast medium (**b**). Facet joints show widening of the joint space bilaterally. This space is hyperintense in T2 (**a**, *arrows*), with no enhancement after contrast medium administration (**b**, *arrows*). These findings indicate joint effusion

P. D'Aprile, A. Tarantino, *MRI of Degenerative Disease of the Spine*, https://doi.org/10.1007/978-3-030-73707-8_5

Case 13: Facet Joint Effusion

- A 68-year old man
- Chronic low back pain, exacerbated by flexion and extension
- History of chronic dorsal and lumbar pain

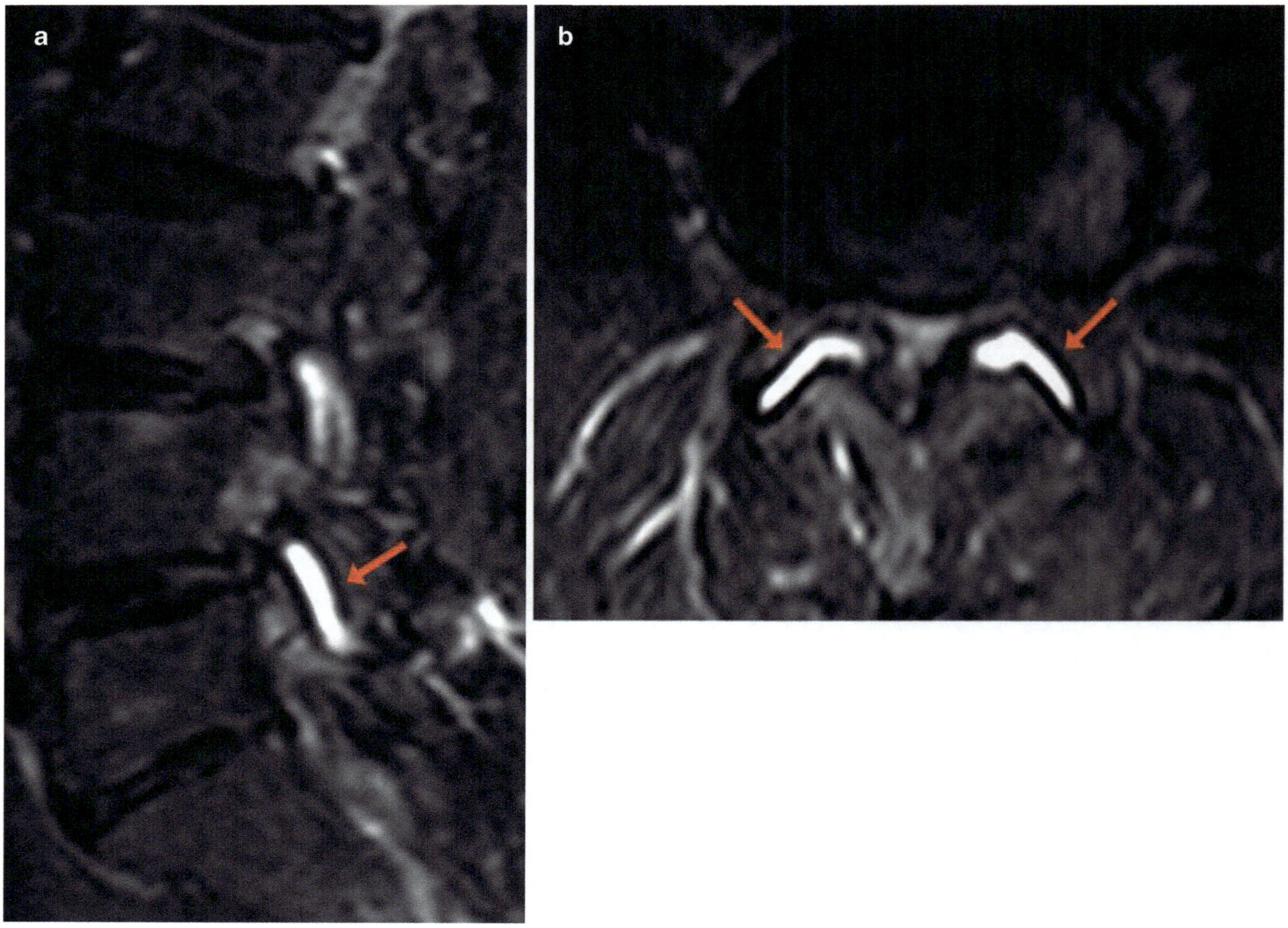

Fig. 2 (**a**, **b**) Sagittal and axial TSE T2-weighted images with fat saturation (**a**, **b**). Facet joint effusion at L4/L5 bilaterally, with widening of the joint spaces (*arrows*)

Case 14: Synovitis. Radiculitis

- A 36-year-old man
- Patient with chronic back pain, exacerbated by flexion and extension
- Radiculopathy on the right side

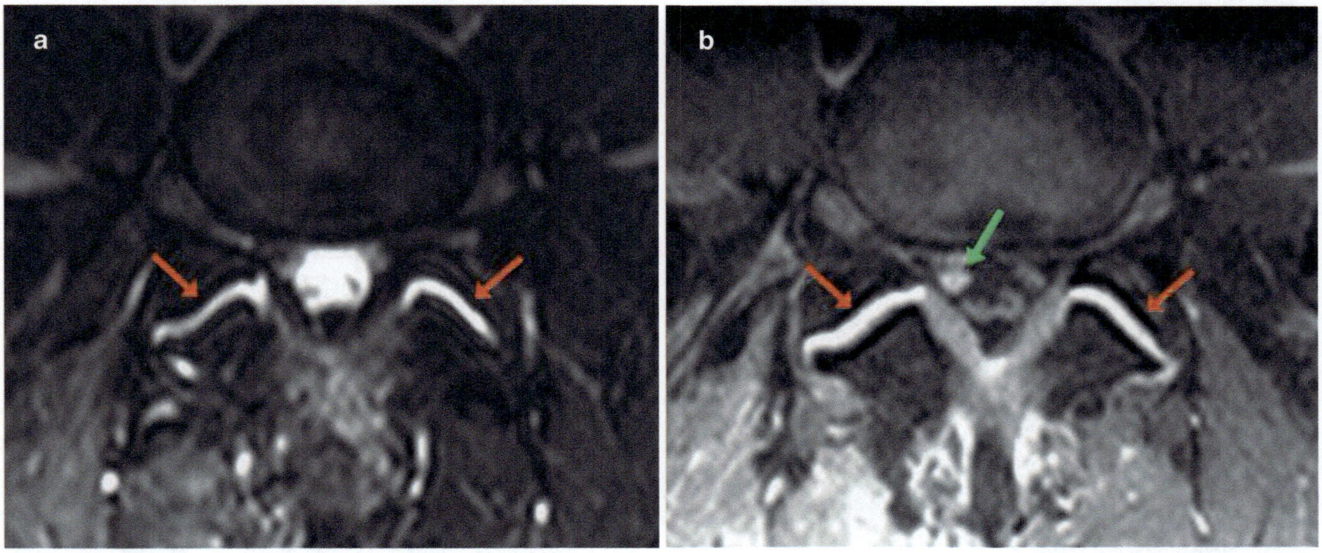

Fig. 3 (**a**, **b**) Axial TSE T2-weighted image with fat saturation (**a**), axial SE T1-weighted image with fat saturation, following contrast medium administration (**b**). Facet joints at L5/S1. Widening of the joint space, with enhancement after contrast medium administration indicating synovitis (*red arrows*). Note also contrast enhancement of a nerve root on the right side, referable to radiculitis (*green arrow*)

Case 15: Facet Joint Osteoarthritis

- A 62-year-old man
- Limitation of motion of the lumbar spine
- Low back pain, more marked on the left side

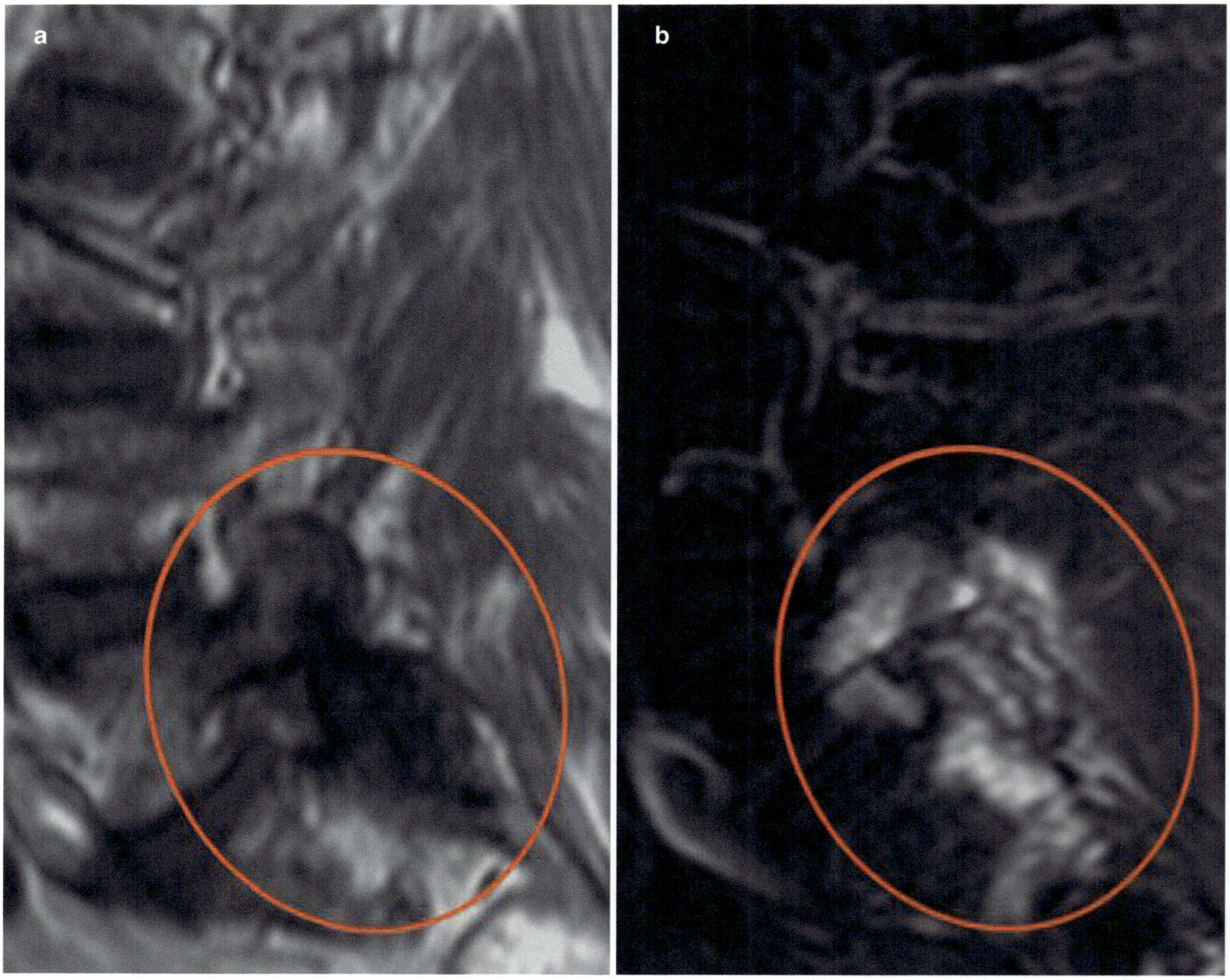

Fig. 4 (**a–f**) Sagittal T1-weighted image (**a**), sagittal and axial T2-weighted images with fat saturation (**b–d**), axial T1-weighted images with fat saturation following administration of contrast medium (**e–f**). Structural and signal changes of the L5/S1 facet joint (**a**, **b** *circle*). The images on the axial plane show T2 hyperintensity (**b–d**, *arrows*) and contrast enhancement (**e**, **f**, *arrows*) of the articular apophyses and pedicles, referable to oedema osteitis. It coexists periapophyseal soft tissue inflammatory reaction, more evident after contrast medium administration (**e**, **f**). Diagnosis: bilateral facet joint osteoarthritis at L5/S1, more marked on the left side, in active inflammatory phase

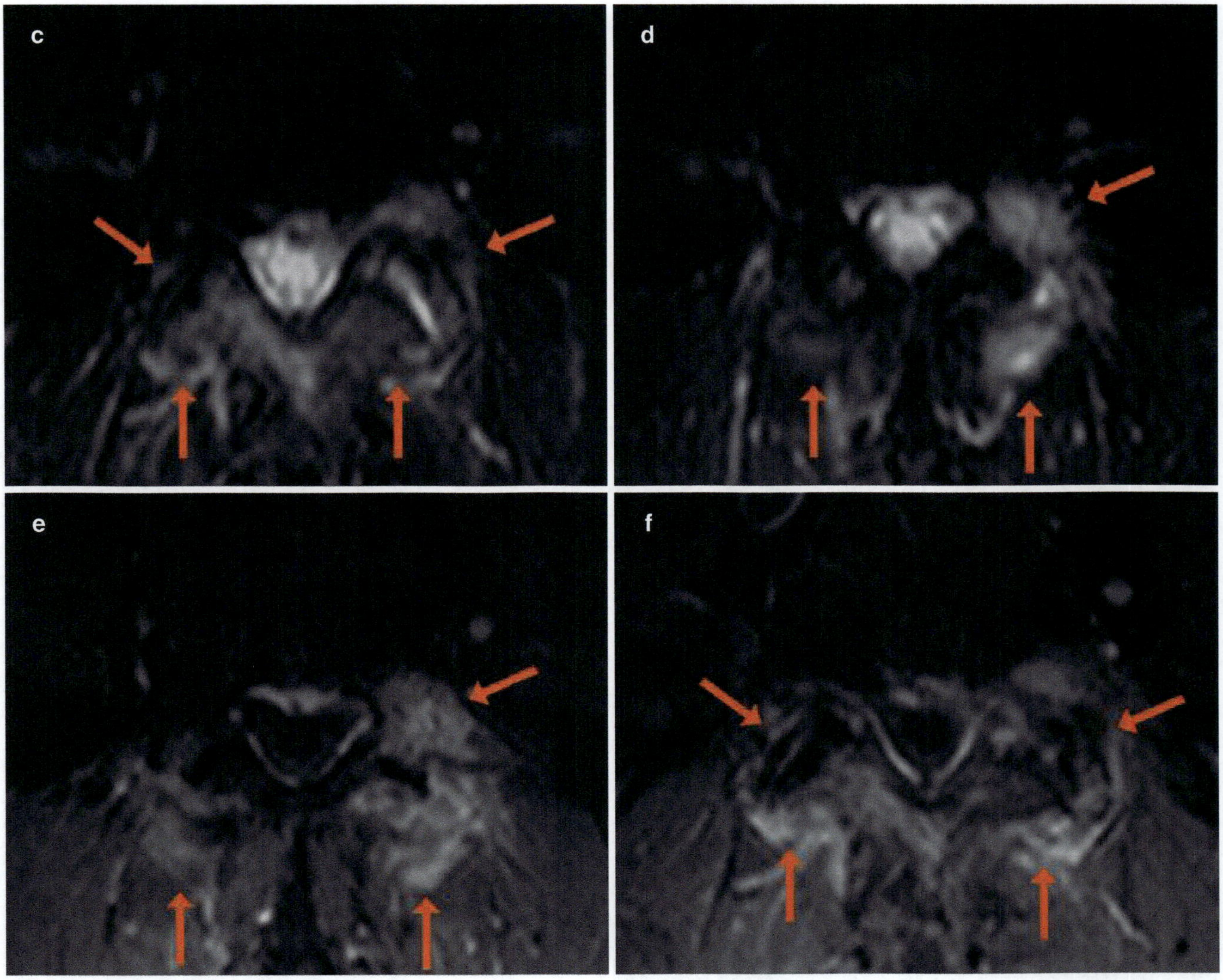

Fig. 4 (continued)

Case 16: Facet Joint Osteoarthritis

- A 67-year-old woman
- Low back pain, more marked on the left side

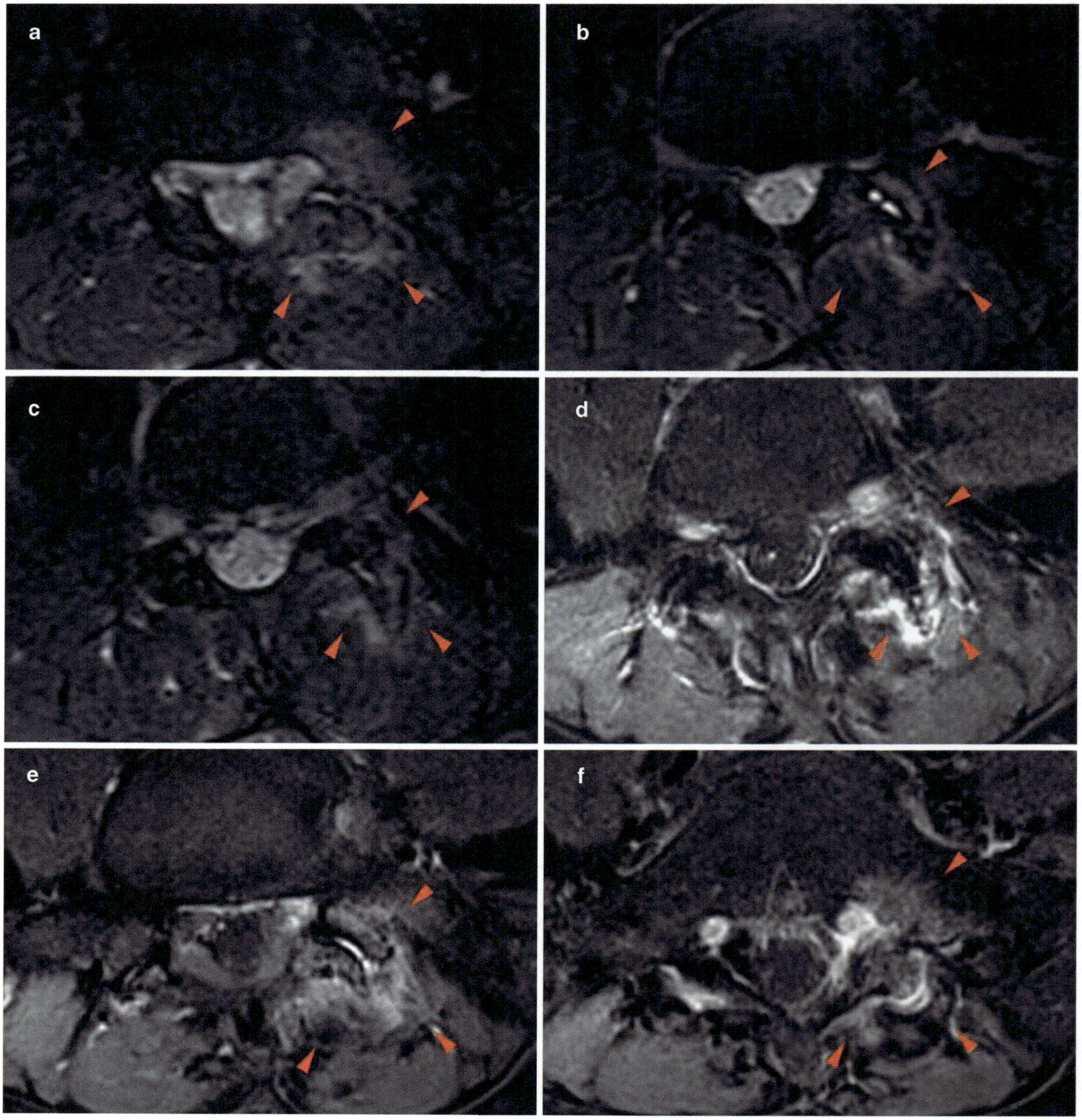

Fig. 5 (**a–f**) Axial TSE T2-weighted images with fat saturation (**a–c**), axial SE T1-weighted images with fat saturation following administration of contrast medium (**d–f**). Left facet joint arthrosis with facet hypertrophy at L5/S1. Hyperintense signal on T2-weighted images in the articular facets and surrounding soft tissues (**a–c**, *arrowheads*). The same areas enhance on T1-weighted images after contrast medium administration (**d–f**, *arrowheads*). There is also contrast enhancement of the facet joint space (**e**). These findings indicate sterile facet joint osteoarthritis in active inflammatory phase, with synovitis and inflammation of the periarticular soft tissues

Case 17: Facet Joint Osteoarthritis

- A 46-year-old man
- Persistent low back pain with focal tenderness on the right side at L5/S1.

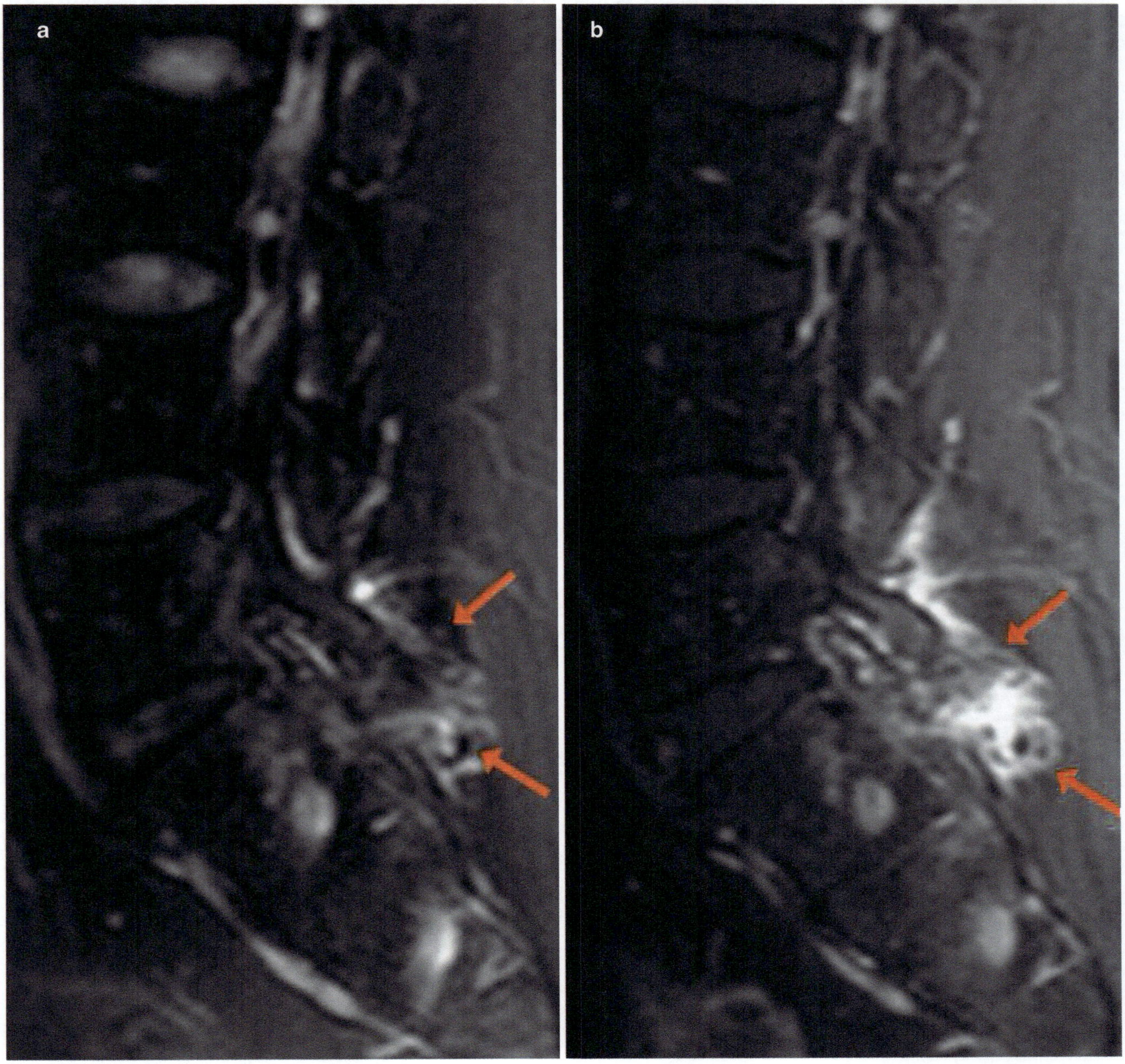

Fig. 6 (**a–h**) Sagittal and axial TSE T2-weighted images with fat saturation (**a**, **d**, **e**), axial SE T1-weighted image (**c**), sagittal and axial SE T1-weighted images with fat saturation images (**b**, **f**, **g**), CT image (**h**). Hyperintense signal in T2 (**a**, *arrow*) and contrast enhancement (**b**, *arrow*) in the articular facets and surrounding soft tissues. Axial images allow a better spatial definition of the lesion, with oedema osteitis of the articular facets, with small erosions of the articular surfaces and with periarticular inflammation (**c–g**, *circle*). CT image shows right facet joint arthrosis, with small articular erosions (**h**, *circle*). Diagnosis: sterile facet joint arthritis in active inflammatory phase

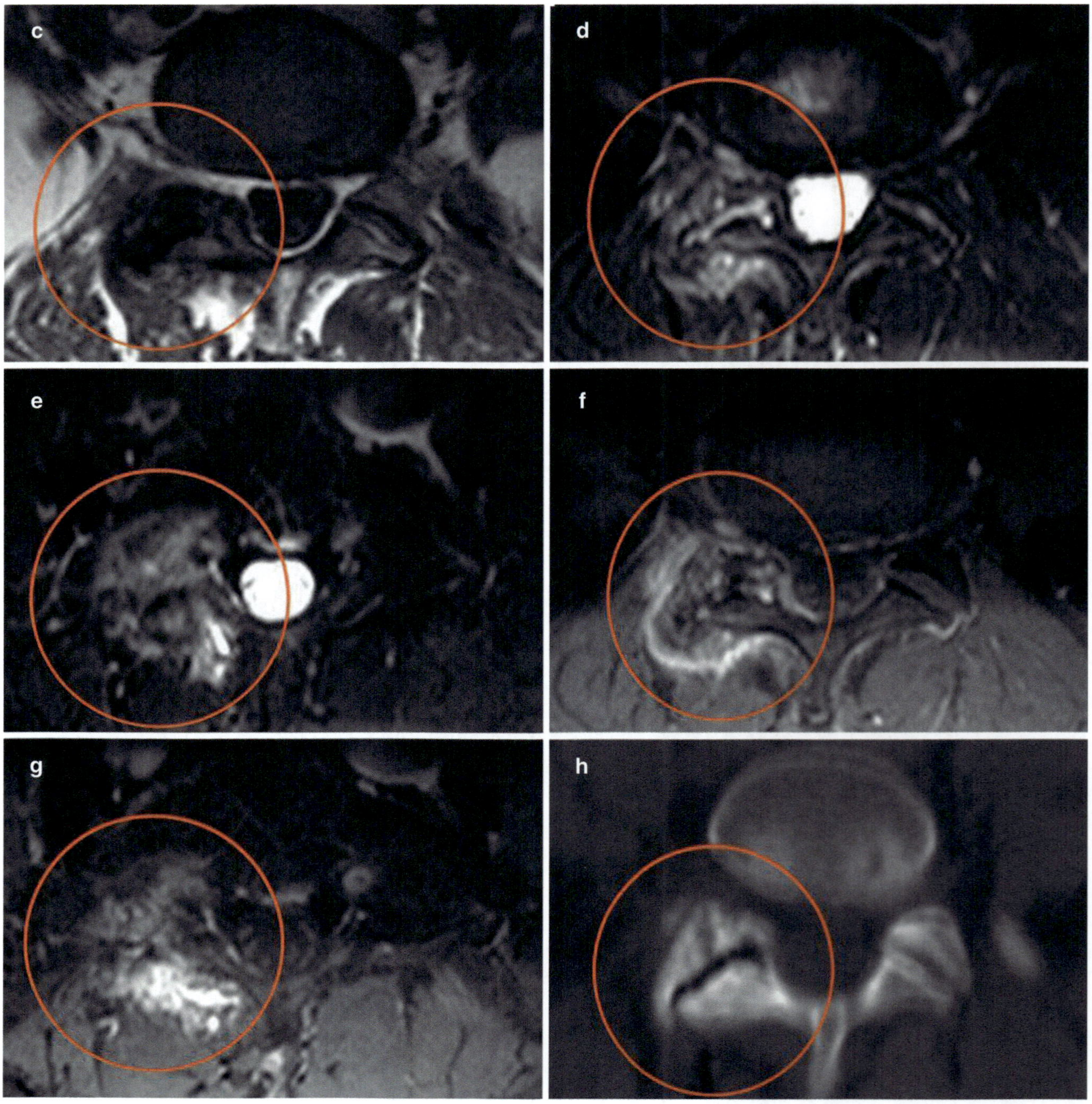

Fig. 6 (continued)

Case 18: C1-C2 Osteoarthritis

- A 70-year-old man
- Neck pain
- Limitation of motion of the cranio-cervical junction

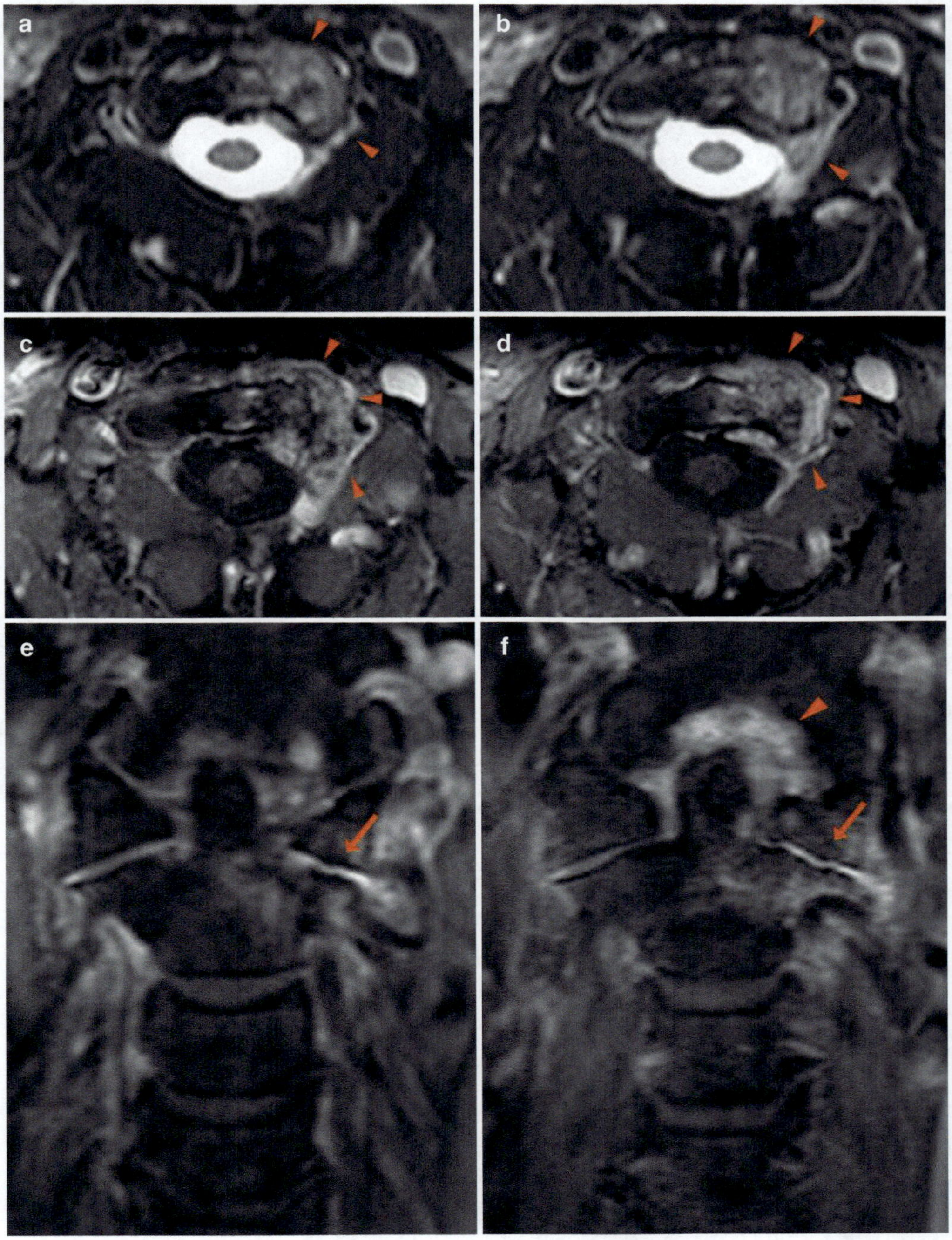

Fig. 7 (**a**–**f**) Axial TSE T2-weighted images with fat saturation (**a**, **b**), axial and coronal SE T1-weighted images with fat saturation following administration of contrast medium (**c**–**f**). Marked atlanto-axial osteoarthritis on the left side. T2 hyperintensity (**a**, **b**, *arrowheads*), and contrast enhancement (**c**, **d**, *arrowheads*) of the left lateral mass of the atlas and axis, indicating oedema-osteitis. The images on coronal plane allow to better highlight contrast enhancement of the joint space, which is reduced in amplitude (**e**, **f**, *arrow*). Note also contrast enhancement of the adjacent periodontoid epidural space, due to inflammatory reaction (**f**, *arrowhead*)

Case 19: Facet Joint Osteoarthritis

- A 67-year-old woman
- Neck pain more marked on the left side

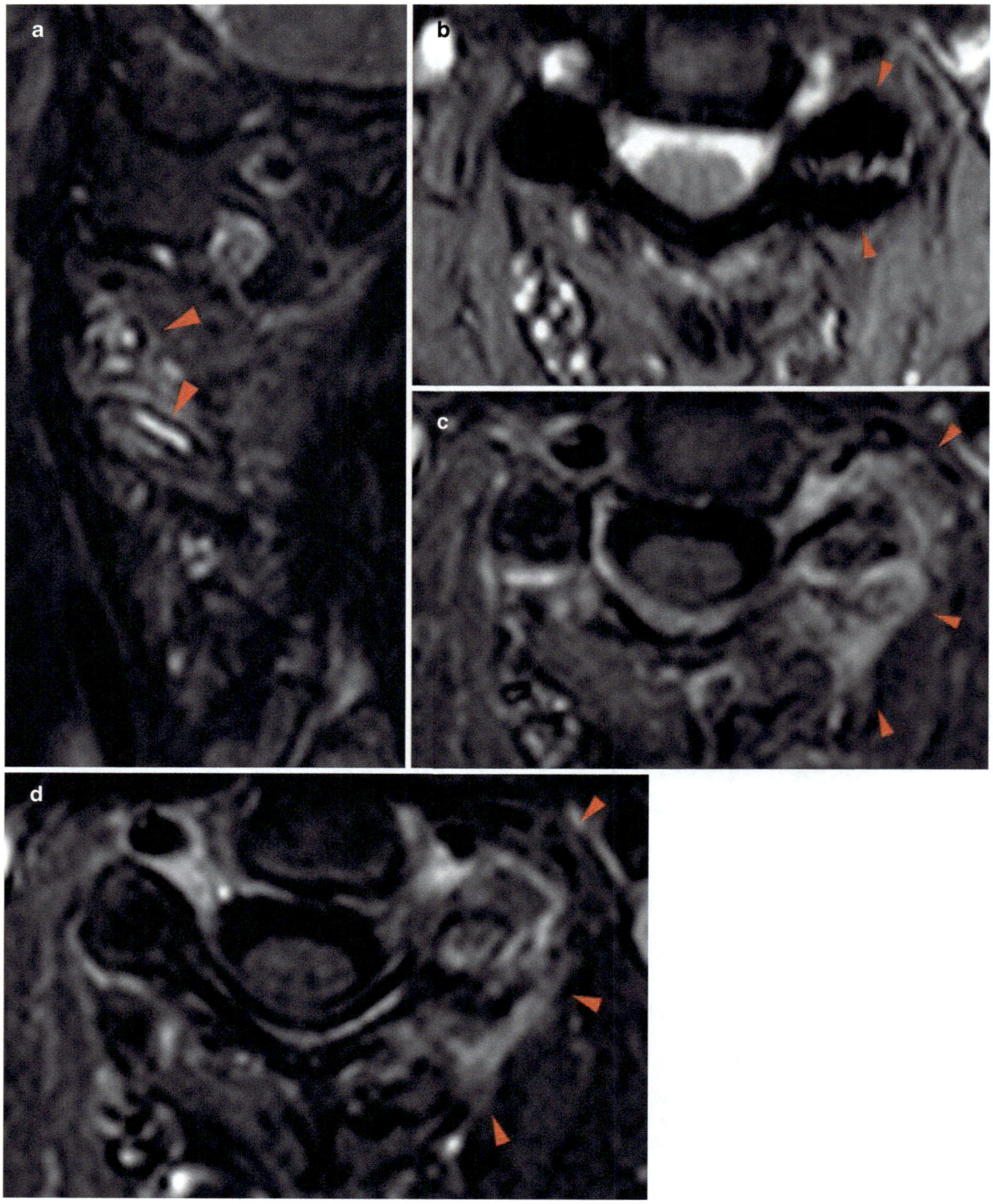

Fig. 8 (**a**–**d**) Sagittal TSE T2-weighted image with fat saturation (**a**), axial GE T2*-weighted image (**b**), axial SE T1-weighted images with fat saturation following administration of contrast medium (**c**, **d**). Oedema of the facet joint at C3/C4, with joint effusion (**a**, *arrowhead*). The axial image confirms a mild joint effusion, with erosion of the articular surfaces (**b**, *arrowhead*). The administration of contrast medium shows enhancement of the facet joint (i.e. osteoarthritis) and periarticular soft tissues (i.e. periapophyseal inflammation) (**c**, **d**, *arrowhead*)

Case 20: Facet Joint Osteoarthritis. Ligamentous Inflammation

- A 43-year-old man
- Neck pain more marked on the right side

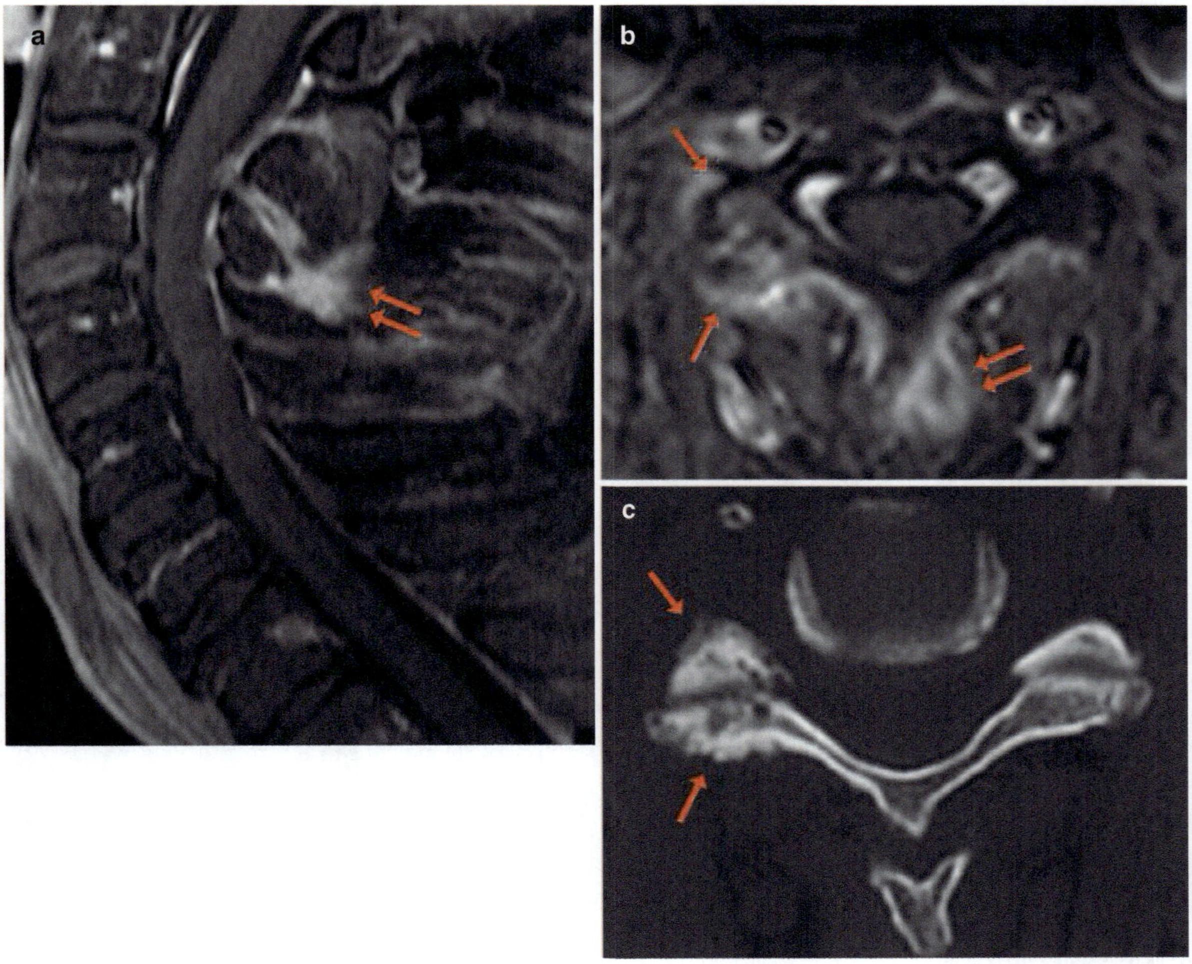

Fig. 9 (**a**–**c**) Sagittal and axial contrast-enhanced T1-weighted images with fat saturation (**a**, **b**), axial CT image (**c**). Contrast enhancement of the interspinous ligaments at C2-C3-C4, due to ligamentous inflammation (**a**, **b**, *double arrow*). Contrast enhancement of the C3/C4 right facet joint and periarticular soft tissues, indicating osteoarthritis and periapophyseal inflammation (**b**, *arrow*). CT image confirms the osteoarthritis, with bone erosions, subchondral cysts and osteosclerosis (**c**, *arrow*)

Case 21: Osteochondrosis. Facet Joint Osteoarthritis

- A 70-year-old man
- Patient with chronic neck pain
- Limited motion
- Point tenderness corresponding to right facet joint at C4/C5

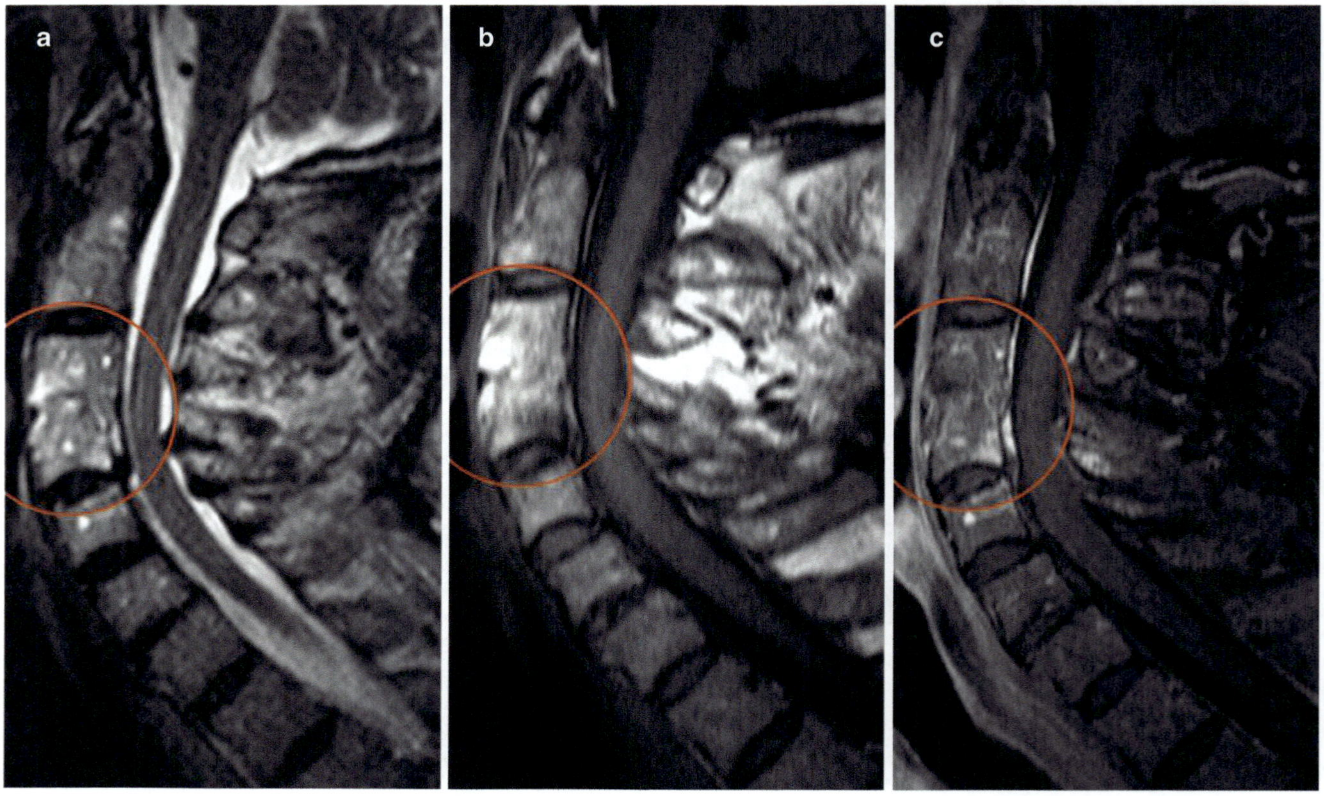

Fig. 10 (**a**–**f**) Sagittal T2-weighted image (**a**), sagittal T1-weighted image (**b**), sagittal and axial T1-weighted images with fat saturation following administration of contrast medium (**c**–**f**). Marked osteochondrosic degeneration at C3/C4, with intervertebral fusion (**a**–**c**, *circle*). The same patient presented a clear C4/C5 facet joint osteoarthritis on the right side, coupled with periapophyseal soft tissue inflammation, well defined by intense contrast enhancement of the same structures (**d**–**f**, *arrowheads*)

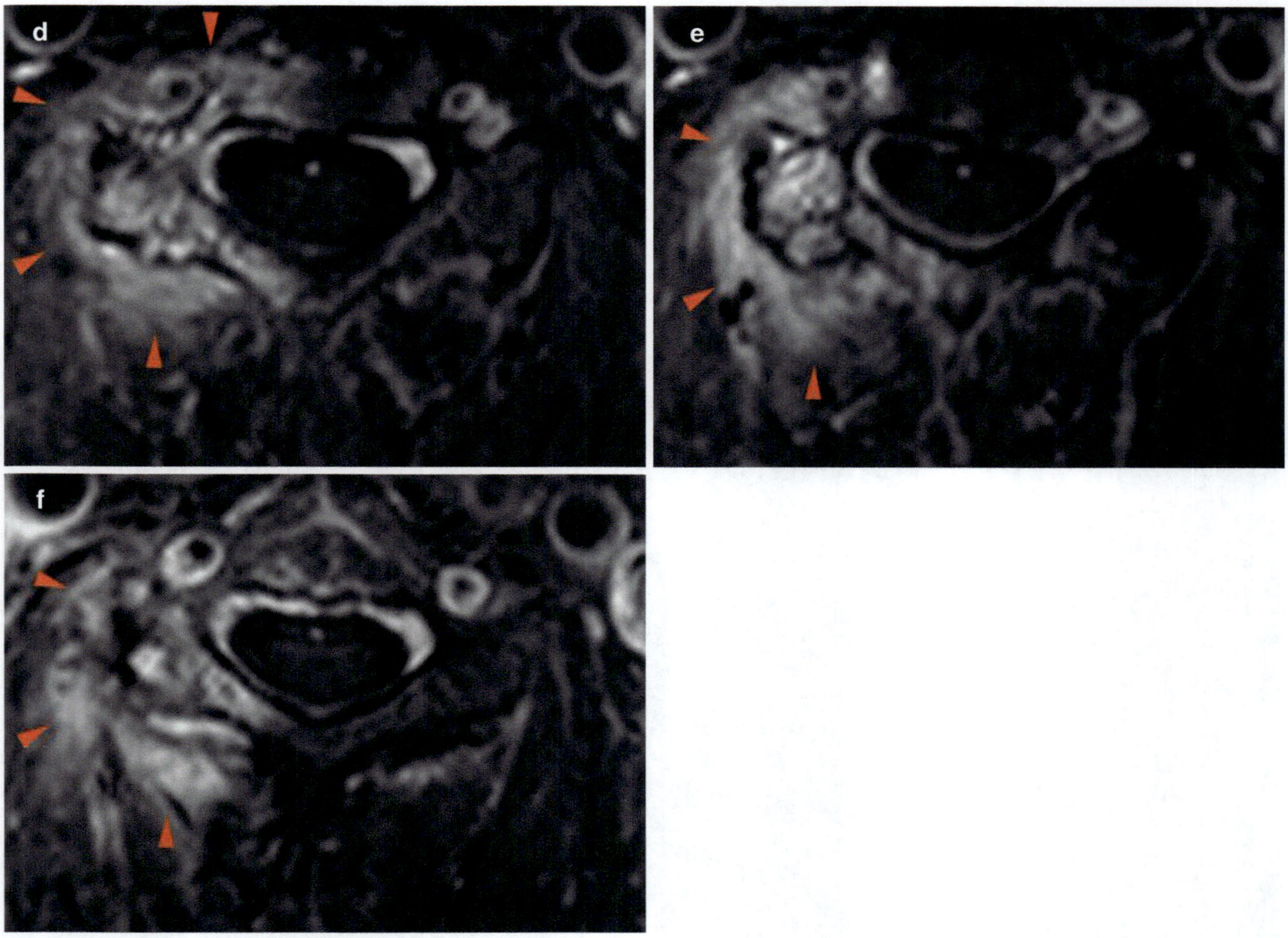

Fig. 10 (continued)

Case 22: Osteochondrosis. Facet Joint Osteoarthritis

- A 48-year-old woman
- Patient with cervical dystonia (the head of the patient was twisted and turned to the left).
- Persistent cervical pain on the left side

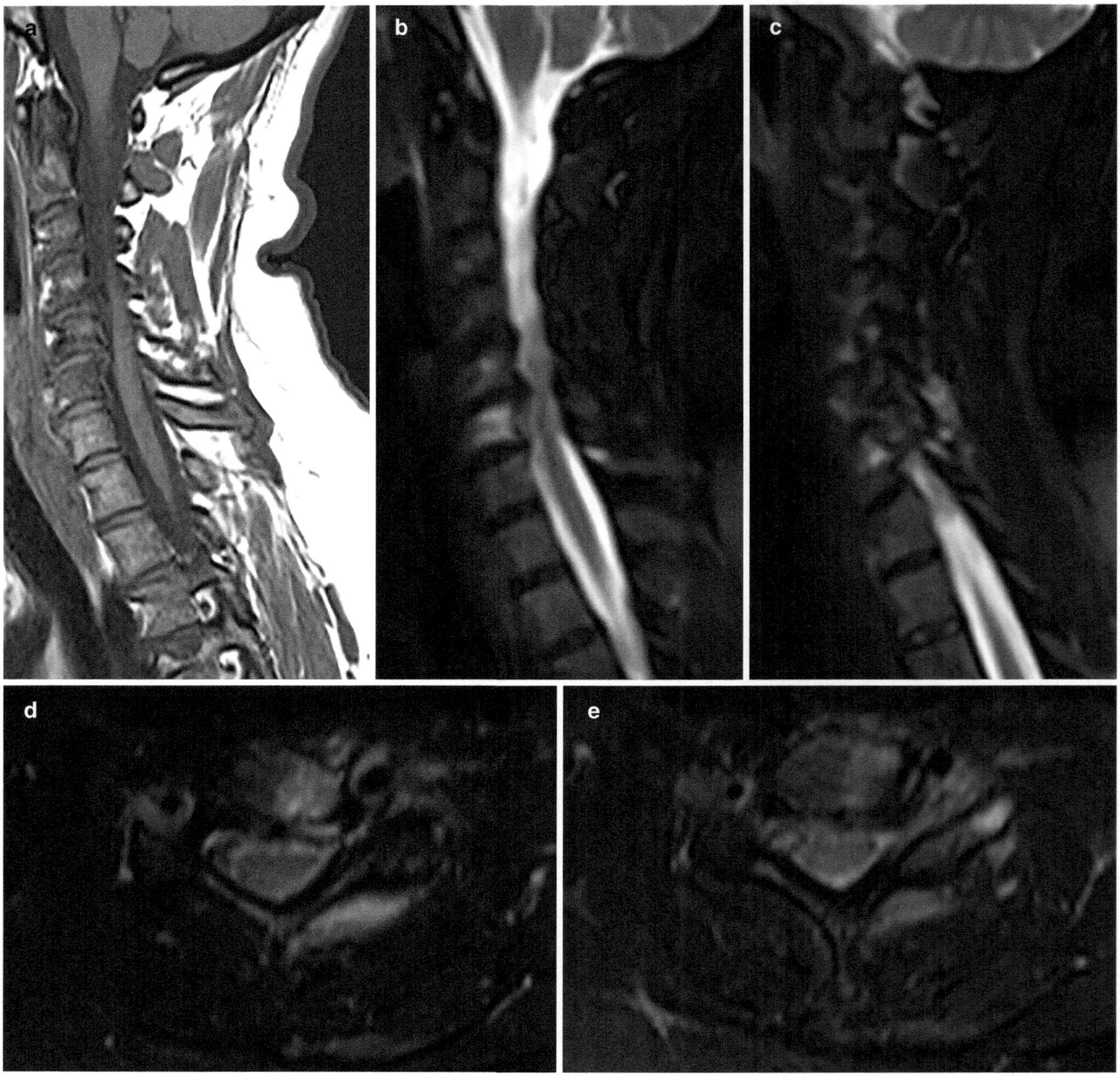

Fig. 11 (**a**–**m**) Sagittal TSE T1-weighted image (**a**), sagittal and axial TSE T2-weighted images with fat saturation (**b**–**f**), sagittal, axial and coronal TSE T1-weighted images with fat saturation after administration of contrast medium (**g**–**m**). Mild hypointensity in T1 (**a**), hyperintensity in T2 (**b**–**f**) with contrast enhancement (**g**–**k**) in the left part of the vertebral bodies C5, C6 and C7, due to osteochondrosis in active-inflammatory phase. Note also hyperintensity in T2 (**c**–**f**) with contrast enhancement (**h**–**m**) of the left facet joint at C6/C7 and periarticular soft tissue, indicating osteoarthritis in active inflammatory phase and reactive inflammation of corresponding periarticular soft tissues. These findings have a degenerative mechanical pathogenesis in consideration of the altered regional static due to cervical dystonia

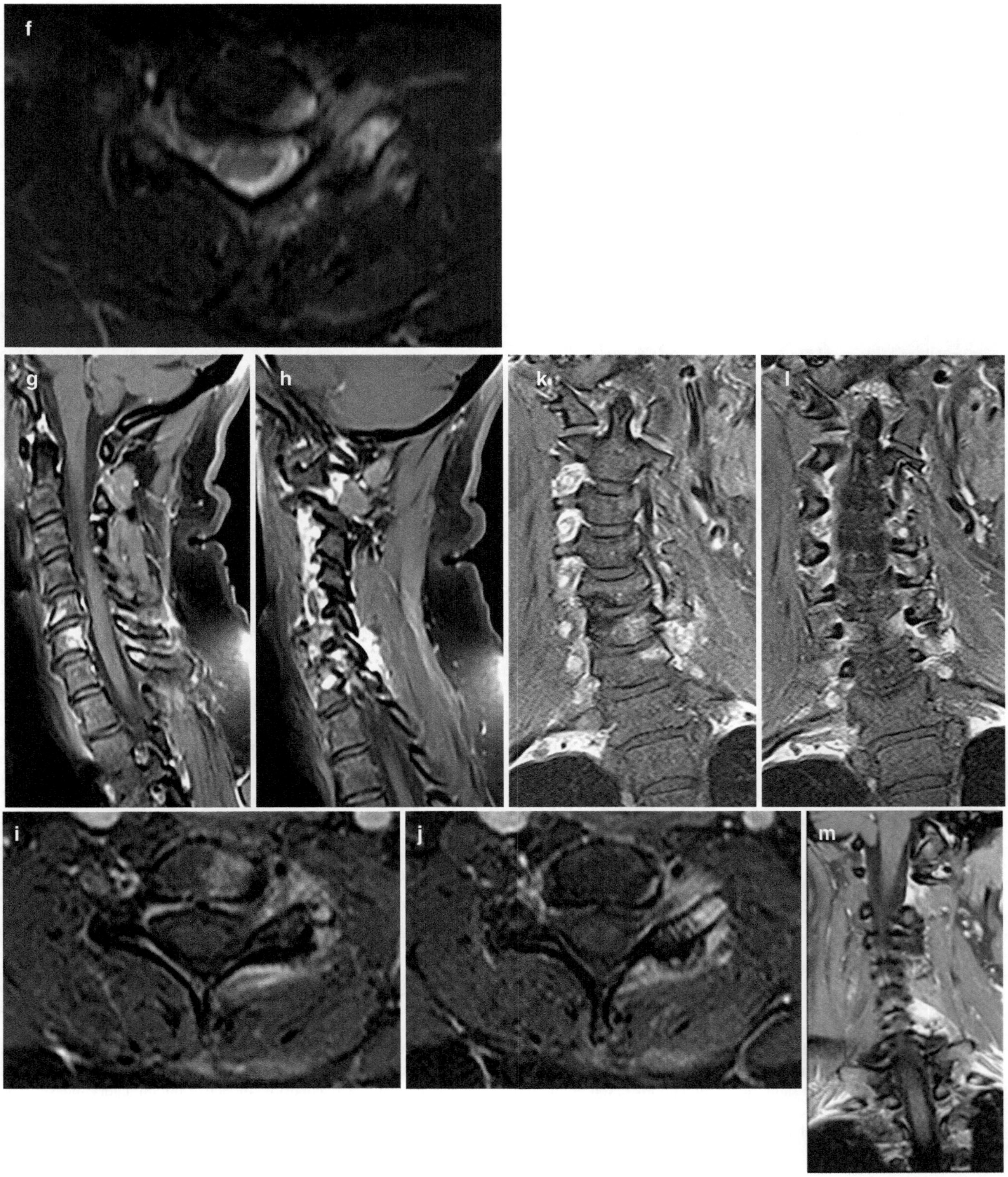

Fig. 11 (continued)

Case 23: Osteochondritis. Facet Joint Osteoarthritis

- A 45-year-old man
- Persistent cervical and low back pain
- Limitation of motion of the cervical and lumbar spine
- Improvement with rest

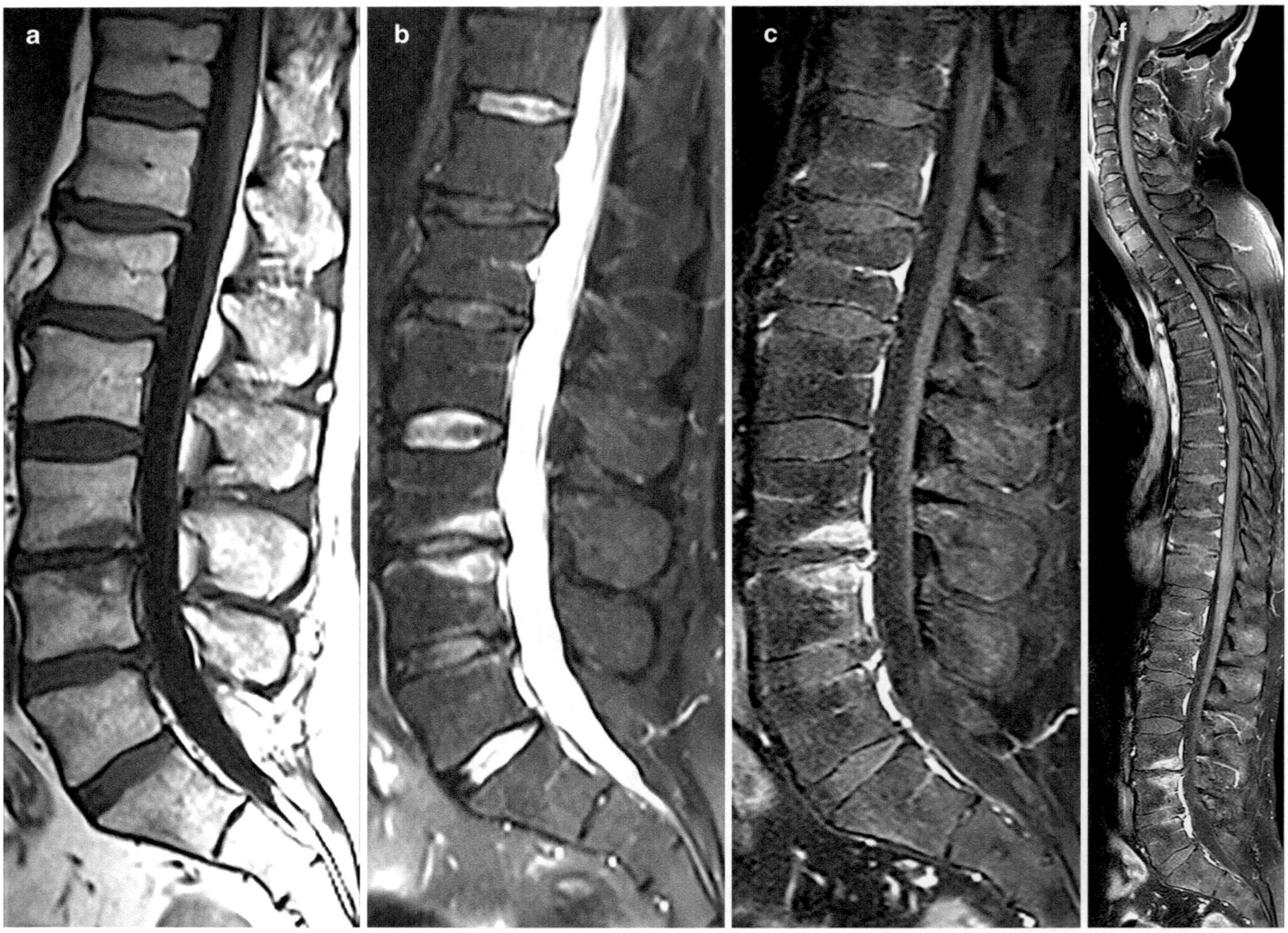

Fig. 12 (**a**–**f**) Sagittal TSE T1-weighted image (**a**), sagittal TSE T2-weighted image with fat saturation (**b**), sagittal and axial TSE T1-weighted images with fat saturation after administration of contrast medium (**c**–**f**). Signal changes (hypointense in T1 and hyperintense in T2) and marked contrast enhancement of the subchondral cancellous bone and part of the chondral surfaces at L3/L4 (**a**–**c**, **f**). Reduction in height of the corresponding L3/L4 intervertebral disc. These findings indicate typical osteochondritis in active-inflammatory phase. The same patient presented bilateral facet joint osteoarthritis at C4/C5, in active inflammatory phase (**d**, **e**)

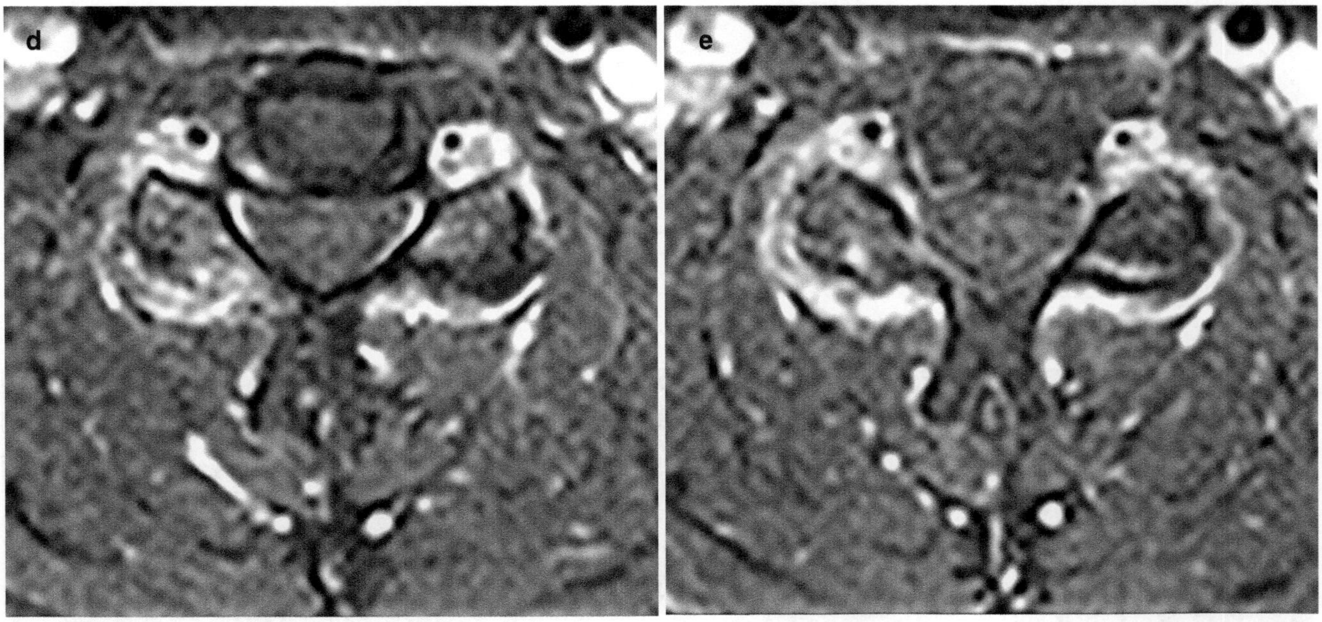

Fig. 12 (continued)

Case 24: Facet Joint Osteoarthritis. Synovitis

- A 60-year-old woman
- Chronic low back pain
- Limited motion of the lumbar spine
- Worsening of pain with motion and improvement with rest

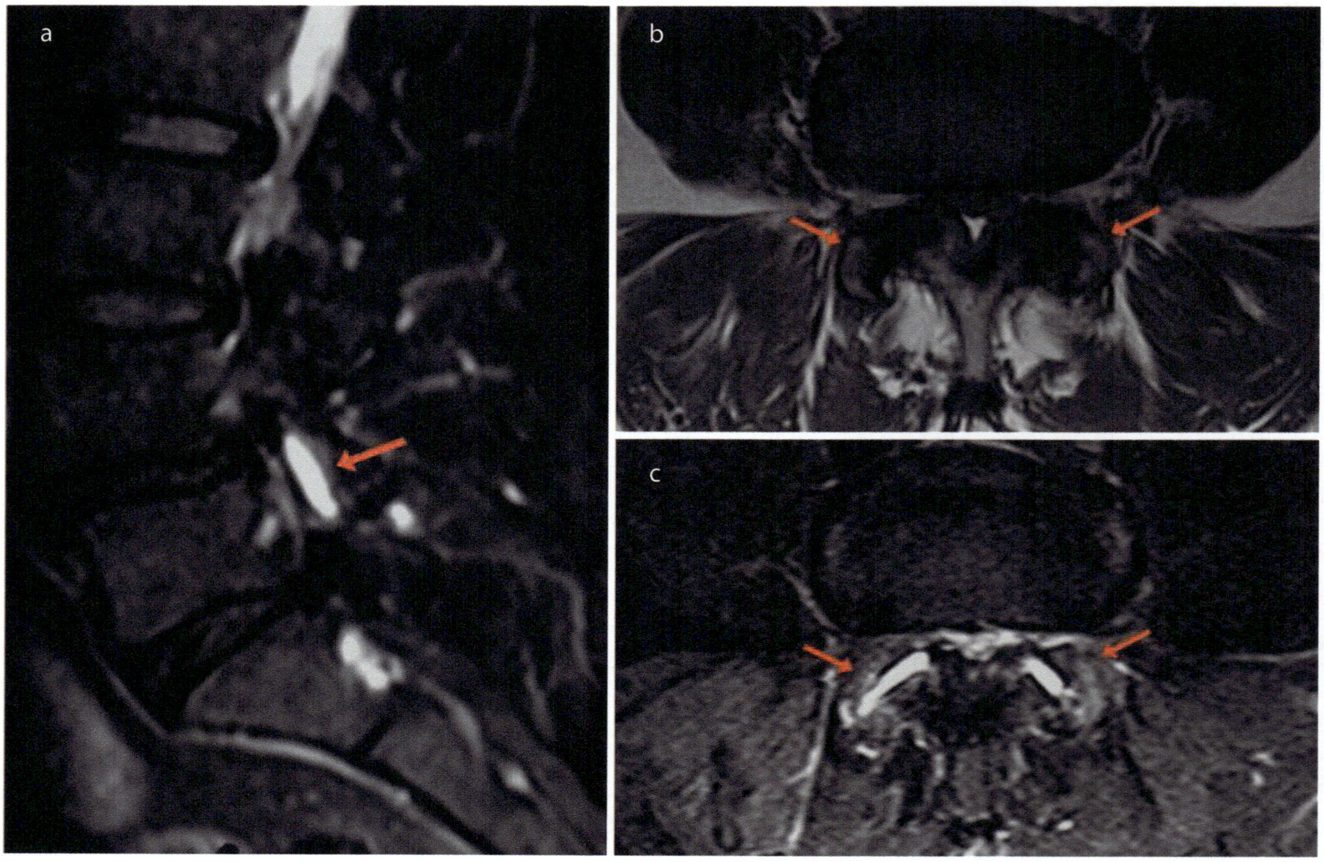

Fig. 13 (**a**–**e**) Sagittal and axial T2-weighted images with fat saturation (**a**, **c**), axial T1-weighted image (**b**), sagittal and axial T1-weighted images with fat saturation following administration of contrast medium (**d**, **e**). Bilateral facet joint osteoarthritis at L4/L5 (**b**, **c**, **e**, *arrows*). Widening of the facet joint spaces (**a**, **c**, *arrows*). Marked contrast enhancement of the synovial membrane, especially postero-inferiorly to the facet joint, indicating synovitis with synovial hypertrophy (**d**, *arrows*). Stenosis of the central spinal canal (**b**, **c**, **e**)

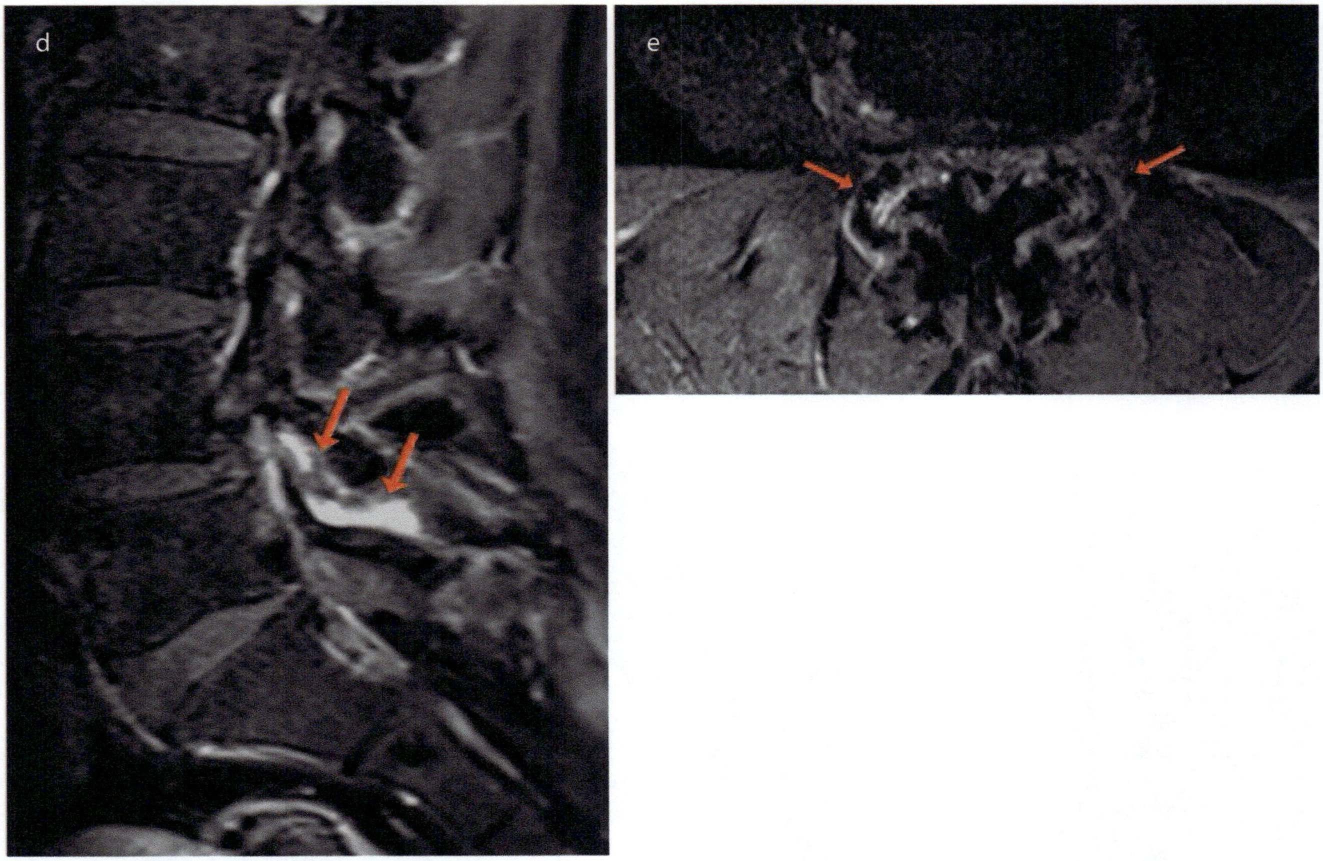

Fig. 13 (continued)

Case 25: Facet Joint Osteoarthritis. Synovitis

- A 61-year-old man
- Chronic low back pain
- Exacerbation of pain by extension and flexion
- Point tenderness corresponding to L4/L5 right facet joint

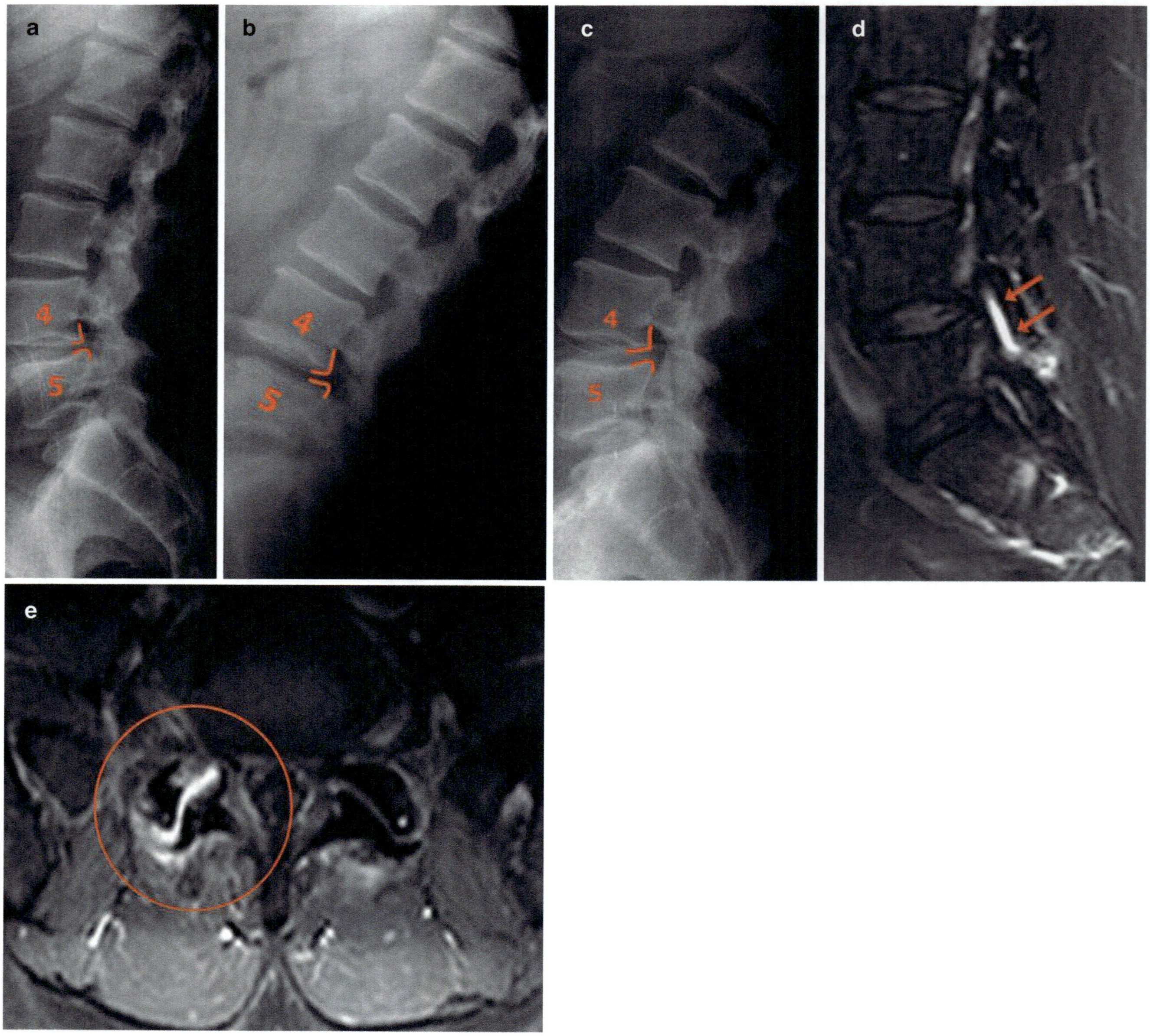

Fig. 14 (**a**–**e**) Dynamic X-ray of the lumbosacral spine (**a**–**c**), sagittal T2-weighted image with fat saturation (**d**), axial SE T1-weighted image with fat saturation following administration of contrast medium (**e**). Mild anterolisthesis of L4 over L5 (**a**–**c**), more evident in hyperflexion (**b**). Right facet joint osteoarthritis, with T2-hyperintensity (**d**, *arrows*) and marked contrast enhancement of the joint space indicating synovitis (**e**, *circle*). The osteoarthritis is clearly an expression of the vertebral instability

Case 26: Atlanto-Axial Osteoarthritis

- A 61-year-old woman
- Deviation of the head
- Chronic cervical pain

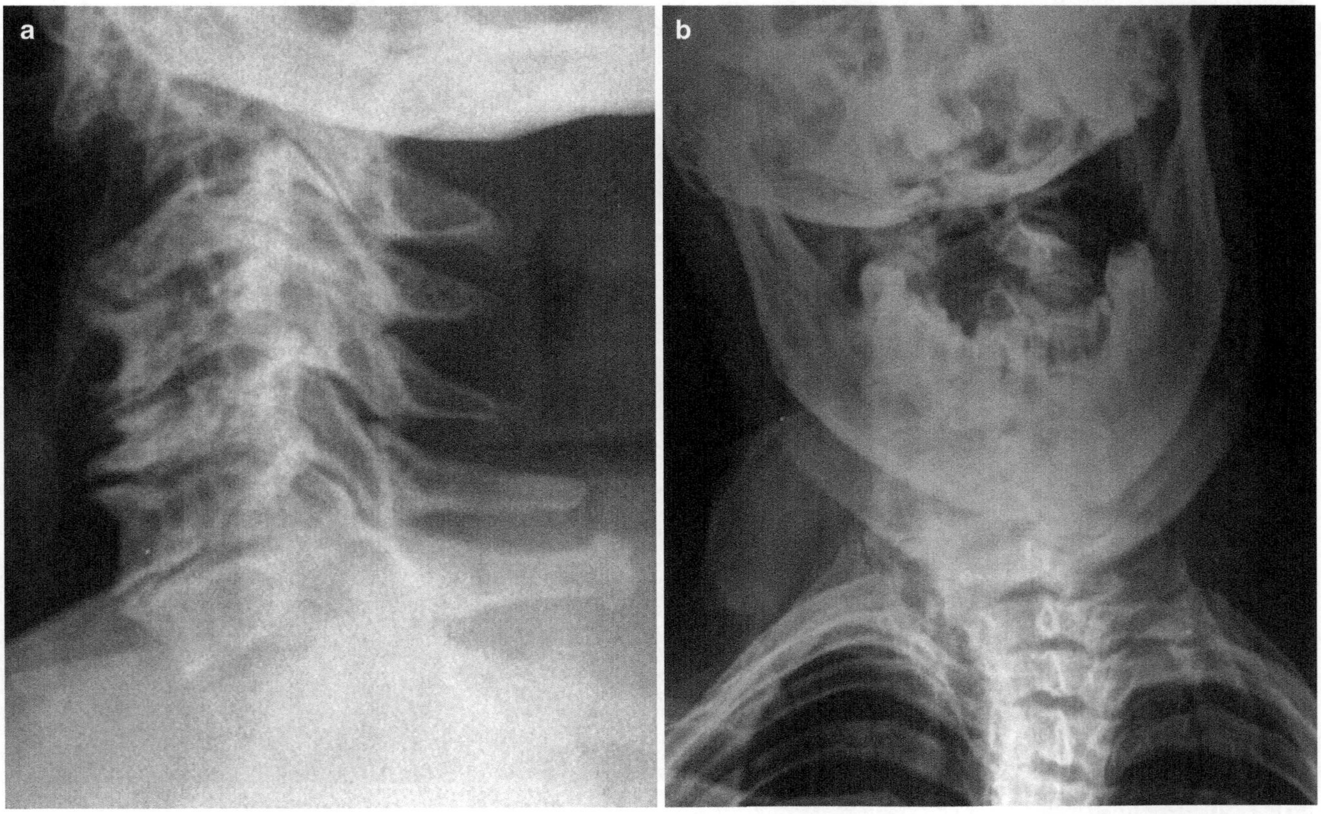

Fig. 15 (**a–g**) Lateral and AP plain film radiographs (**a**, **b**), axial SE T1-weighted images with fat saturation after contrast medium administration (**c–e**), CT images (**f**, **g**). Diffuse spondylotic and osteochondrotic degenerative changes (**a**). Right deviation of the head in malformation of the craniocervical junction (**b**). MRI shows marked contrast enhancement of the atlanto-axial and atlanto-odontoid joint on the right side, indicating osteoarthritis in active inflammatory phase (**c–e**, *arrows*). Note also diffuse epidural contrast enhancement at the same level, indicating a reactive epidural inflammation (**e**). CT images show widening of the distance between the right lateral mass of the atlas and the odontoid process (**f**, **g**, *arrow*)

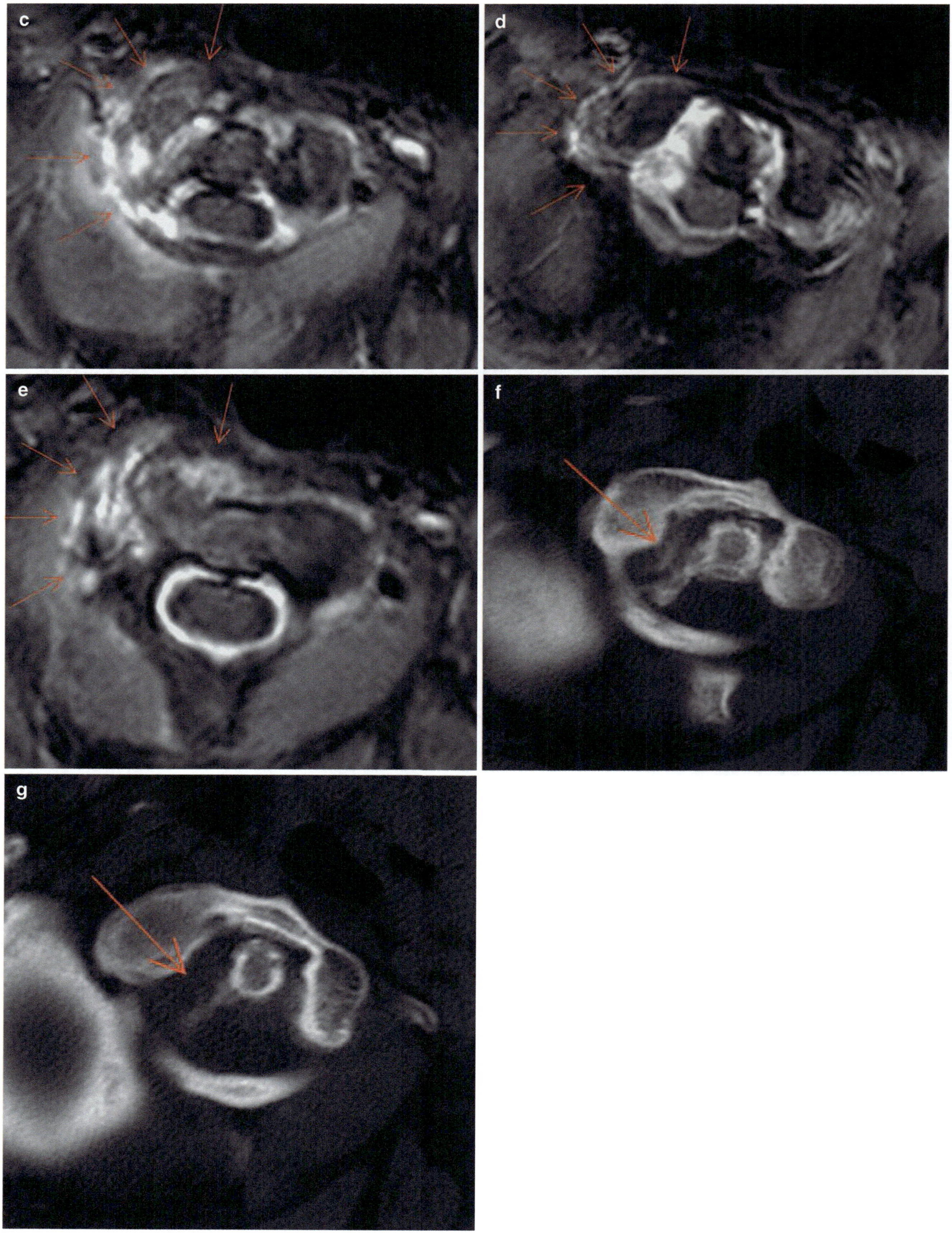

Fig. 15 (continued)

Case 27: Peridiscal Inflammation. Synovitis. Bone Collision

- A 74-year-old patient
- Chronic low back pain
- Radiculopathy on the right side
- Exacerbation of pain with lateral flexion on the right side

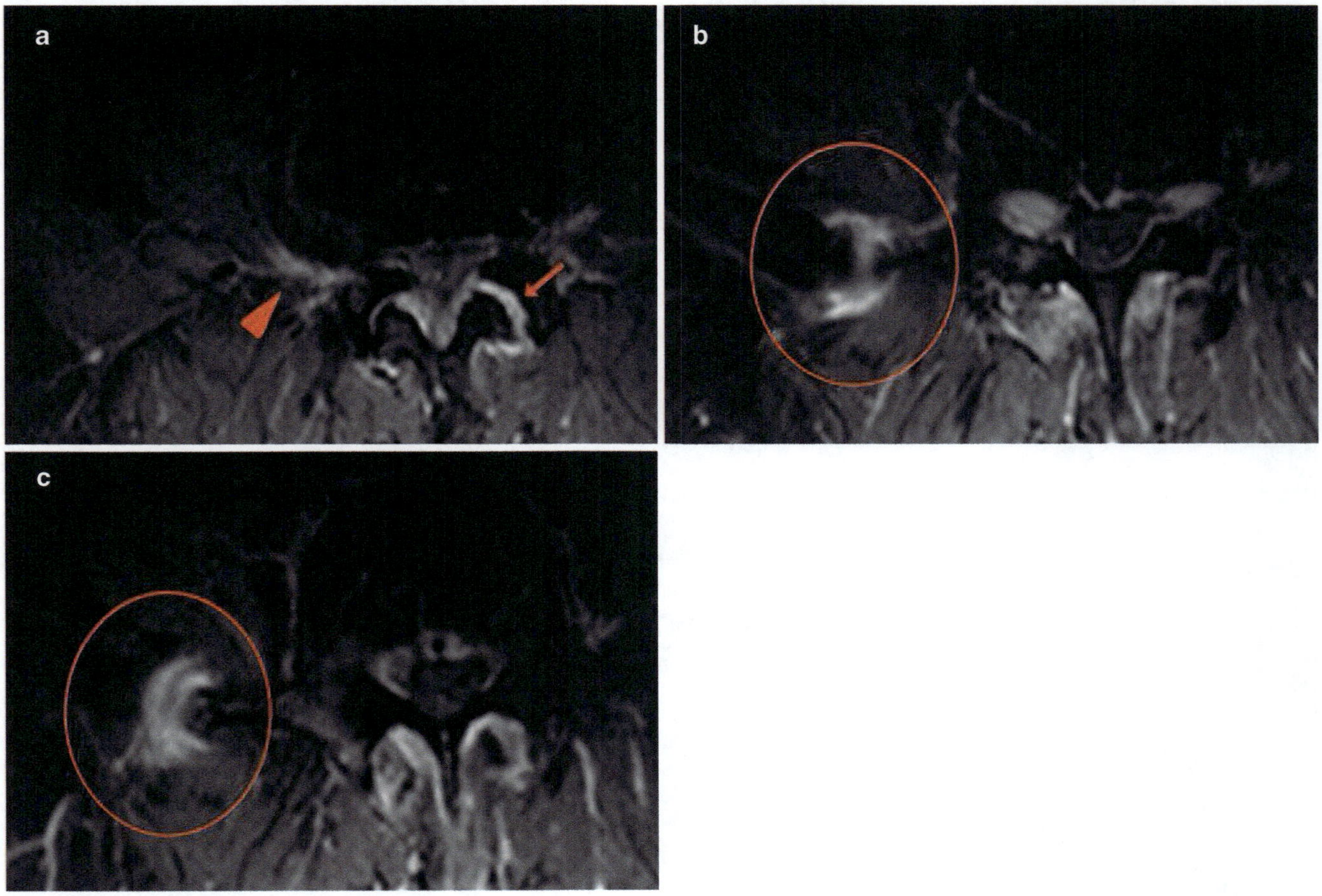

Fig. 16 (**a–c**) Axial SE T1-weighted images with fat saturation following administration of contrast medium (**a–c**). Extraforaminal disc protrusion with surrounding contrast enhancement due to peridiscal inflammation (**a**, *arrowhead*). Contrast enhancement of the left facet joint space, indicating synovitis (**a**, *arrow*). Bone collision between the right trans-verse process of L4 and ipsilateral iliac wing, with contrast enhancement at the same level indicating reactive inflammatory phenomena (**b**, **c**, *circle*)

Case 28: Atlanto-Axial Osteoarthritis

- A 68-year-old woman
- Cervical pain
- Limitation of motion of the head

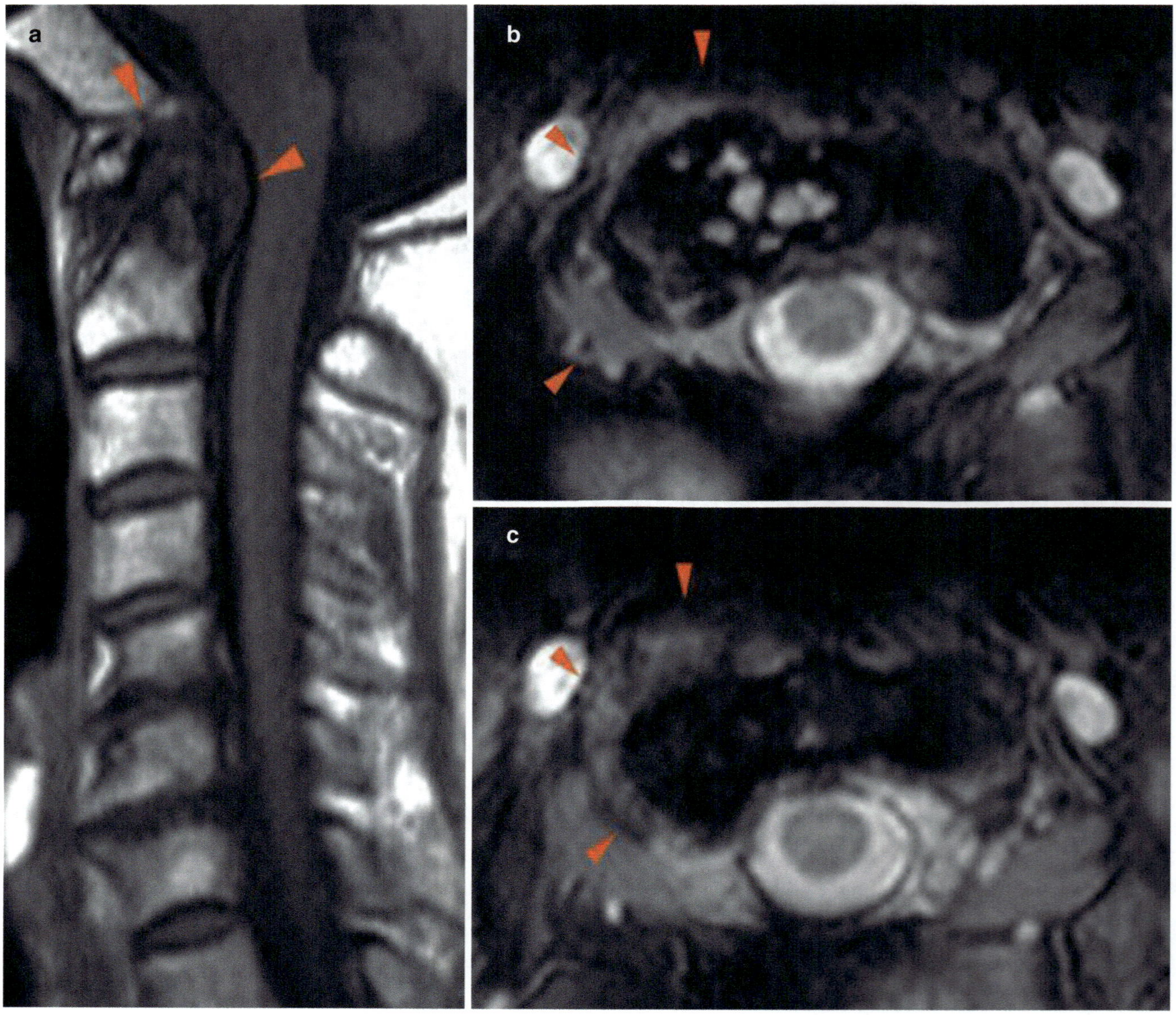

Fig. 17 Sagittal SE T1-weighted image (**a**), axial GE T2*-weighted images (**b**, **c**), sagittal and axial SE T1-weighted images with fat saturation after the administration of contrast medium (**d–g**), axial CT images (**h**, **i**). Malformation of the cranio-cervical junction, with posterior atlanto-occipital fusion (**a**). T1-weighted imaging shows pathological tissue at C1/C2 (**a**, *arrowheads*). Multiple small hyperintense areas in T2 at the level of atlanto-axial and atlanto-odontoid joints on the right side and periarticular soft tissues (**b**, **c**, *arrowheads*). The same areas enhance after administration of contrast medium (**e–g**, *arrowheads*). CT images show osteosclerosis, joint erosions and cysts (**h**, **i**, *arrowheads*). These findings indicate osteoarthritis in active inflammatory phase, with periarticular soft tissue inflammation

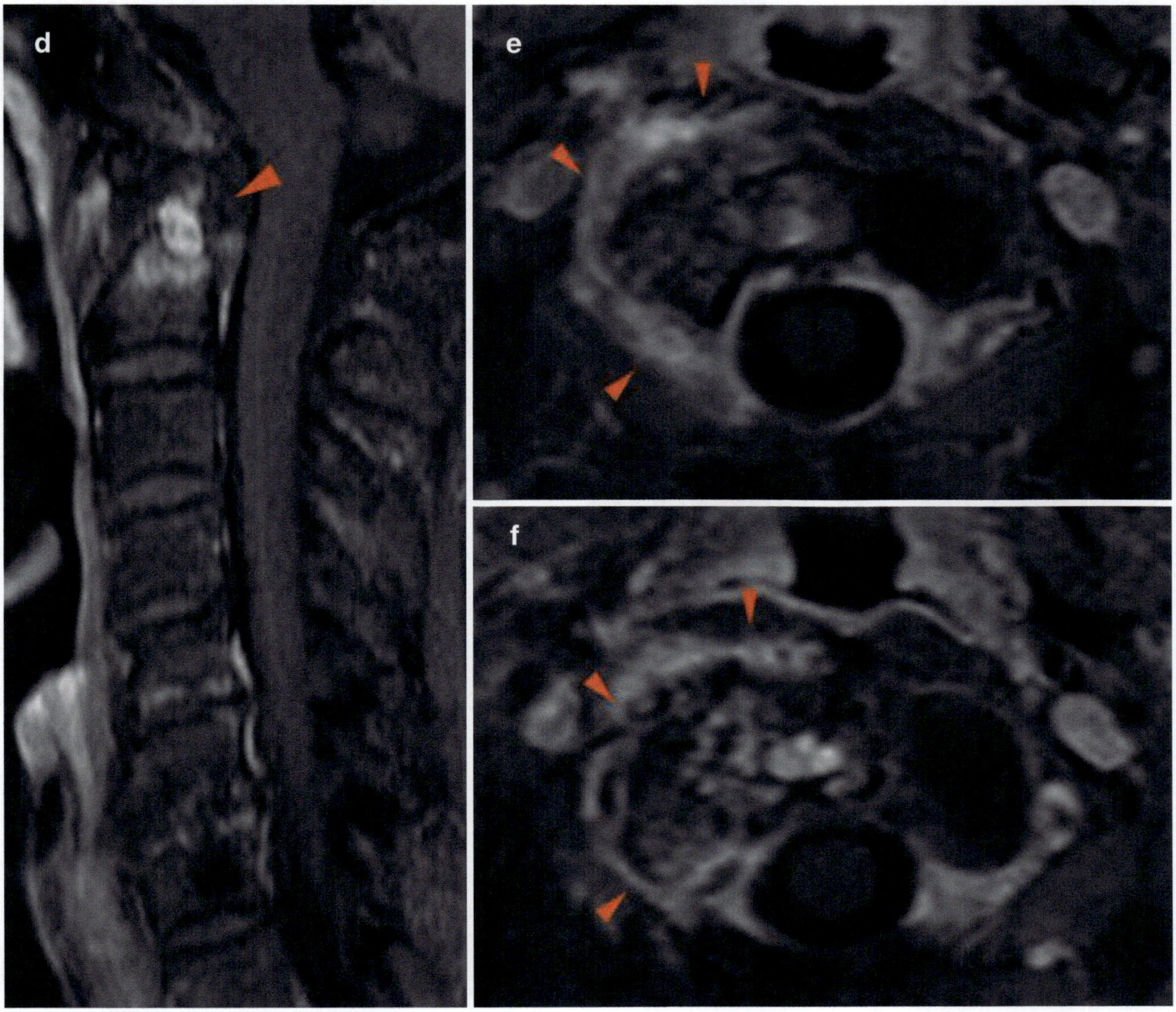

Fig. 17 (continued)

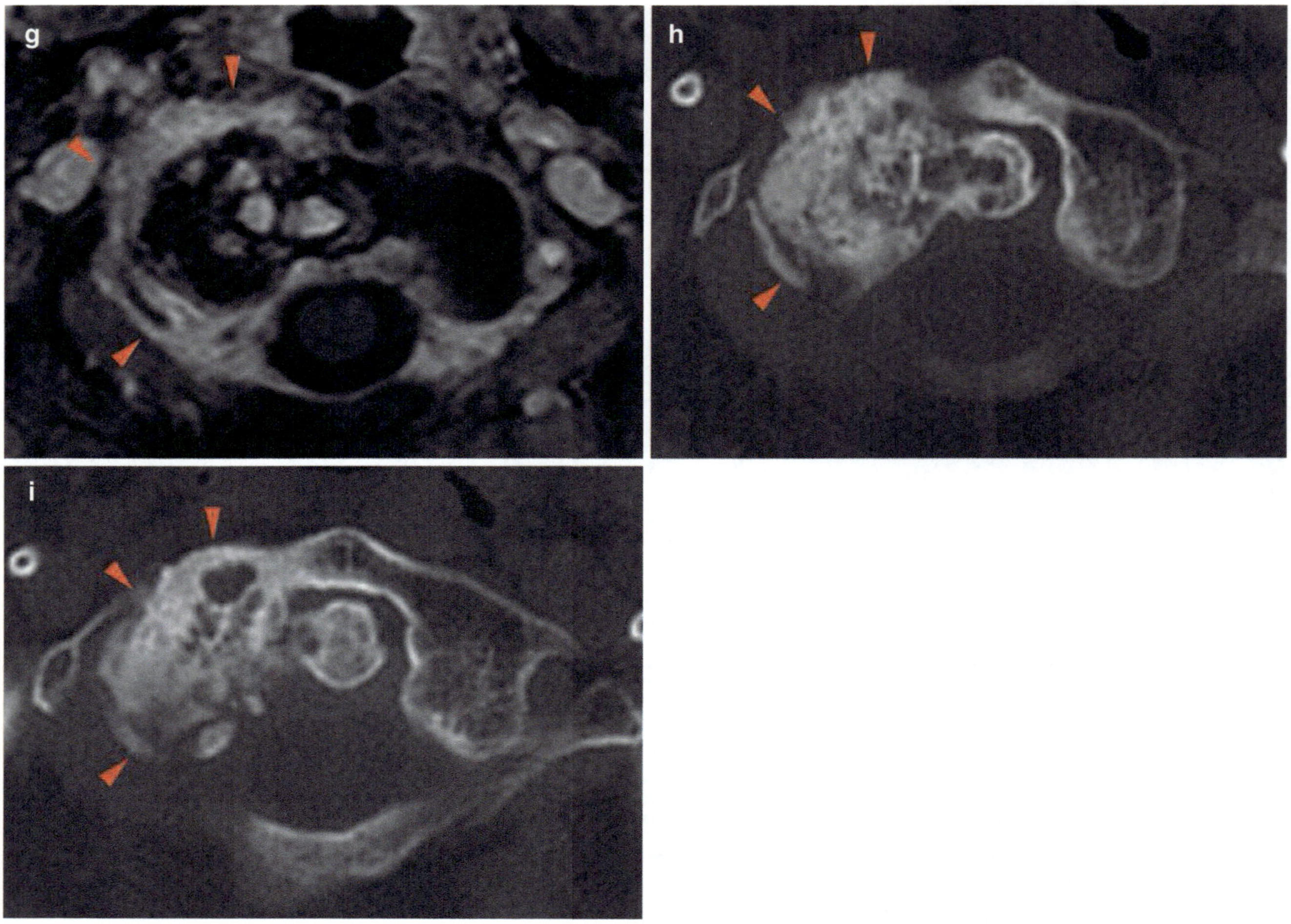

Fig. 17 (continued)

Case 29: Spine Instability. Facet Joint Osteoarthritis

- A 57-year-old man
- Low back pain exacerbated by flexion
- Point tenderness corresponding to L4/L5 right facet joint

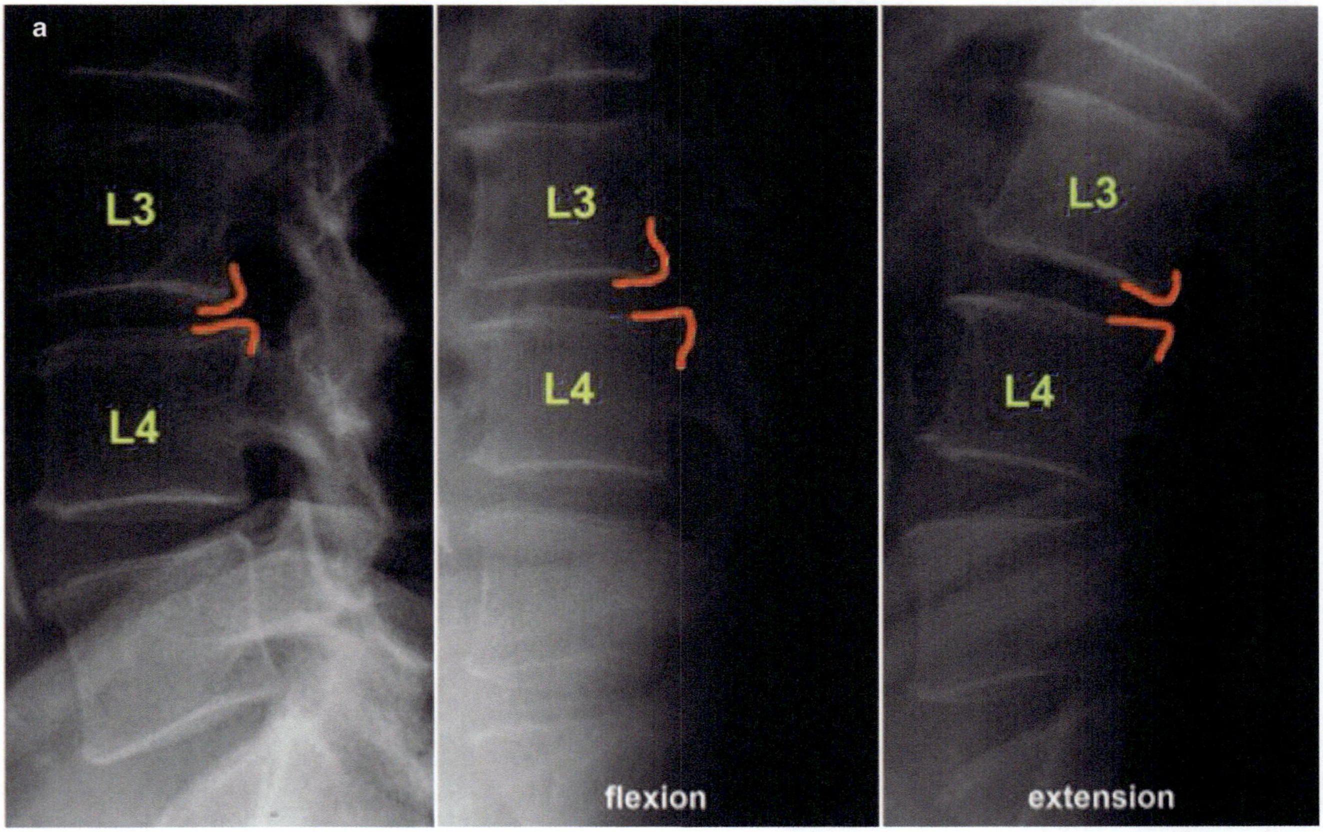

Fig. 18 Dynamic lumbar radiography (**a**), sagittal SE T1-weighted image (**b**), sagittal and axial SE T2-weighted images with fat saturation (**c–f**), axial SE T1-weighted images with fat saturation following the administration of contrast medium (**g–i**). Anterolisthesis of L3 over L4, more marked in flexion (**a**). MRI confirms the spinal instability L3/L4 (**b**). The same patient presented right facet joint osteoarthritis at L5/S1, with bone oedema and intra-articular effusion (**c–f**, *arrow*). The administration of contrast medium shows enhancement of the same apophyseal processes, confirming the aseptic inflammation of the bone marrow, i.e. osteitis in the context of osteoarthritis (**g**, *arrow*). Note also synovial hypertrophy of the same joint, well delineated after contrast medium administration (**h**, **i**, *arrow*)

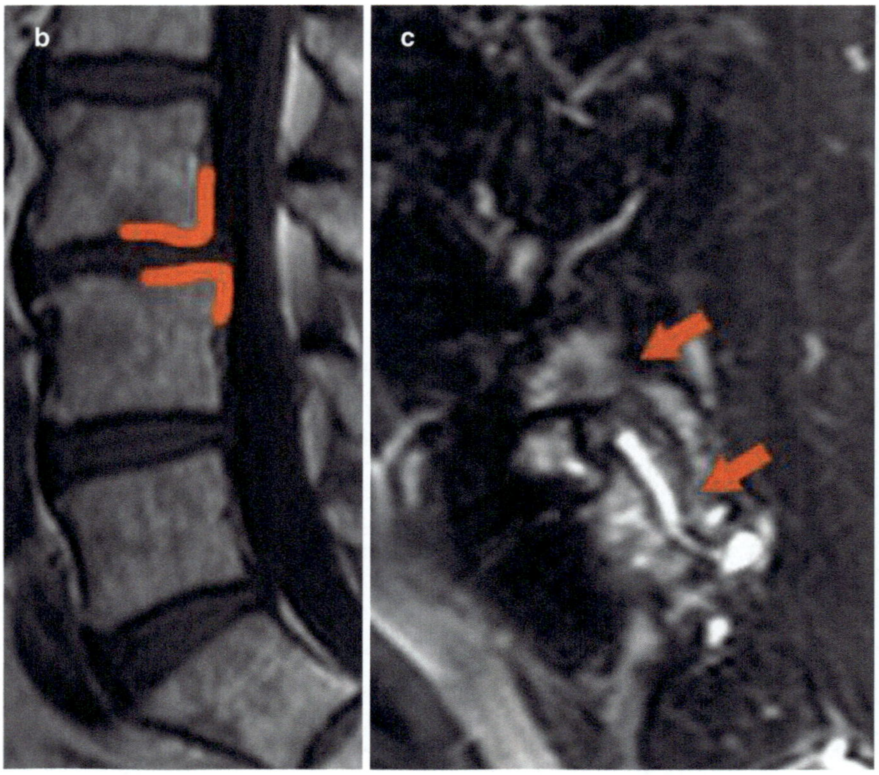

Fig. 18 (continued)

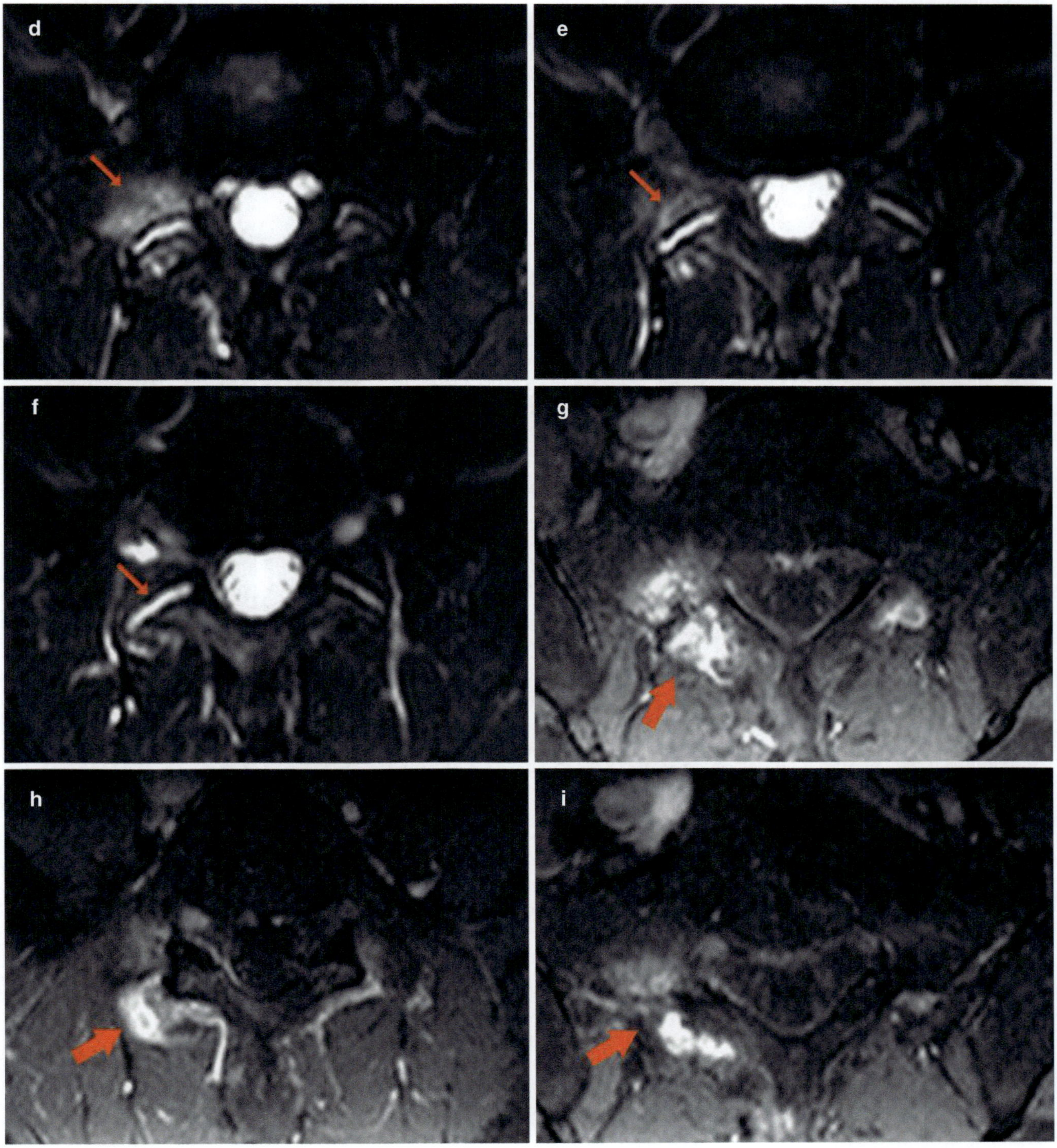

Fig. 18 (continued)

Case 30: Synovitis. Inflammation of Ligaments

- A 61-year-old man
- Persistent low back pain
- Tenderness on palpation of the lumbar interspinous spaces

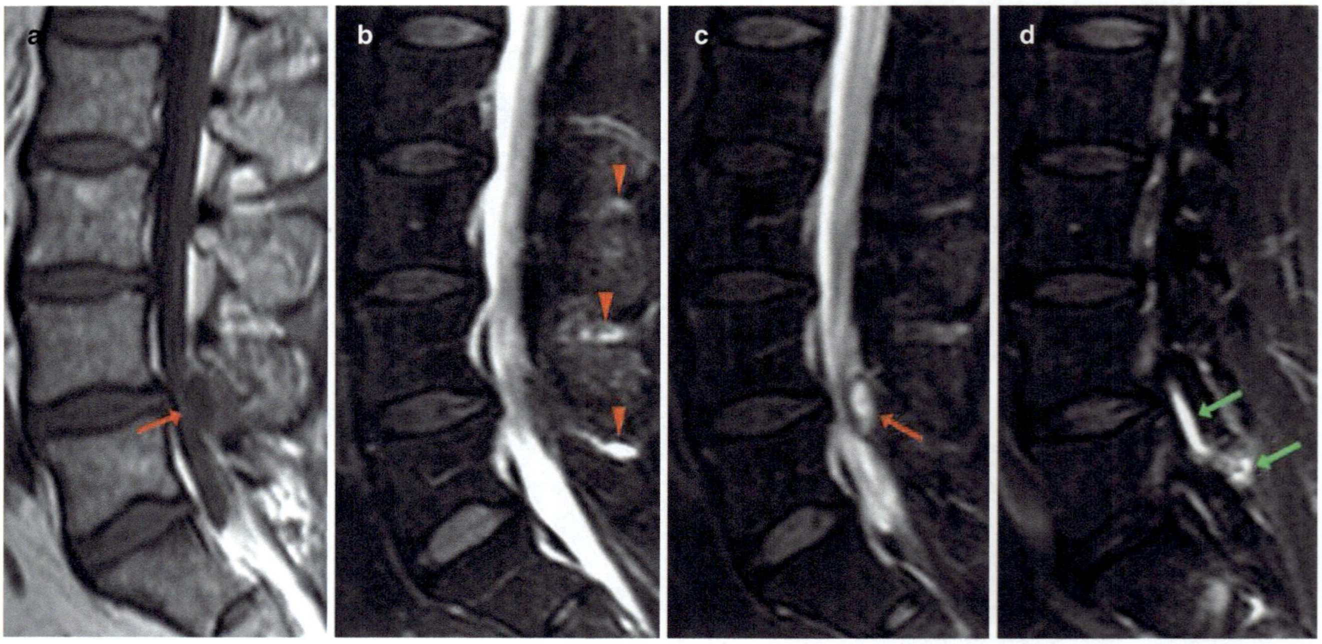

Fig. 19 Sagittal SE T1-weighted image (**a**), sagittal TSE T2-weighted images with fat saturation (**b–d**), sagittal and axial SE T1-weighted images with fat saturation following administration of contrast medium (**e–g**, **i**, **j**), axial CISS T2-weighted image (**h**). Mild anterolisthesis of L4 over L5 (**a–g**). Hypertrophy and contrast enhancement of the L4/L5 left flavum ligament, due to inflammation with cystic component (**a**, **c**, **e**, **f**, **l**, *red arrow*). T2 hyperintensity and contrast enhancement of the interspinous ligament from L2 to L5, indicating ligamentous degenerative inflammatory changes (**b**, **e**, **i**, *arrowhead*). The L4/L5 left facet joint space is widened (**d**, **h**, *green arrows*) and enhances after contrast medium administration (**g**, **l**, *green arrows*), indicating synovitis; note also synovial hypertrophy postero-inferiorly to the same joint (**g**)

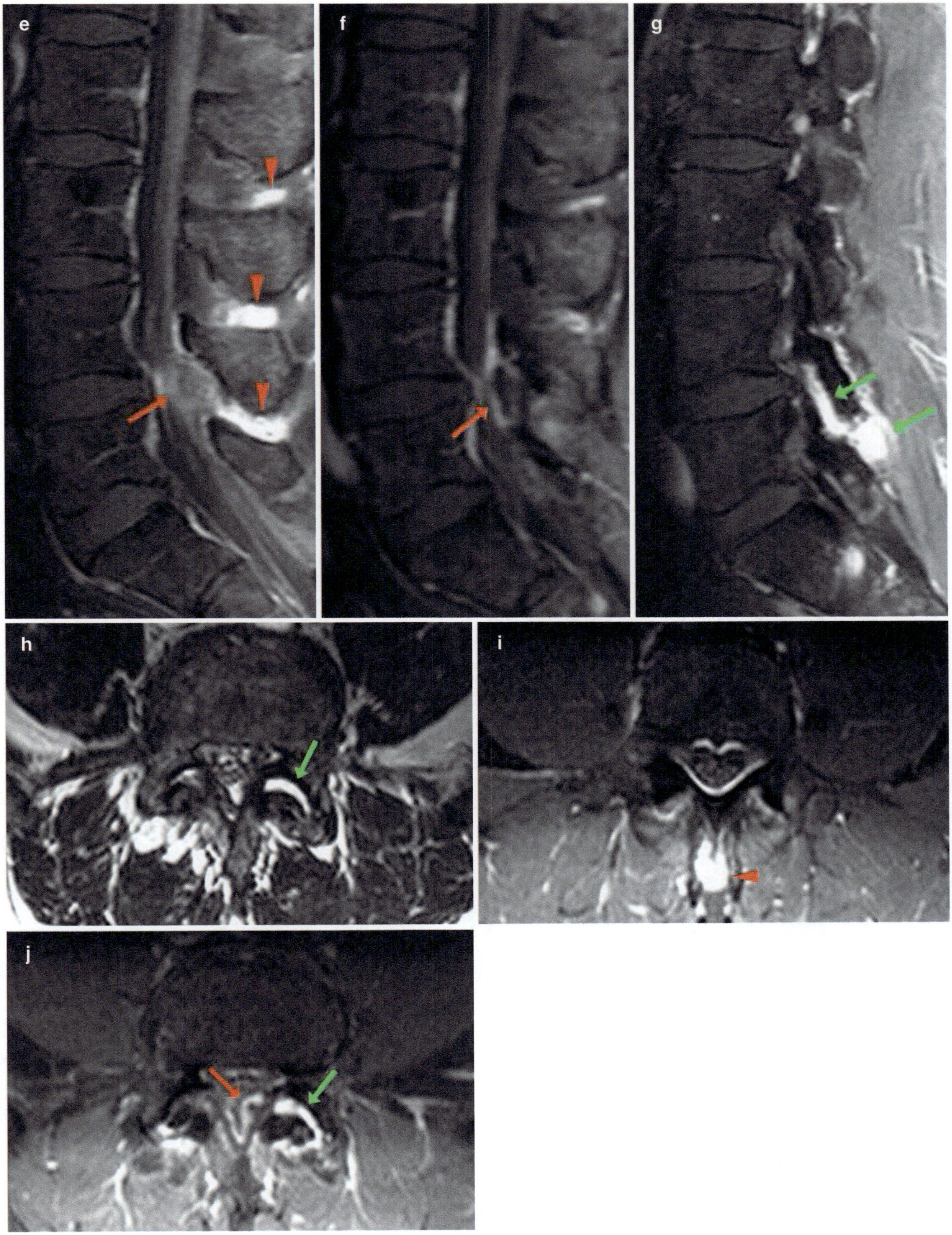

Fig. 19 (continued)

Case 31: Synovial Cyst

- A 59-year-old man
- Neck pain with radiculopathy on the left side

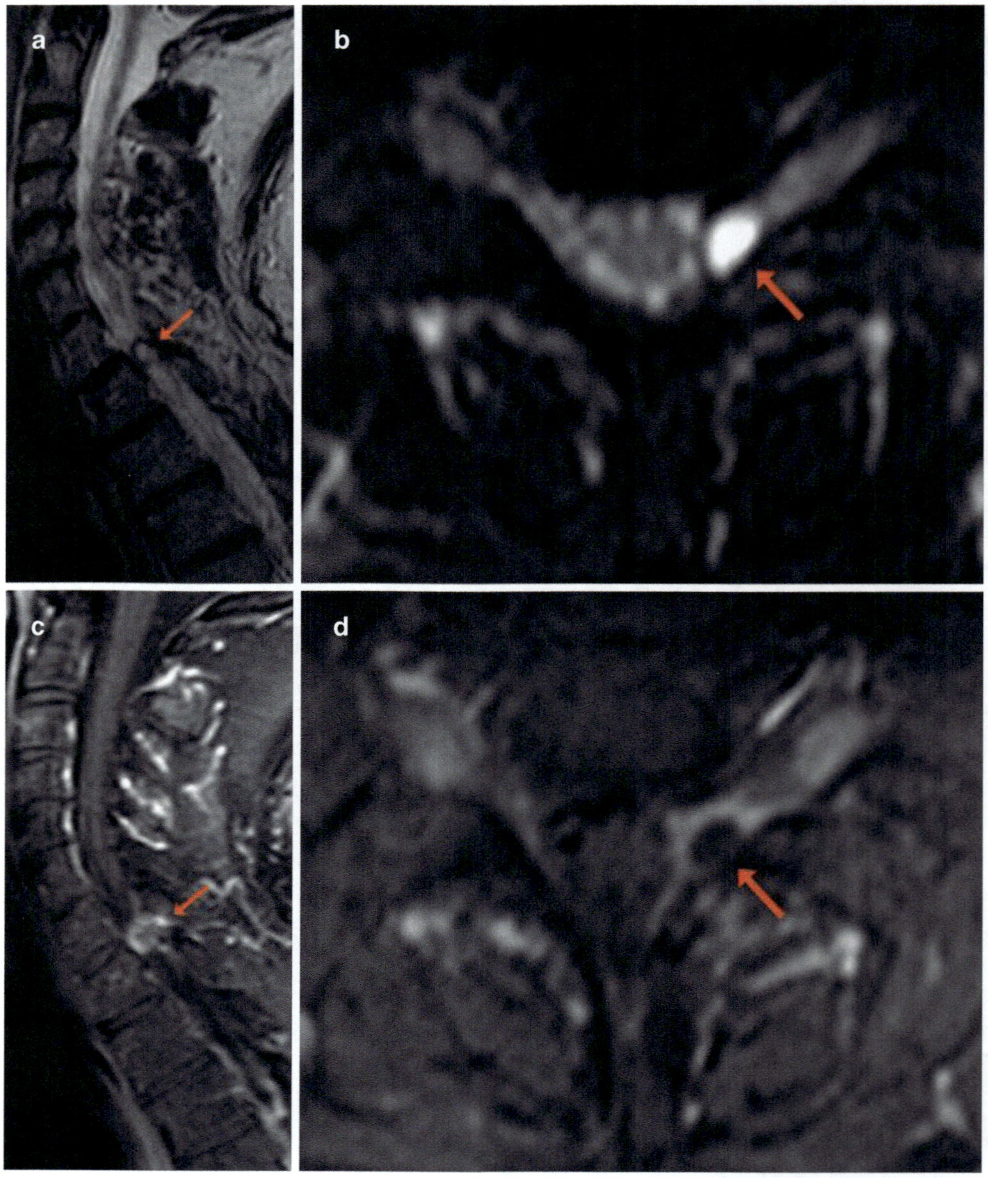

Fig. 20 Sagittal TSE T2-weighted image (**a**), axial TSE T2-weighted image with fat saturation (**b**), sagittal and axial SE T1-weighted images with fat saturation following administration of contrast medium (**c**, **d**). Presence of synovial cyst in the left lateral recess of the spinal canal at C7/D1 (**a**–**d**, *arrow*). The cyst is hyperintense on T2-weighted images (**a**, **b**) and hypointense in T1, with peripheral enhancement after contrast medium administration (**c**, **d**)

Case 32: Synovial Cyst. Facet Joint Osteoarthritis

- A 74-year-old woman
- Patient with persistent neck pain, more marked on the right side

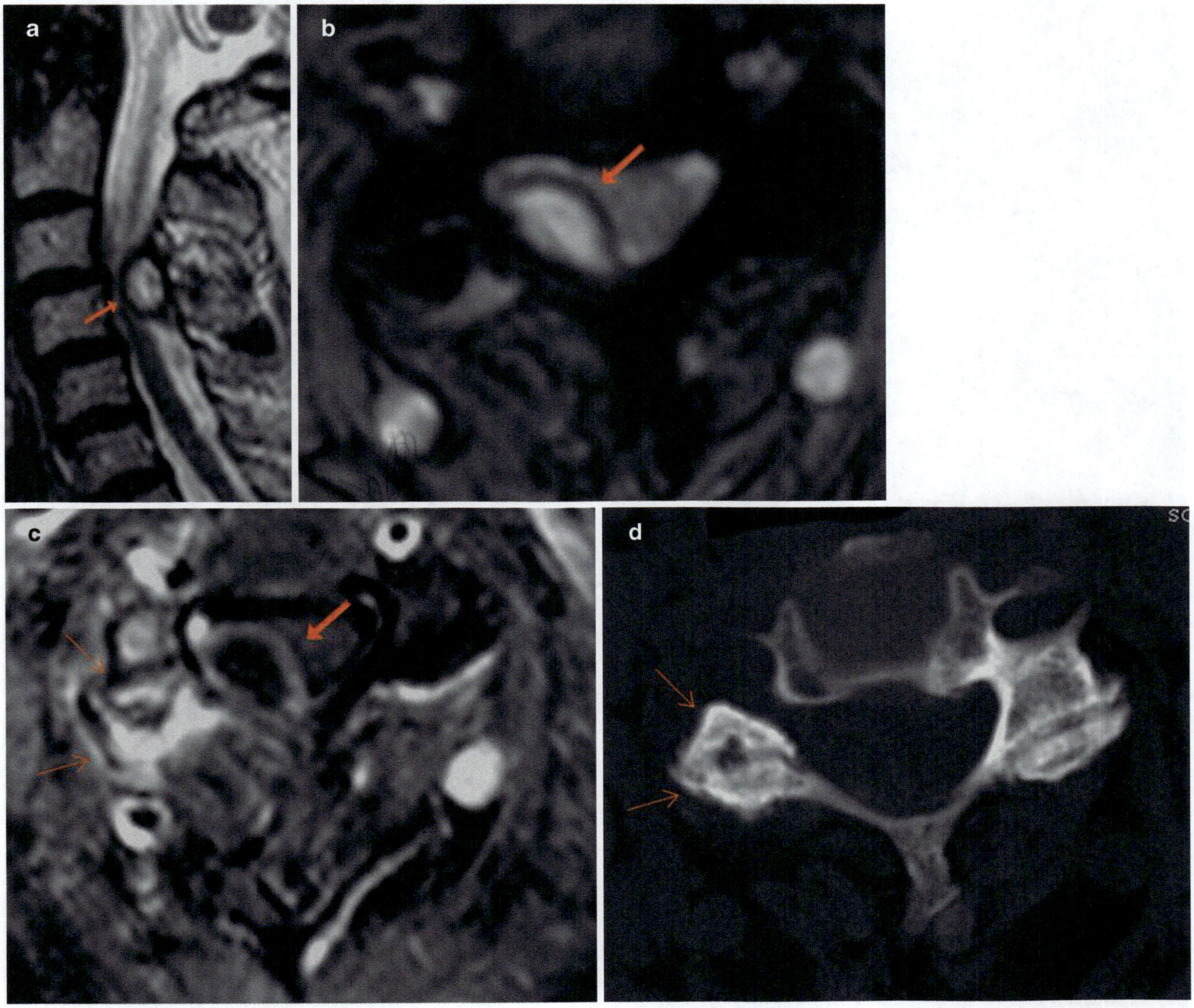

Fig. 21 Sagittal TSE T2-weighted image (**a**), axial GE T2*-weighted image (**b**), axial SE T1-weighted image with fat saturation after administration of contrast medium (**c**), axial CT scan (**d**). Anterolisthesis of C3 over C4 and C4 over C5. Cystic lesion in the right part of the vertebral canal (*arrow*), hyperintense in T2 (**a**, **b**) and hypointense in T1, with peripheral contrast enhancement (**c**). The cyst compresses and displaces the spinal cord. This is a typical intracanal synovial cyst. Note also a right facet joint osteoarthritis, with contrast enhancement of the apophyses and periapophyseal soft tissues, indicating active inflammation (**c**, *thin arrows*). CT scan shows osteosclerosis of the apophyses and erosions of the articular surfaces (**d**, *thin arrows*). Most probably the synovial cyst is an epiphenomenon of the adjacent osteoarthritis and vertebral instability

Case 33: Synovial Cyst

- A 64-year-old man
- Chronic cervical pain

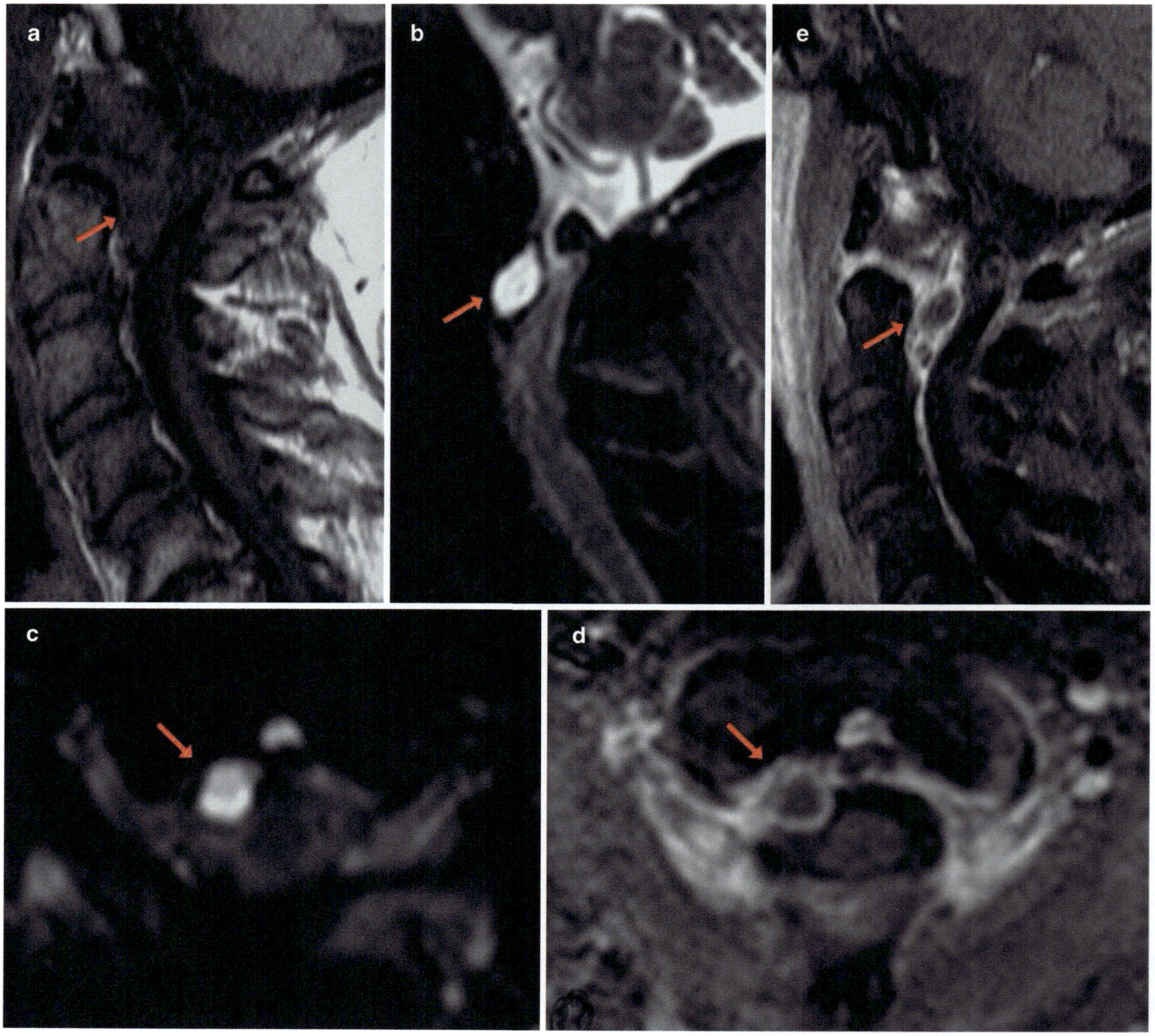

Fig. 22 Sagittal SE T1-weighted image (**a**), sagittal and axial TSE T2-weighted images with fat saturation (**b**, **c**), sagittal and axial SE T1-weighted images with fat saturation after administration of contrast medium (**d**, **e**). Extradural cystic lesion in the right part of the vertebral canal (*arrow*), hypointense in T1 (**a**) and hyperintense in T2 (**b**, **c**), with peripheral contrast enhancement (**d**, **e**). Diagnosis: intracanal synovial cyst

Case 34: Synovial Cyst

- A 43-year-old woman
- Low back pain with radiculopathy on the right side

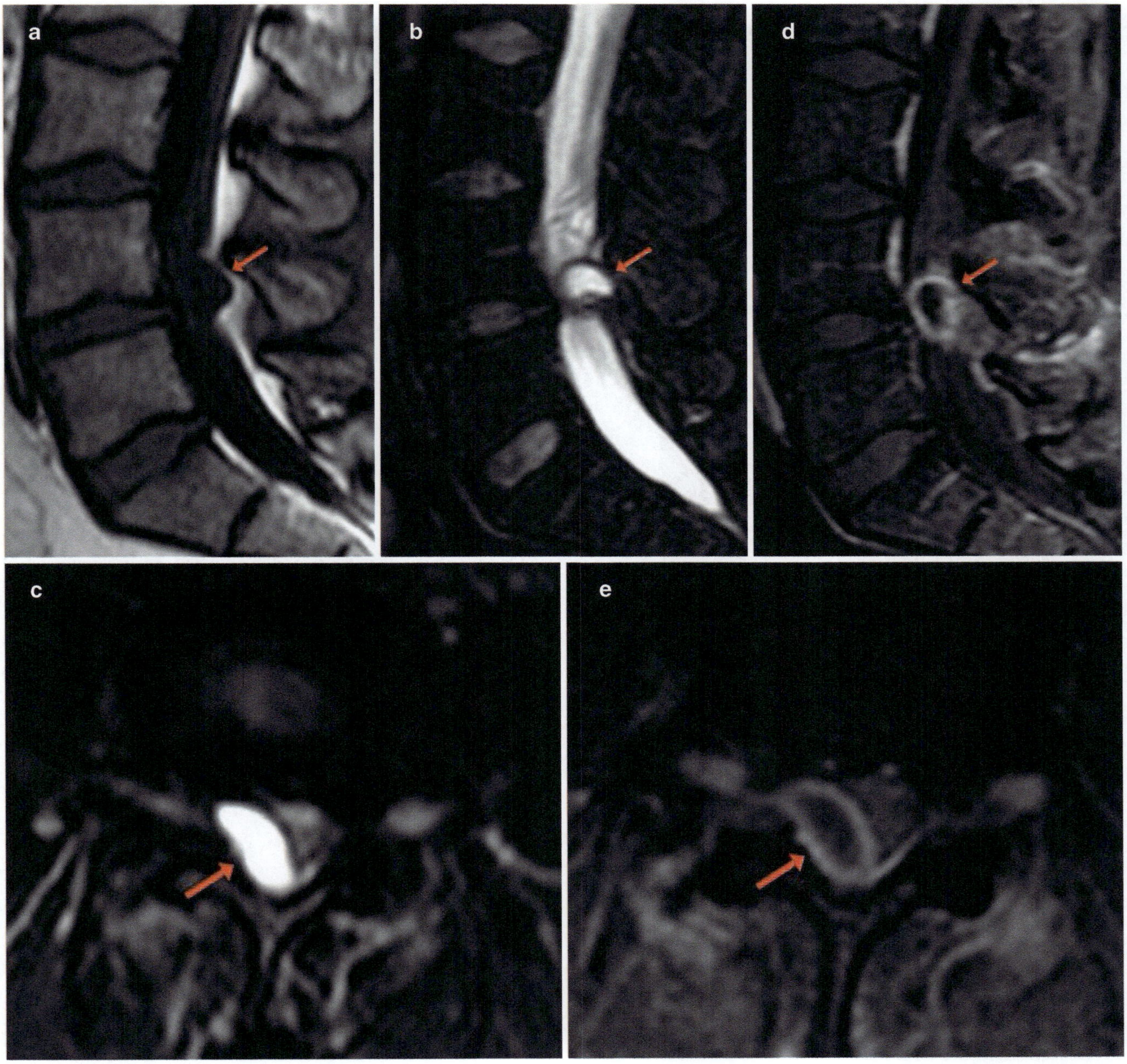

Fig. 23 Sagittal SE T1-weighted image (**a**), sagittal and axial TSE T2-weighted images with fat saturation (**b**, **c**), sagittal and axial SE T1-weighted images with fat saturation following administration of contrast medium (**d**, **e**). Endocanal synovial cyst at L4/L5 on the right side (**a**–**e**, *arrow*). The cyst displaces the thecal sac. Cystic content resembles CSF in all sequences (**a**–**c**). Cyst capsule enhances following contrast administration (**d**, **e**)

Case 35: Synovial Cyst

- A 45-year-old man
- Left L5 radiculopathy

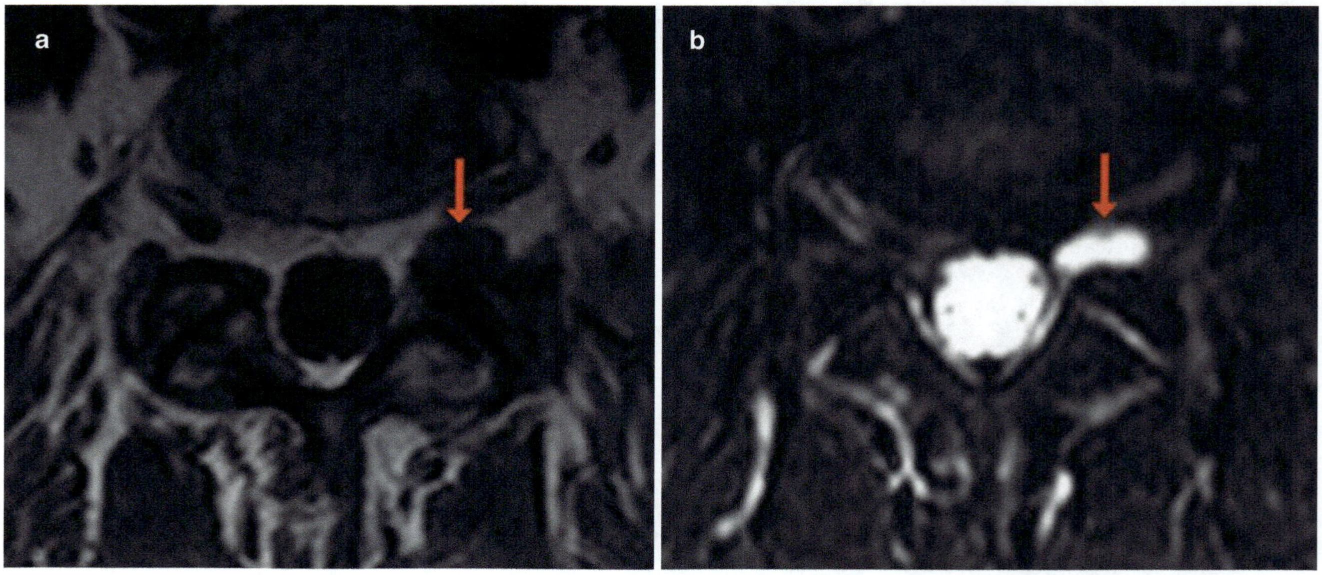

Fig. 24 Axial SE T1-weighted image (**a**), axial TSE T2-weighted image with fat saturation (**b**), sagittal and axial SE T1-weighted images with fat saturation following administration of contrast medium (**c–e**). Intraforaminal cystic lesion at L5/S1 on the left side (**a–c**, **e**, *arrow*). Cystic content resembles CSF. The wall of the cyst shows a thin and regular contrast enhancement (**c**, **e**). The L5 root is clearly separated and located anteriorly to the cyst (**d**, *arrow*). Diagnosis: intraforaminal synovial cyst. The major differential diagnosis of synovial cyst is a free disc fragment and cystic nerve root tumour. Signal characteristics and position of the lesion allow the proper diagnosis

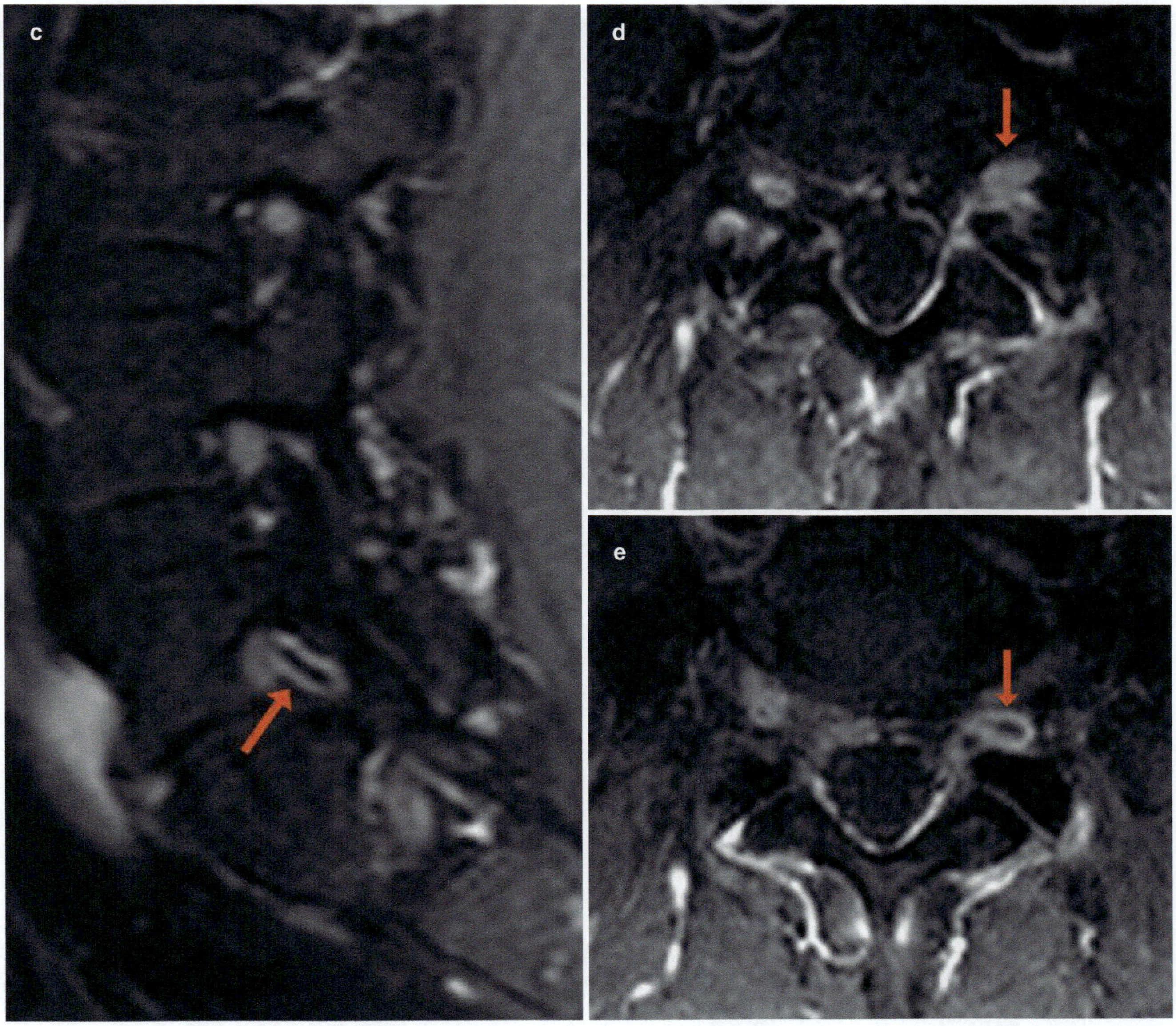

Fig. 24 (continued)

Case 36: Facet Joint Osteoarthritis. Synovial Cyst

- A 54-year-old man
- Chronic low back pain, more marked in flexion and extension

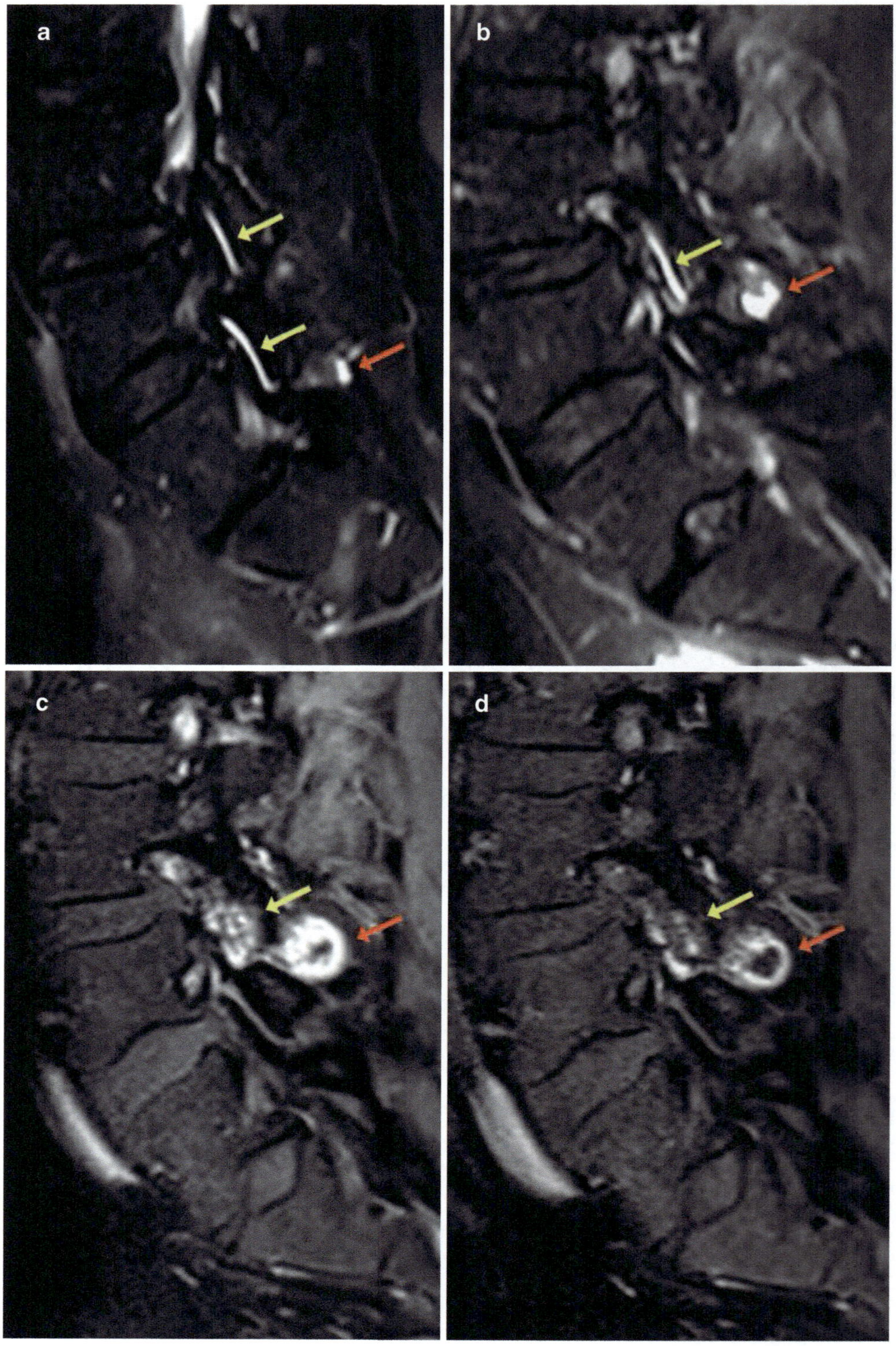

Fig. 25 Sagittal TSE T2-weighted images with fat saturation (**a**, **b**), sagittal and axial SE T1-weighted images with fat saturation following administration of contrast medium (**c**–**f**). Facet joint arthritis (*yellow arrow*, **a**–**d**). Extracanal synovial cyst, adjacent to degenerated facet joint (*orange arrow*, **a**–**f**). The cyst is more delineated on the left side after contrast medium administration (**d**, **f**)

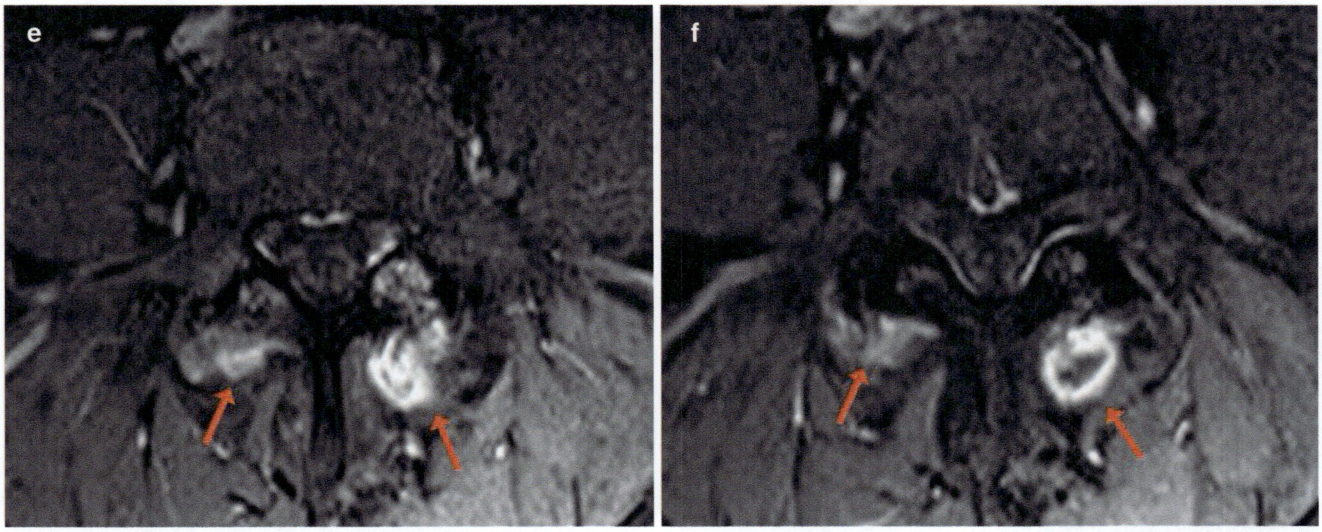

Fig. 25 (continued)

Case 37: Facet Joint Osteoarthritis. Synovial Cyst

- A 46-year-old woman
- Low back pain
- Pain exacerbated by flexion and extension

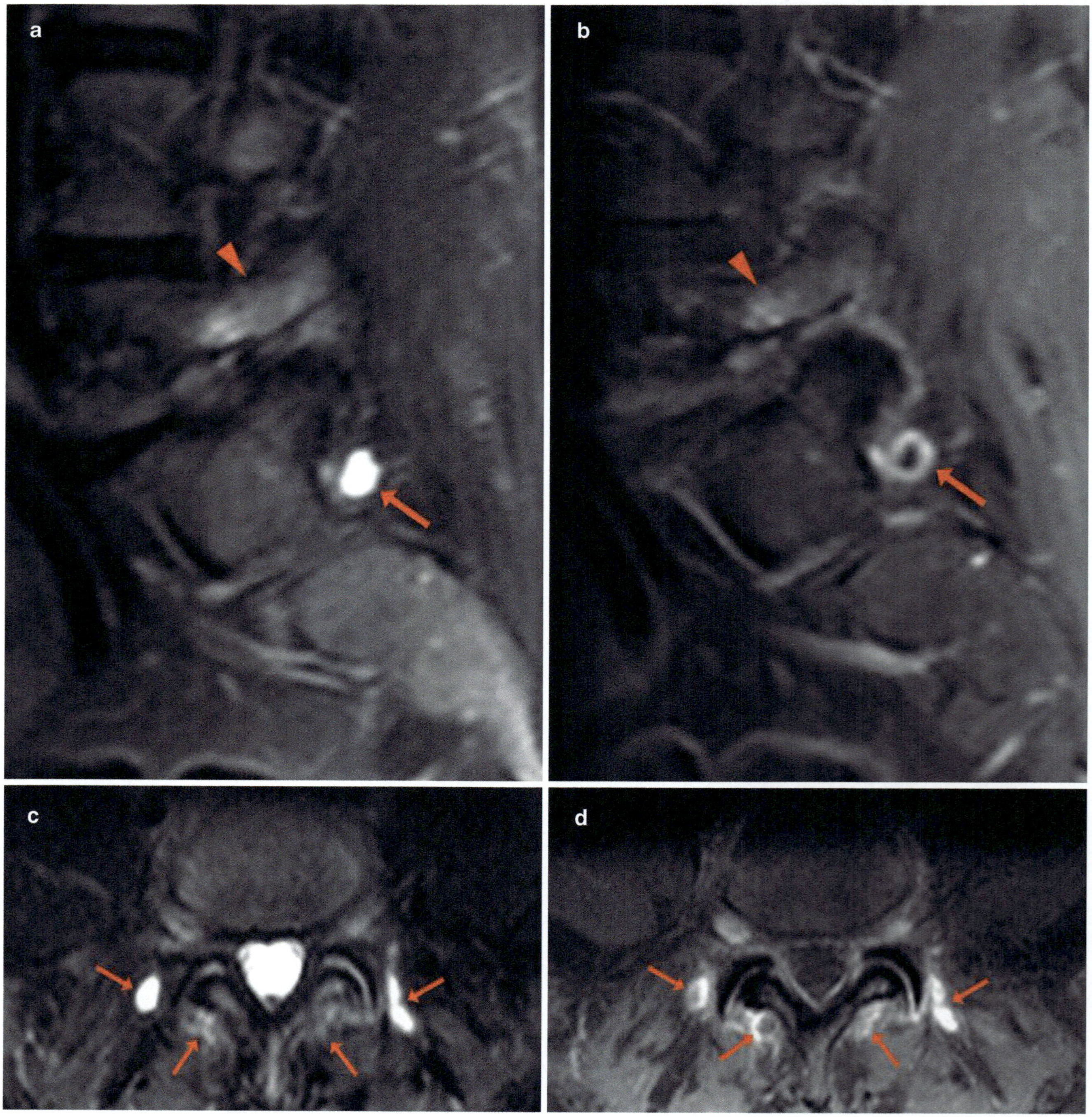

Fig. 26 Sagittal and axial T2-weighted images with fat saturation (**a**, **c**), sagittal and axial SE T1-weighted images with fat saturation after contrast medium administration (**b**, **d**). Facet joint osteoarthritis with oedema osteitis that extends to the left pedicle of L5 (**a**, **b**, *arrowheads*). Extracanal synovial cysts and synovial "hypertrophy" adjacent to the facet joints bilaterally (**a**–**d**, *arrows*). Synovial cysts typically show peripheral enhancement after contrast medium administration (**b**, **d**)

6 Spondylolysis

Case 38: Spondylolysis

- A 18-year-old man
- Acute-subacute low back pain in a young athlete

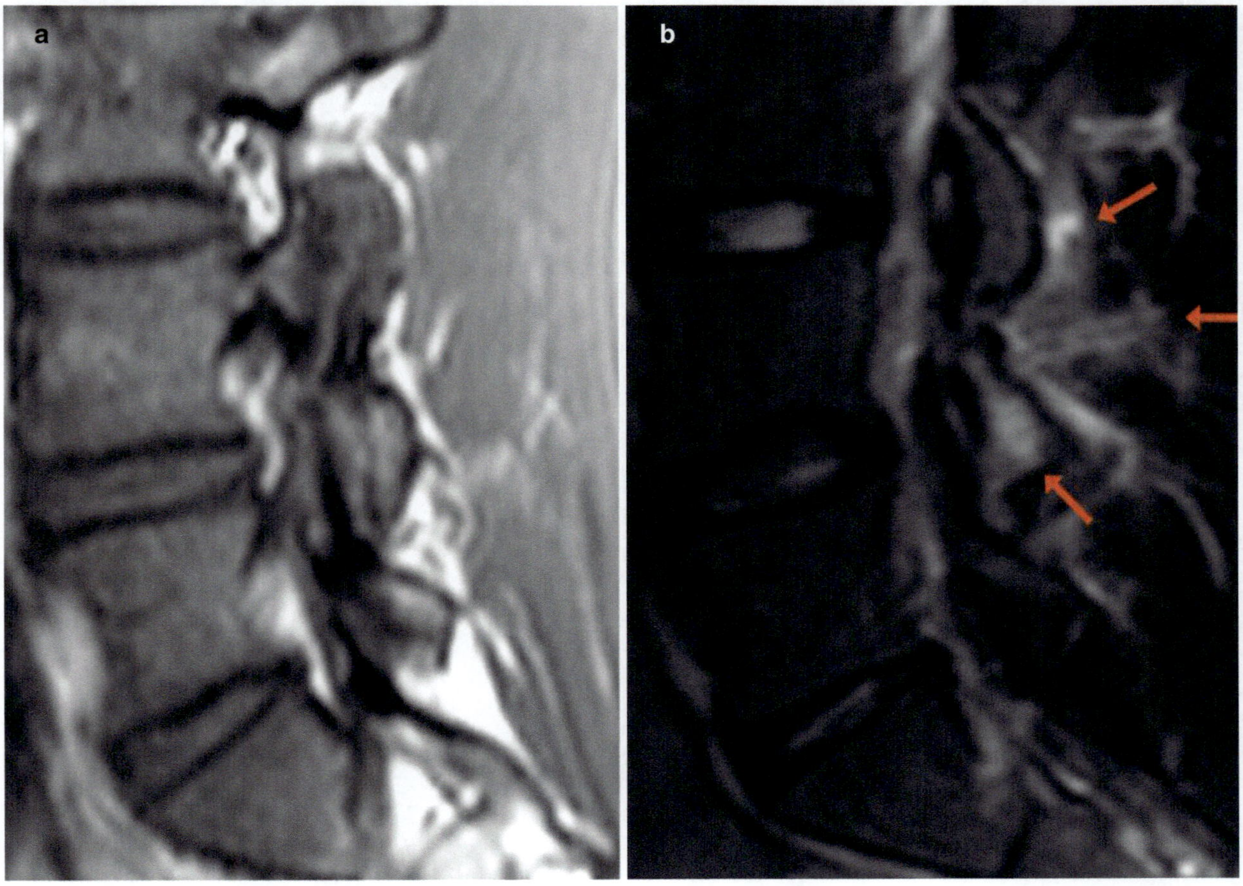

Fig. 1 Sagittal SE T1-weighted image (**a**), sagittal and axial T2-weighted images with fat saturation (**b–d**), axial SE T1-weighted images with fat saturation after administration of contrast medium (**e–g**). T1-weighted image shows no abnormalities (**a**). T2-weighted image shows hyperintensity of the periapophyseal soft tissue, bilaterally, indicating oedema (**b–d**, *arrows*). The administration of contrast medium shows bilateral spondylolysis of L4, with enhancement of the pars fracture (**e–g**) and periapophyseal enhancement indicating inflammation of the soft tissue (**e–g**, *arrows*)

P. D'Aprile, A. Tarantino, *MRI of Degenerative Disease of the Spine*, https://doi.org/10.1007/978-3-030-73707-8_6

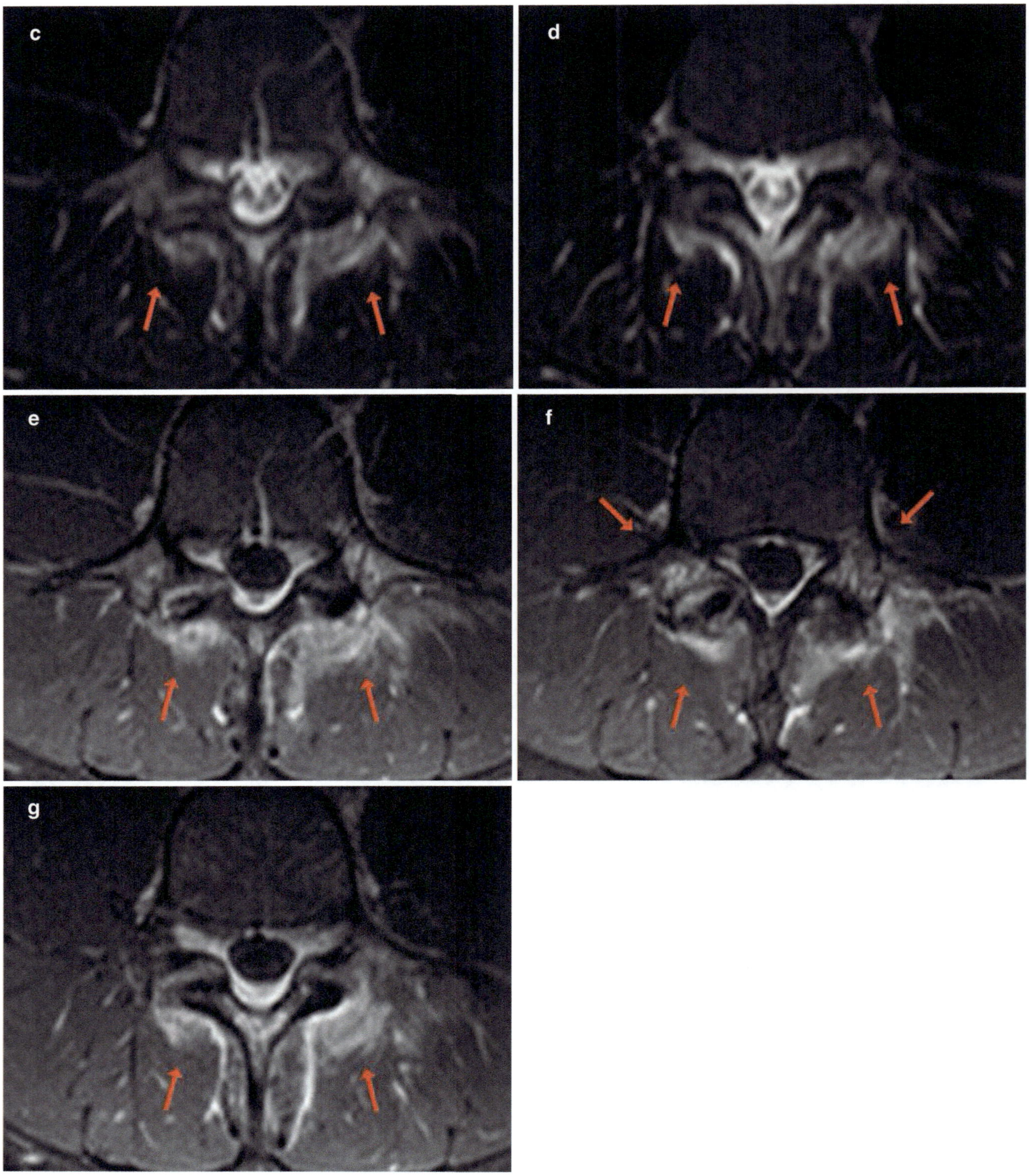

Fig. 1 (continued)

Case 39: Spondylolysis

- A 42-year-old man
- Persistent low back pain, more marked in flexion and extension

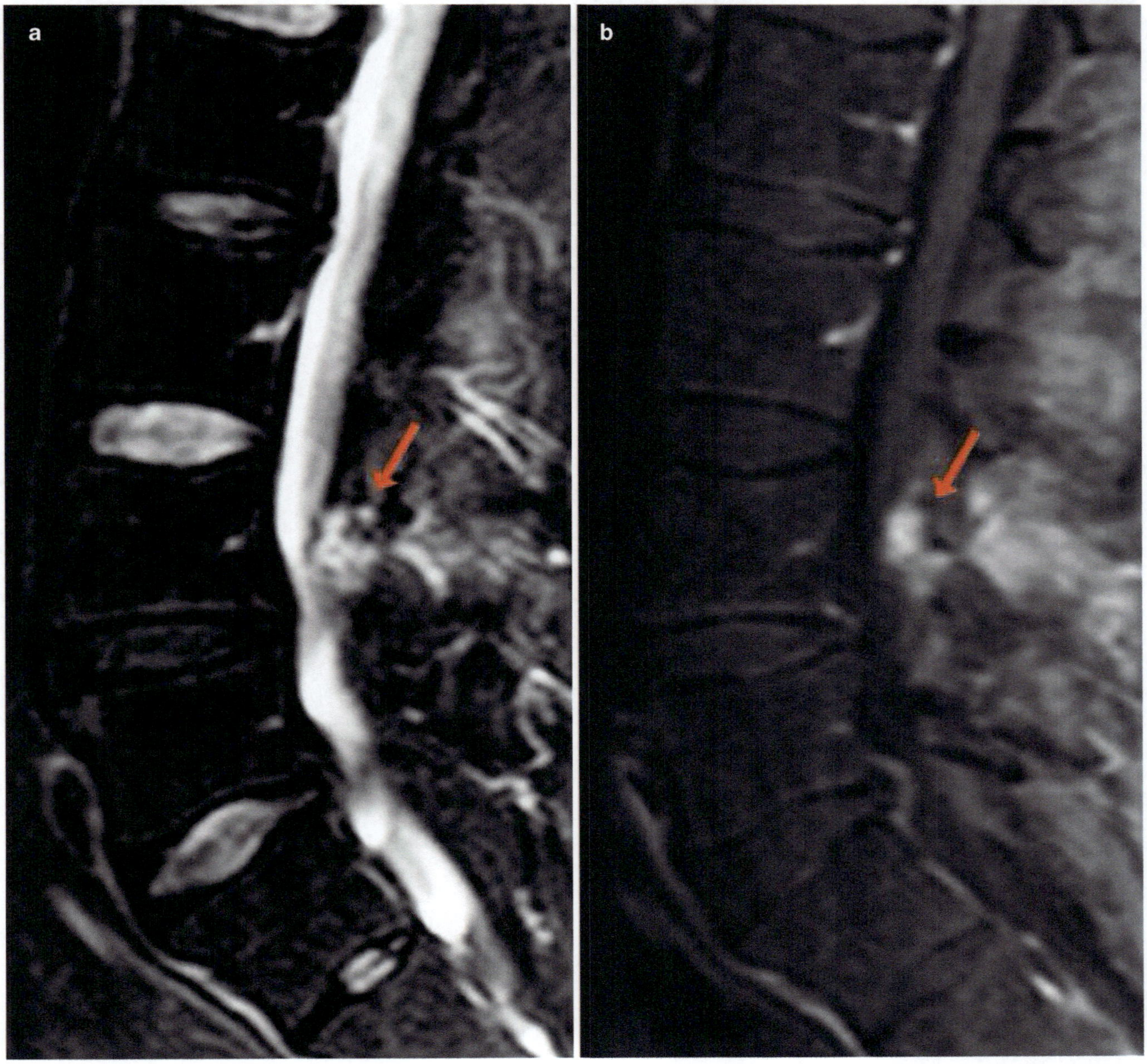

Fig. 2 Sagittal and axial T2-weighted images with fat saturation (**a**, **c**), sagittal and axial T1-weighted images with fat saturation following contrast medium administration (**b**, **d**, **e**), axial CT scan (**f**). Hyperintense areas in T2 (**a**, **c**, *arrows*), with contrast enhancement (**b**, **d**, **e**, *arrows*), at the level of the pars interarticularis of L4, bilaterally. These findings are referable to spondylolysis with reactive inflammation of the adjacent soft tissues. Axial CT scan confirm bilateral spondylolysis of L4 (**f**, *arrows*)

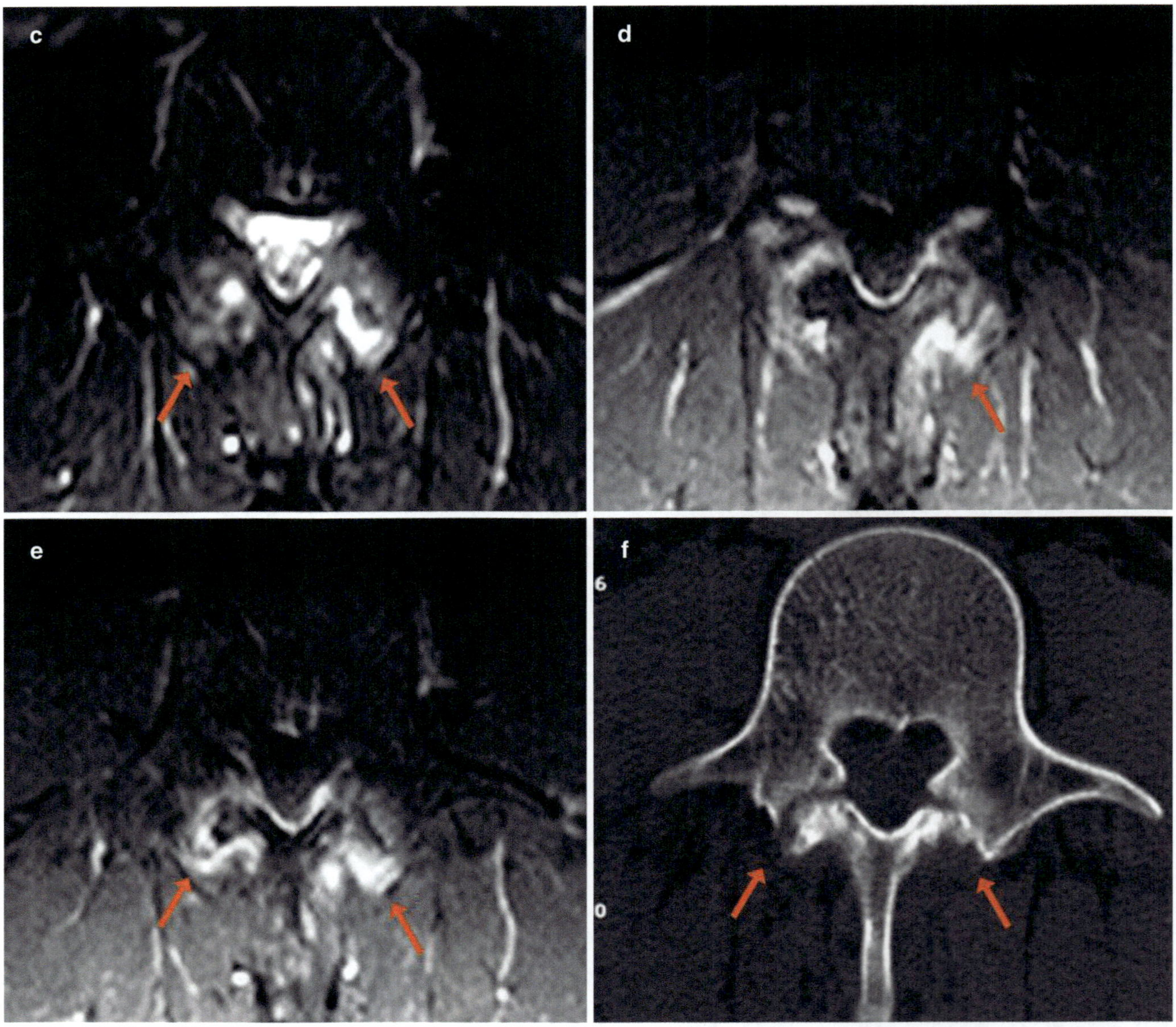

Fig. 2 (continued)

Case 40: Spondylolysis

- A 41-year-old man
- Persistent right low back pain

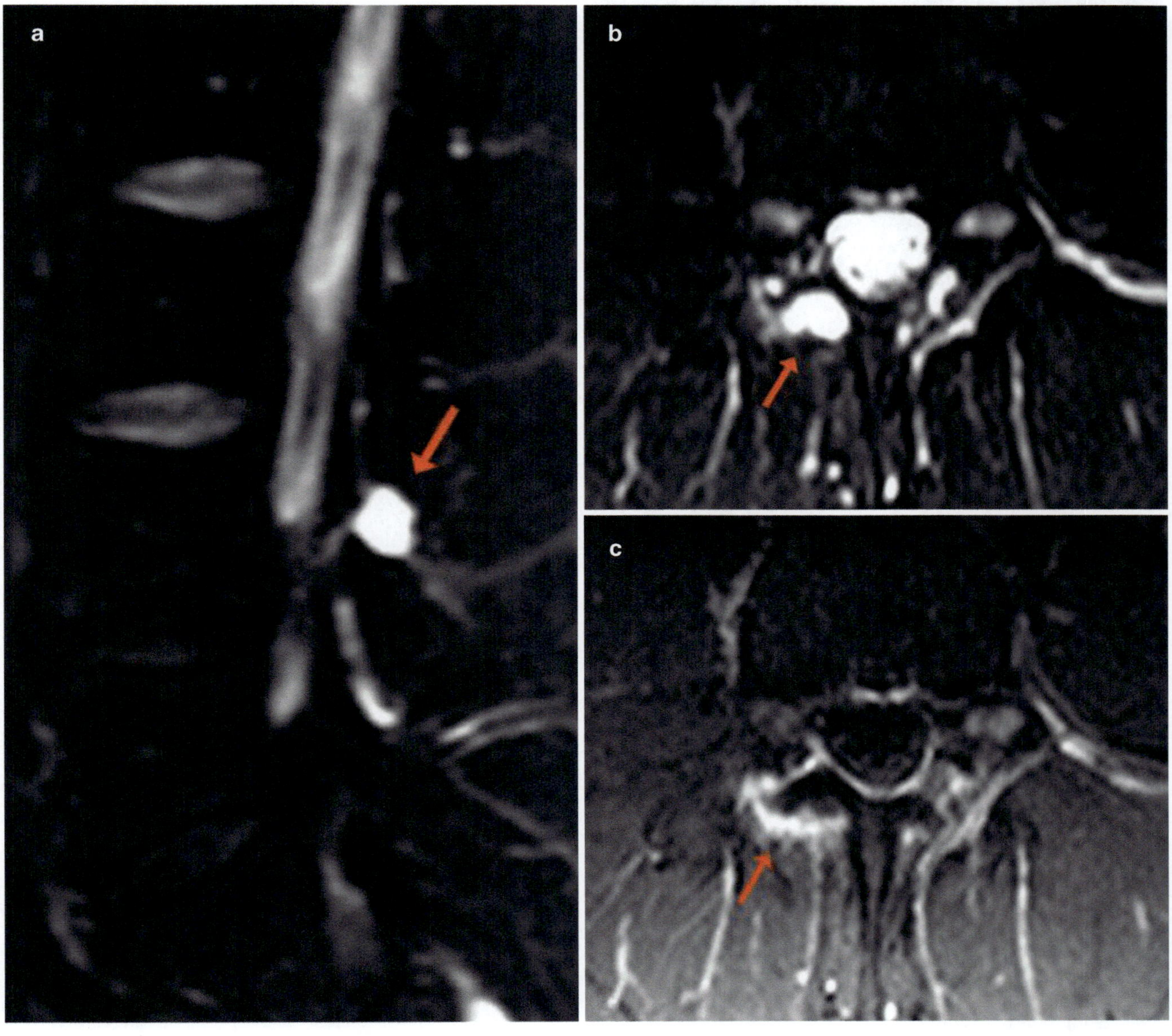

Fig. 3 Sagittal and axial TSE T2-weighted images with fat saturation (**a**, **b**), axial contrast-enhanced SE T1-weighted image with fat saturation (**c**), axial CT scan (**d**). Right spondylolysis of L4, with neocyst formation (**a**, **b**, *arrow*). Contrast enhancement of the pars and adjacent soft tissue, due to reactive infl ammation (**c**, *arrow*). CT scan confirms the fracture of the pars interarticularis (**d**, *arrow*)

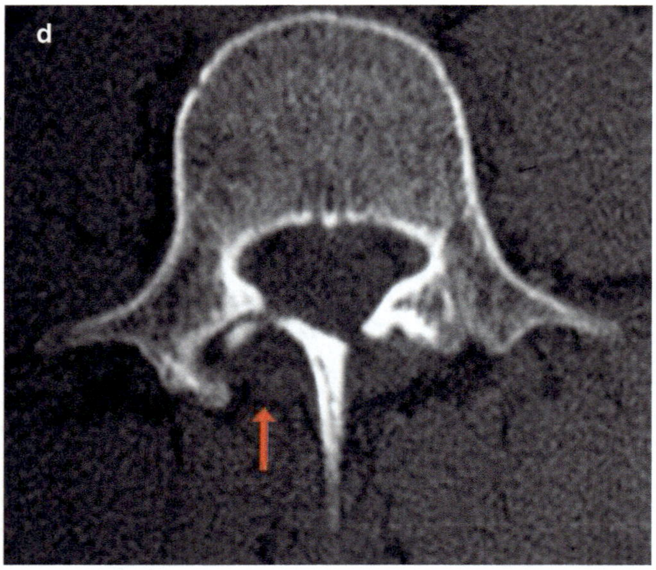

Fig. 3 (continued)

Case 41: Spondylolysis. Muscular Inflammation

- An 18-year-old man
- Persistent right low back pain
- Tenderness at examination of posterior perispinal muscles at L3-L4-L5 on the right side

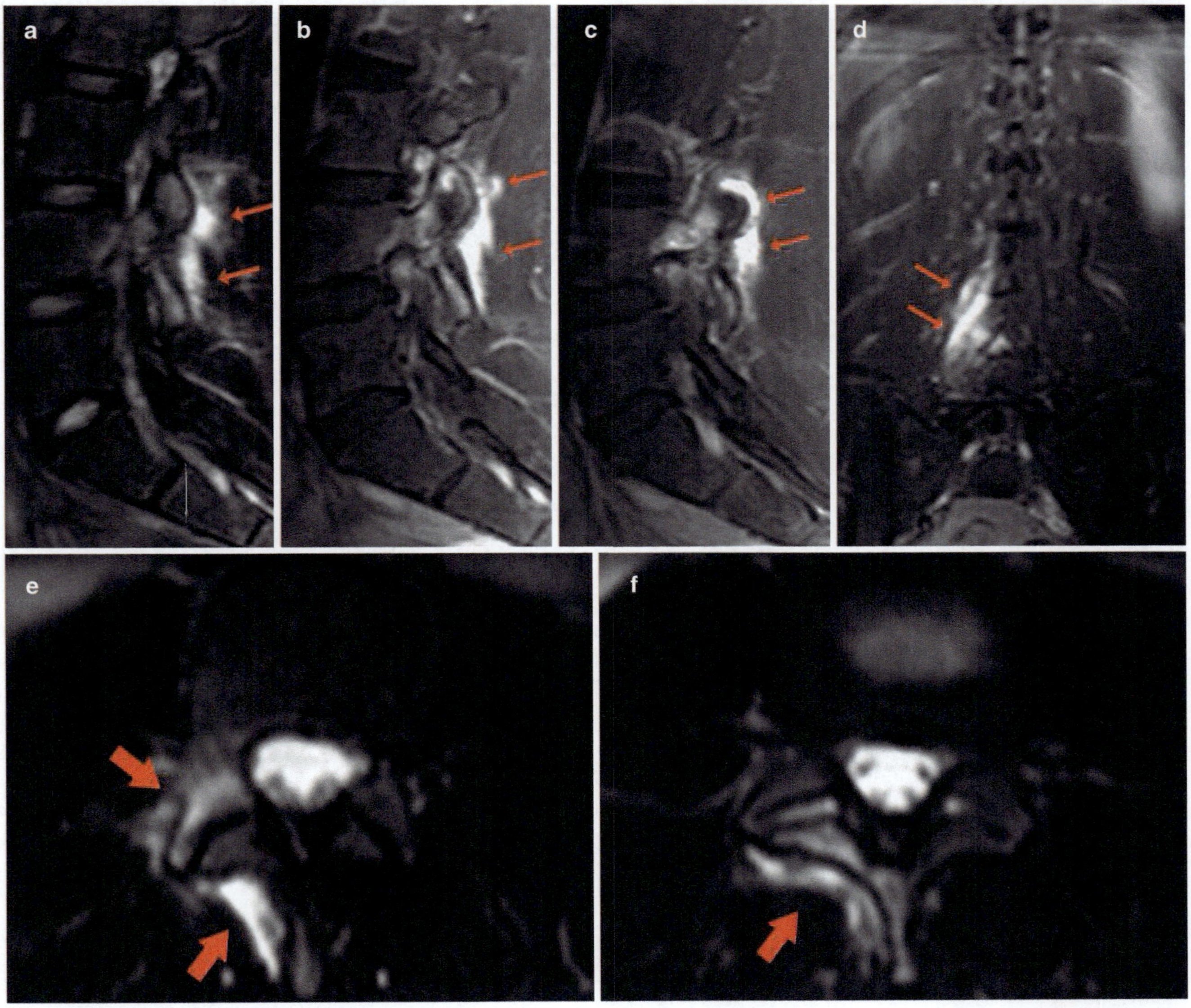

Fig. 4 Sagittal and axial SE T2-weighted images with fat saturation (**a**, **e–h**), sagittal and axial SE T1-weighted images with fat saturation after the administration of contrast medium (**b–d**, **i–k**), axial CT scan (**l**). T2 hyperintensity and contrast enhancement of the right posterior arch of L4 and adjacent periapophyseal soft tissues, indicating oedema inflammation (**a–c**, *arrow*). The images on the axial plane allow a better spatial resolution of the lesion (**e–k**, *arrows*). Oedema of the perispinal muscles is well defined in coronal image (**d**, *arrows*). CT image shows right spondylolysis of L4, which is the cause of the above-mentioned oedematous lesions (**l**, *arrow*)

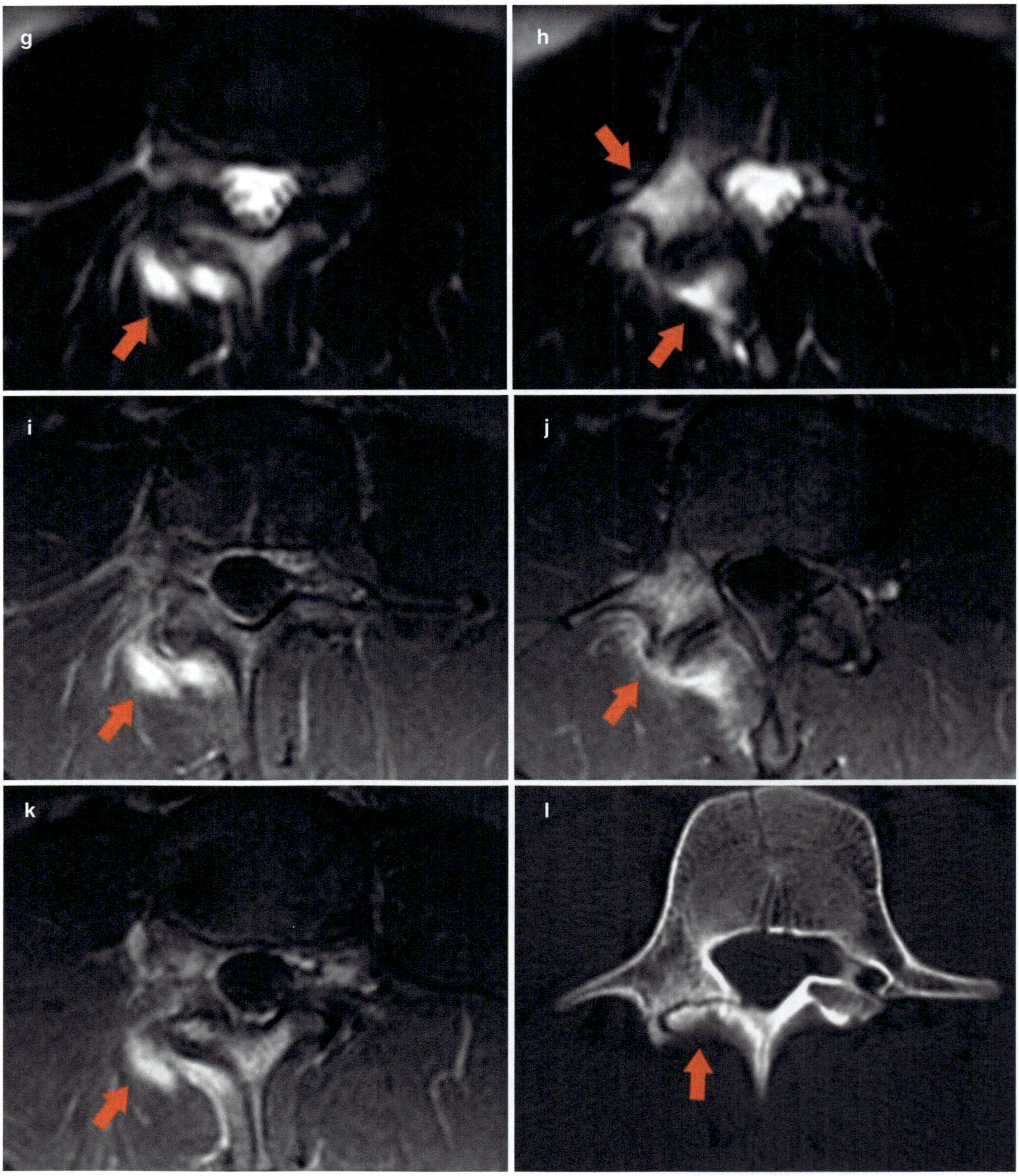

Fig. 4 (continued)

Case 42: Spondylolysis

- An 18-year-old man
- Patient with persistent low back pain after sports activity

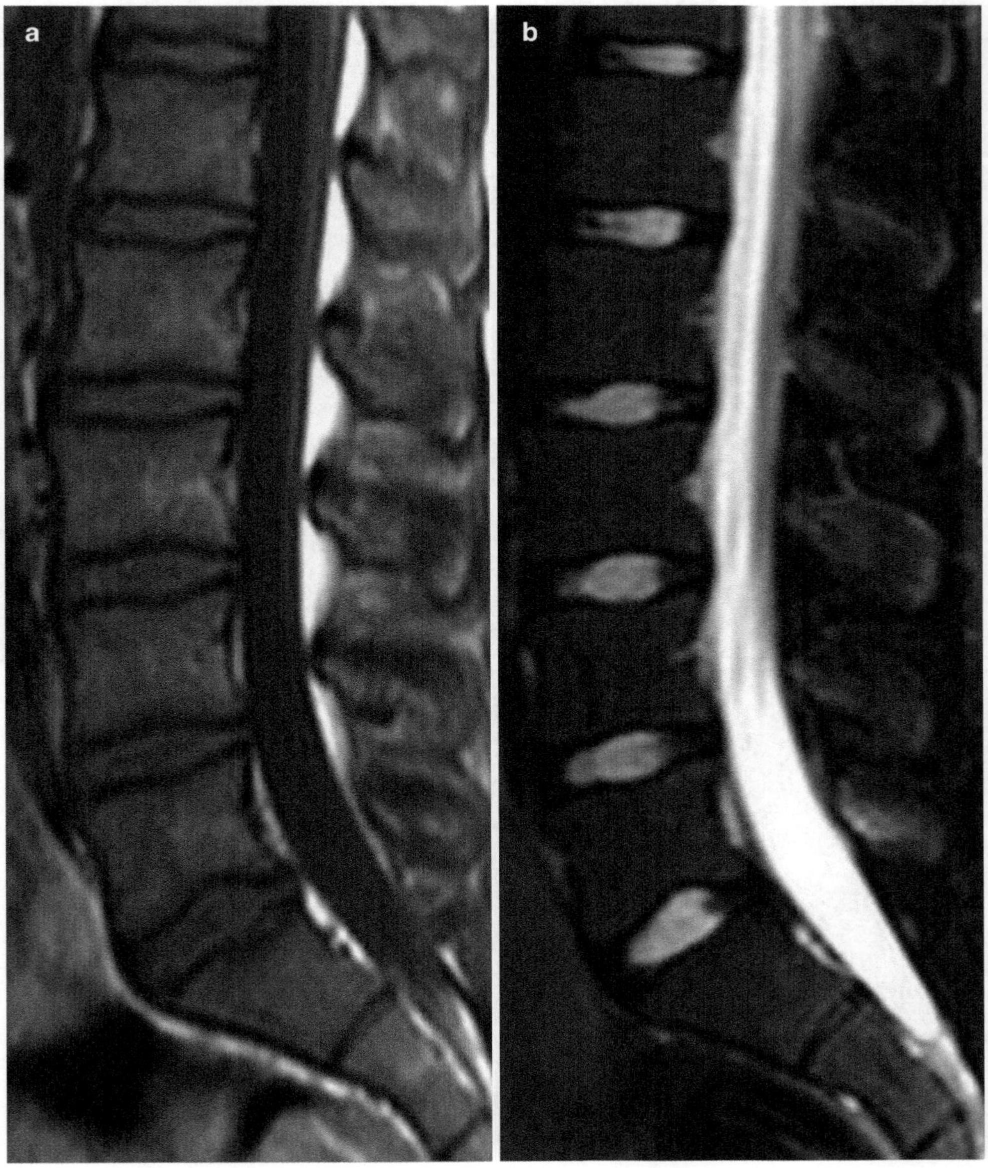

Fig. 5 Sagittal T1-weighted image (**a**), sagittal and axial TSE T2-weighted images with fat saturation (**b**, **c**), axial SE T1-weighted images with fat saturation following administration of contrast medium (**d**, **e**), axial CT images (**f**, **g**). The images on the sagittal plane do not show significant changes. Oedematous pattern of the left pedicle at L5 and adjacent soft tissues (**c**, *arrow*). Fractures of the right pars interarticularis and left lamina; the lines of fractures are well defined after contrast medium administration (**d**, **e**, *thin arrows*). Contrast enhancement of the adjacent soft tissue, due to reactive inflammation (**d**, **e**, *large arrows*). CT examination confirmed the lines of fracture (**f**, **g**, *arrows*)

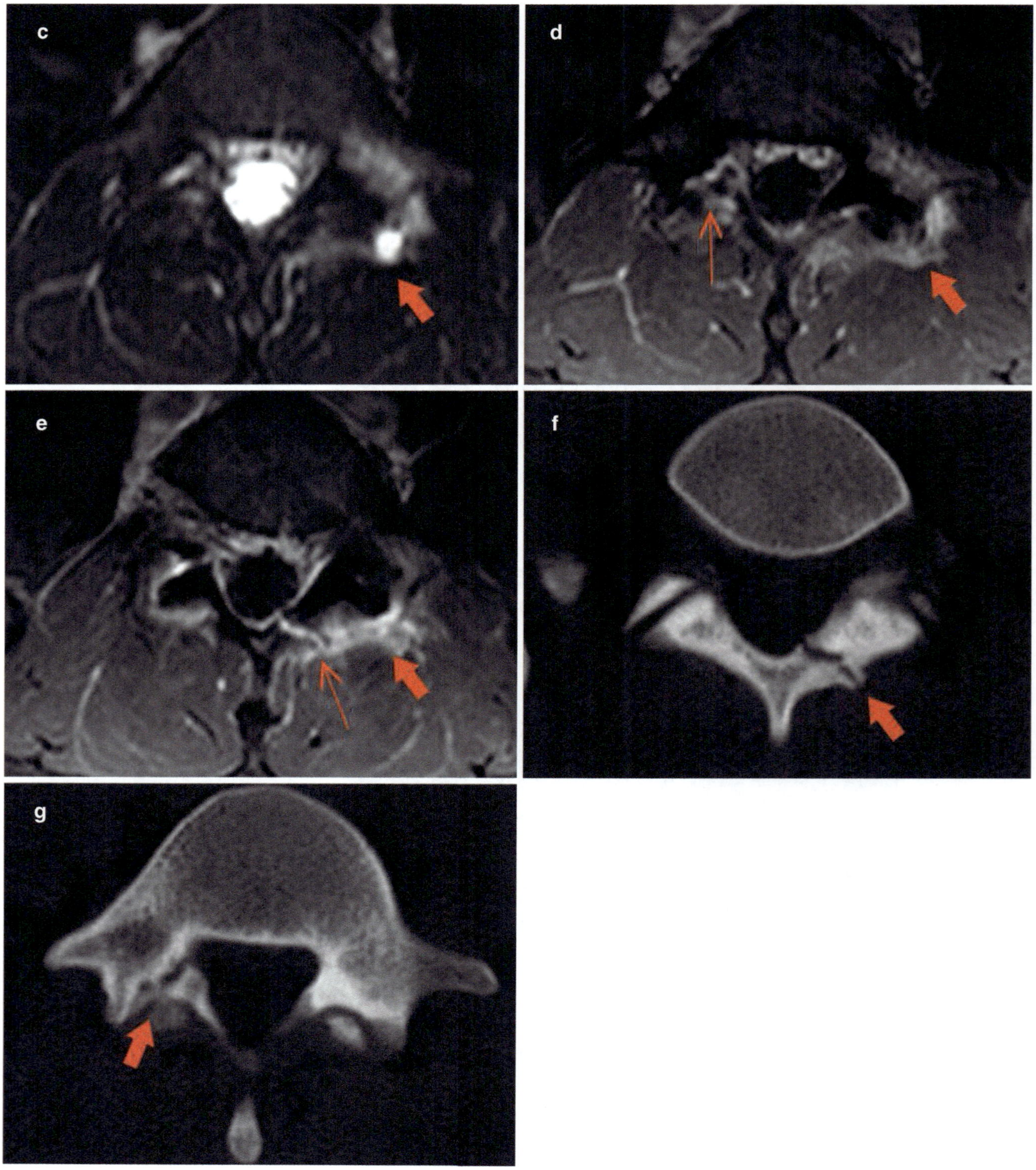

Fig. 5 (continued)

Case 43: Spondylolysis. Degenerative Inflammatory Changes of Ligaments

- A 44-year-old man
- Patient with low back pain, more marked in flexion and extension, and focal tenderness Qon palpation of the interspinous space

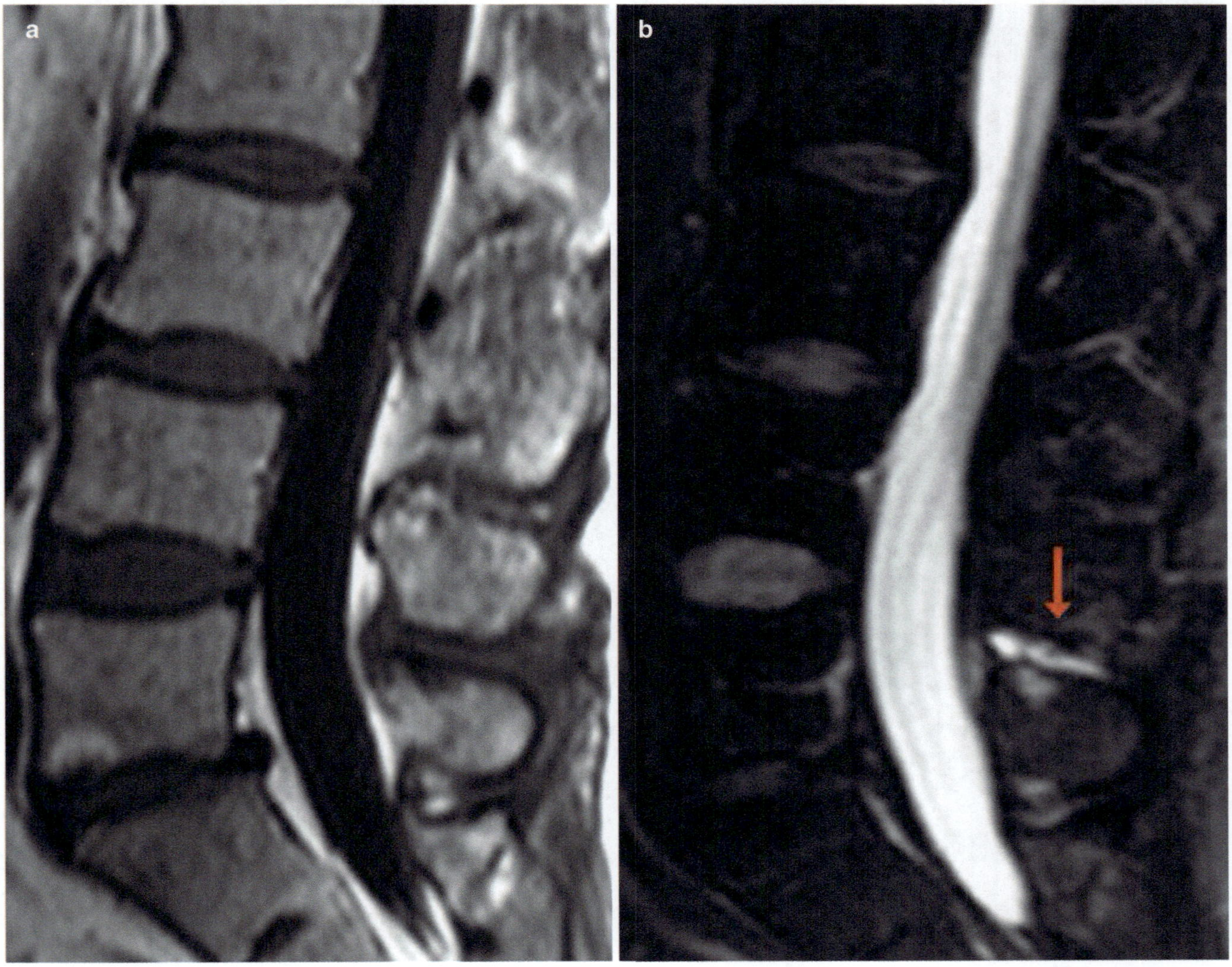

Fig. 6 Sagittal T1-weighted image (**a**), sagittal and axial TSE T2-weighted images with fat saturation (**b**, **c**), sagittal and axial SE T1-weighted images with fat saturation following administration of contrast medium (**d**, **e**), axial CT image (**f**). Mild anterolisthesis of L5 over S1. The interspinous ligament at L4/L5 is hyperintense on T2-weighted imaging (**b**, **c**, *posterior arrow*) and enhances after contrast medium administration (**d**, **e**, *posterior arrow*); these findings indicate degenerative inflammatory changes of the ligament. The images on the axial plane show bilateral spondylolysis of L5. The pars defect is well seen as hyperintense both in T2-weighted images with fat saturation and contrast enhanced T1-weighted images with fat saturation (**c**, **e**, *lateral arrows*). CT image confirms the lines of fractures of the pars interarticularis (**f**, *arrows*)

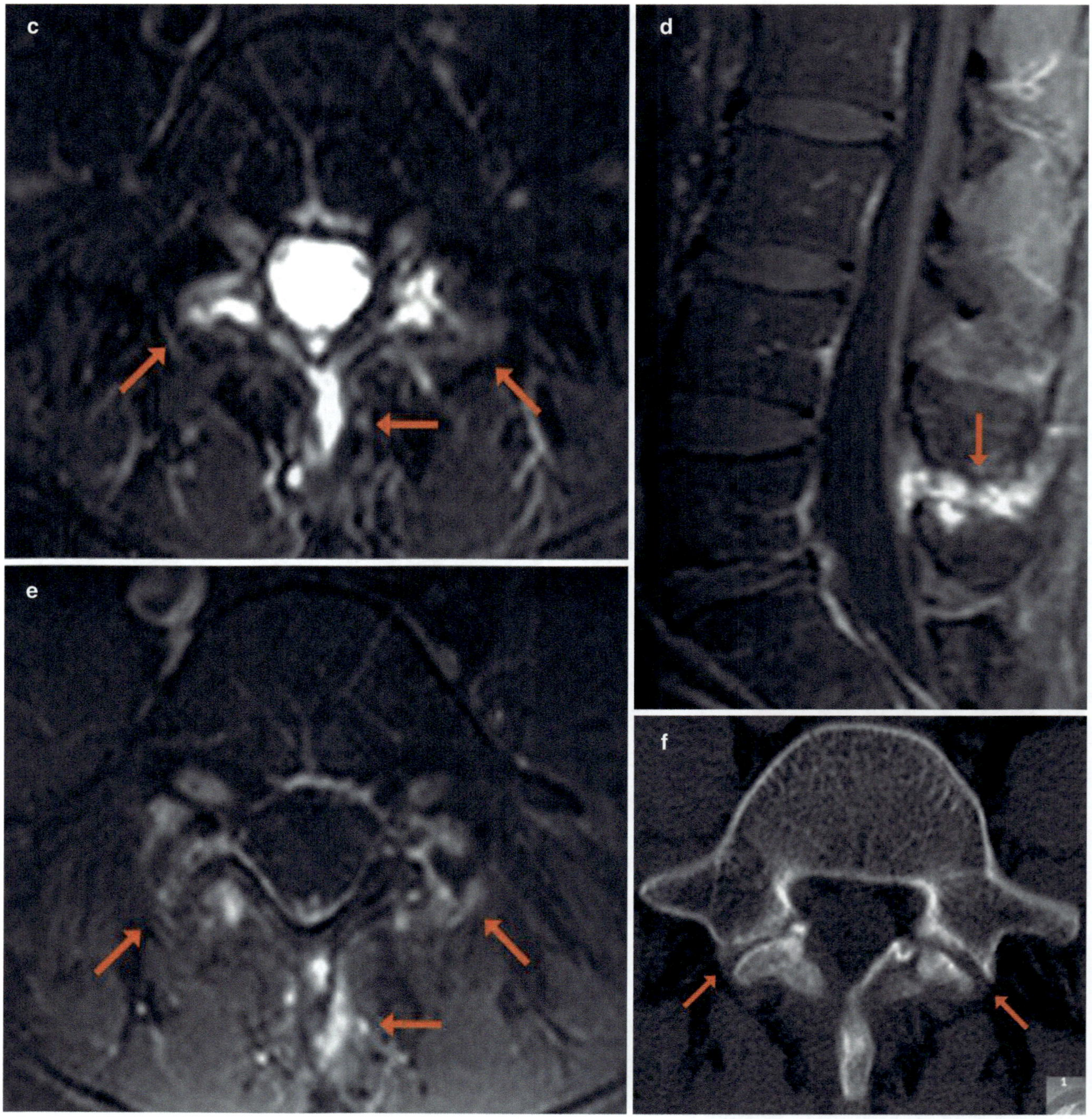

Fig. 6 (continued)

Case 44: Spondylolysis

- A 19-year-old man
- Patient with persistent low back pain arising after sports activity

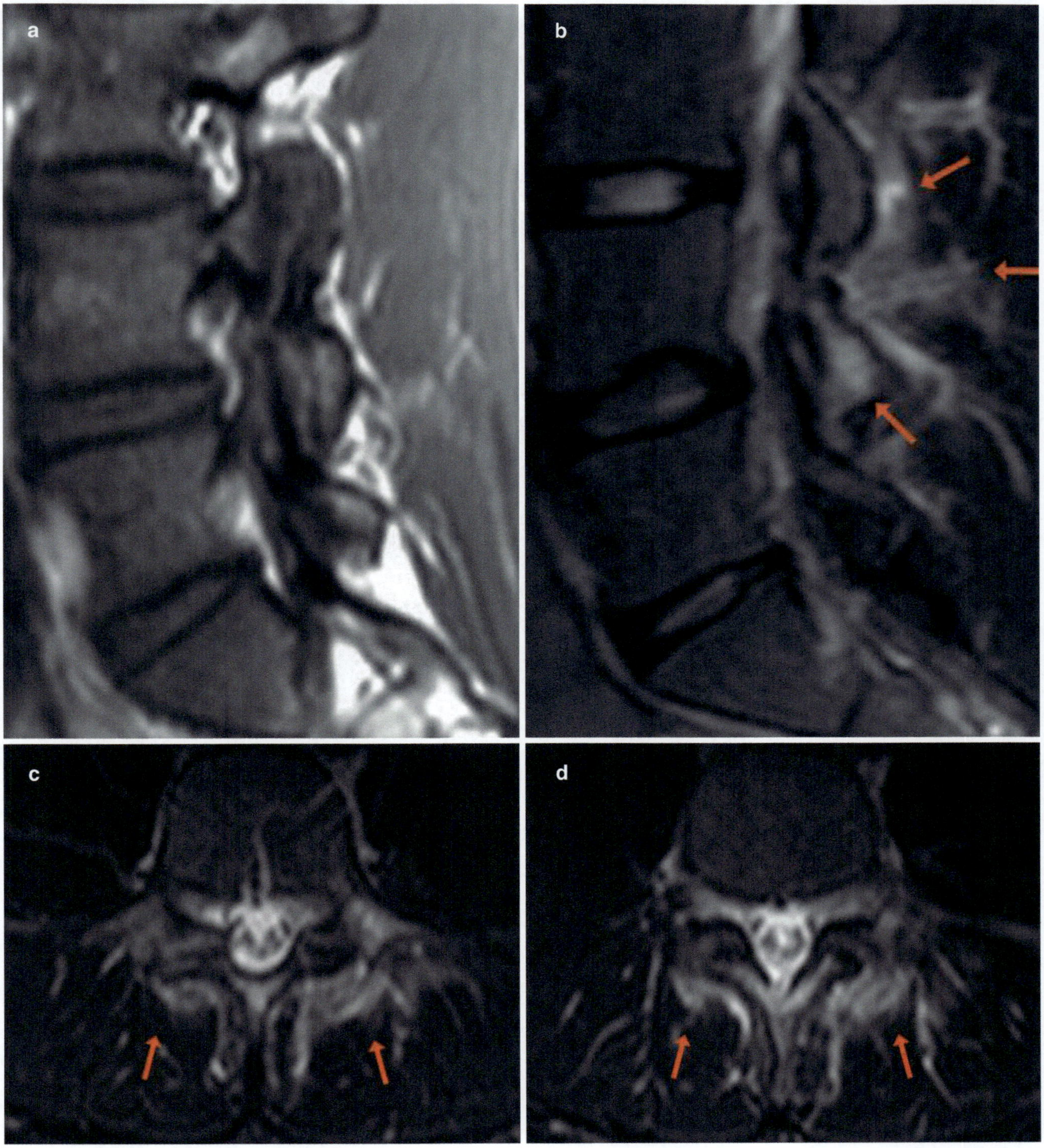

Fig. 7 Sagittal T1-weighted image (**a**), sagittal and axial TSE T2-weighted images with fat saturation (**b–d**), axial SE T1-weighted images with fat saturation following administration of contrast medium (**e–g**). Oedema of the posterior vertebral arch of L4 and periapophyseal soft tissues (**b–d**, *arrows*). The administration of contrast medium reveals bilateral spondylolysis of L4 (**e–g**, *arrowhead*) and reactive inflammation of the adjacent soft tissues (**e–g**, *arrows*). Note also peridural contrast enhancement at the same level (**e–g**)

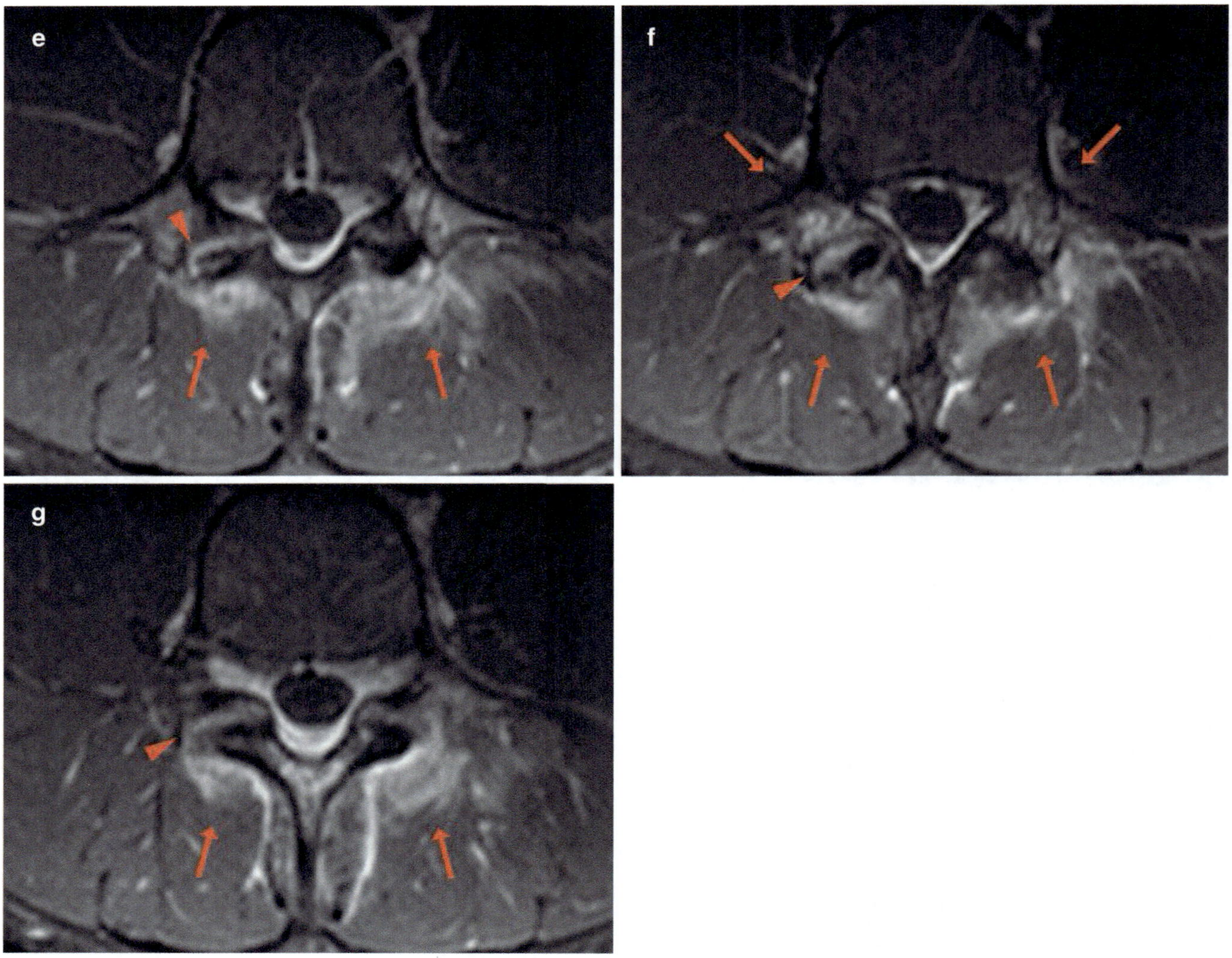

Fig. 7 (continued)

Degeneration-Inflammation of Ligaments and Muscles

7

Case 45: Degeneration-Inflammation of Ligaments

- A 47-year-old patient
- Chronic low back pain, more marked in flexion and extension

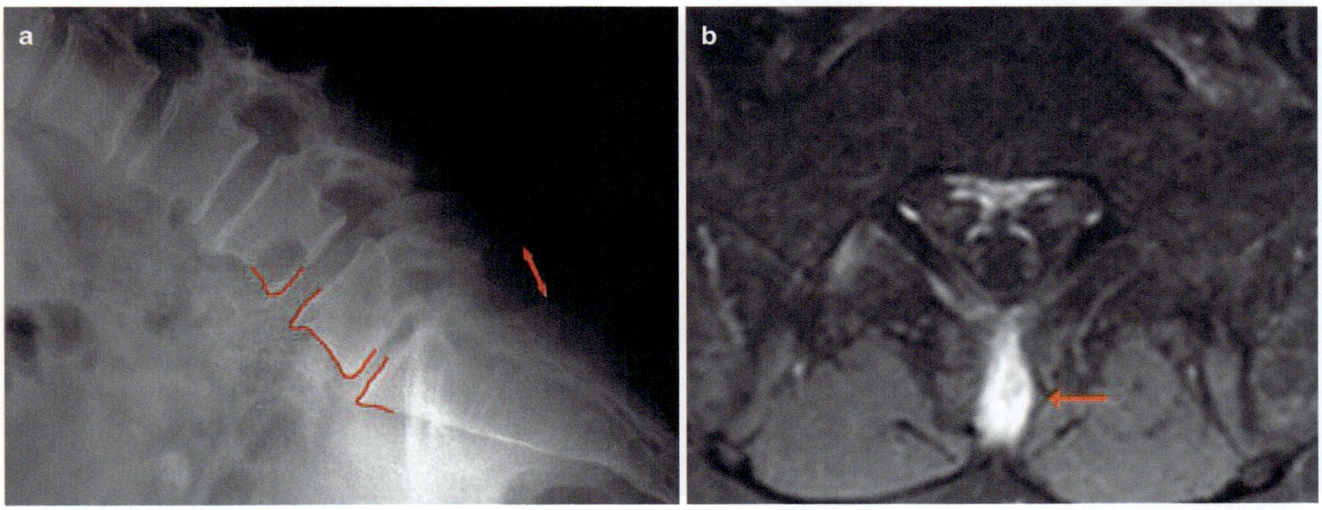

Fig. 1 Lateral radiography in hyperflexion (**a**), sagittal and axial SE T1-weighted images with fat saturation following administration of contrast medium (**b**, **c**). The radiography shows mild retrolisthesis of L5 over S1 and widening of the corresponding interspinous space (**a**). MRI confirms the spinal instability and shows marked contrast enhancement of the interspinous ligament at L5/S1 (**b**, **c**, *arrows*), due to rupture degeneration and inflammation of the same ligament

P. D'Aprile, A. Tarantino, *MRI of Degenerative Disease of the Spine*, https://doi.org/10.1007/978-3-030-73707-8_7

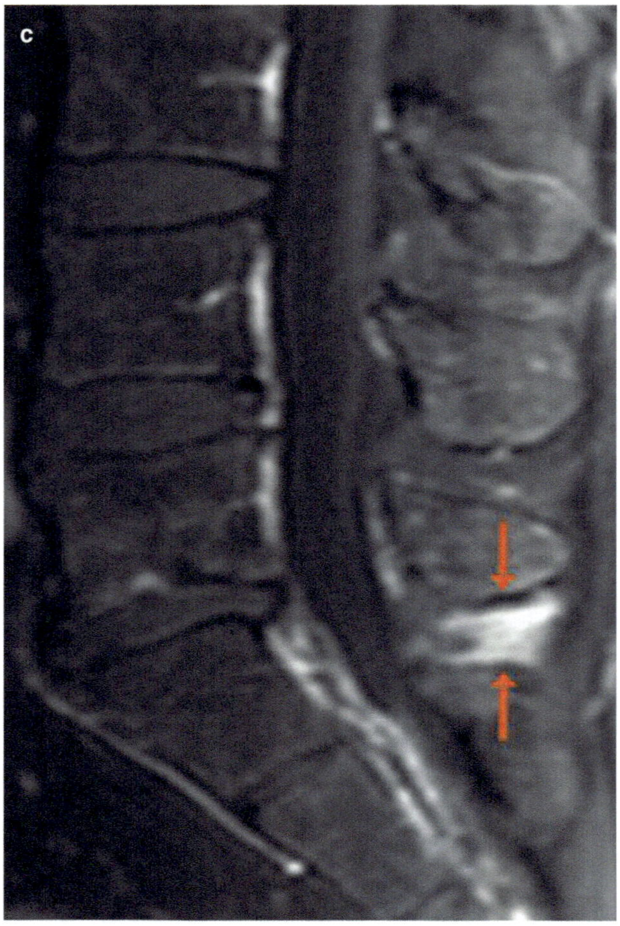

Fig. 1 (continued)

Case 46: Degeneration-Inflammation of Ligaments

- A 68-year-old woman
- Low back pain
- Tenderness on palpation of the lumbar interspinous spaces

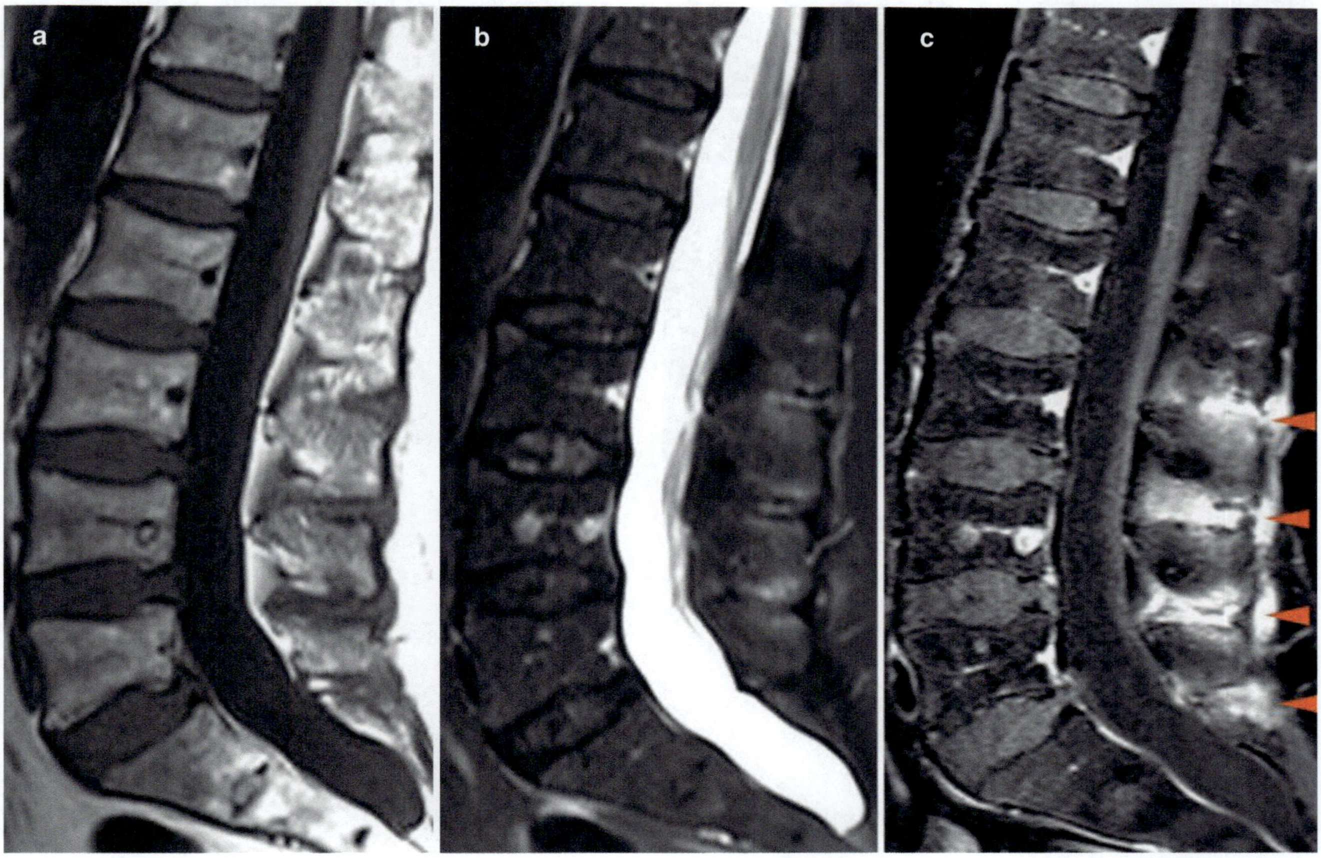

Fig. 2 Sagittal SE T1-weighted image (**a**), sagittal TSE T2-weighted image with fat saturation (**b**), sagittal and axial T1-weighted images with fat saturation following administration of contrast medium (**c**–**f**). Mild hyperintensity in T2 of the interspinous ligaments from L2 to S1 (**b**). Contrast medium administration reveals marked enhancement of the interspinous and supraspinous ligaments from L2 to S1 (**c**–**e**, *arrowheads*). It is also evident that there is contrast enhancement of the ligamenta flava at L4/L5 and L5/S1 (**d**, **f**, *arrows*). These findings indicate degenerative inflammatory ligamentous changes. Note that such ligamentous changes are clearly detectable after the administration of contrast medium coupled with fat-suppressed T1-weighted imaging

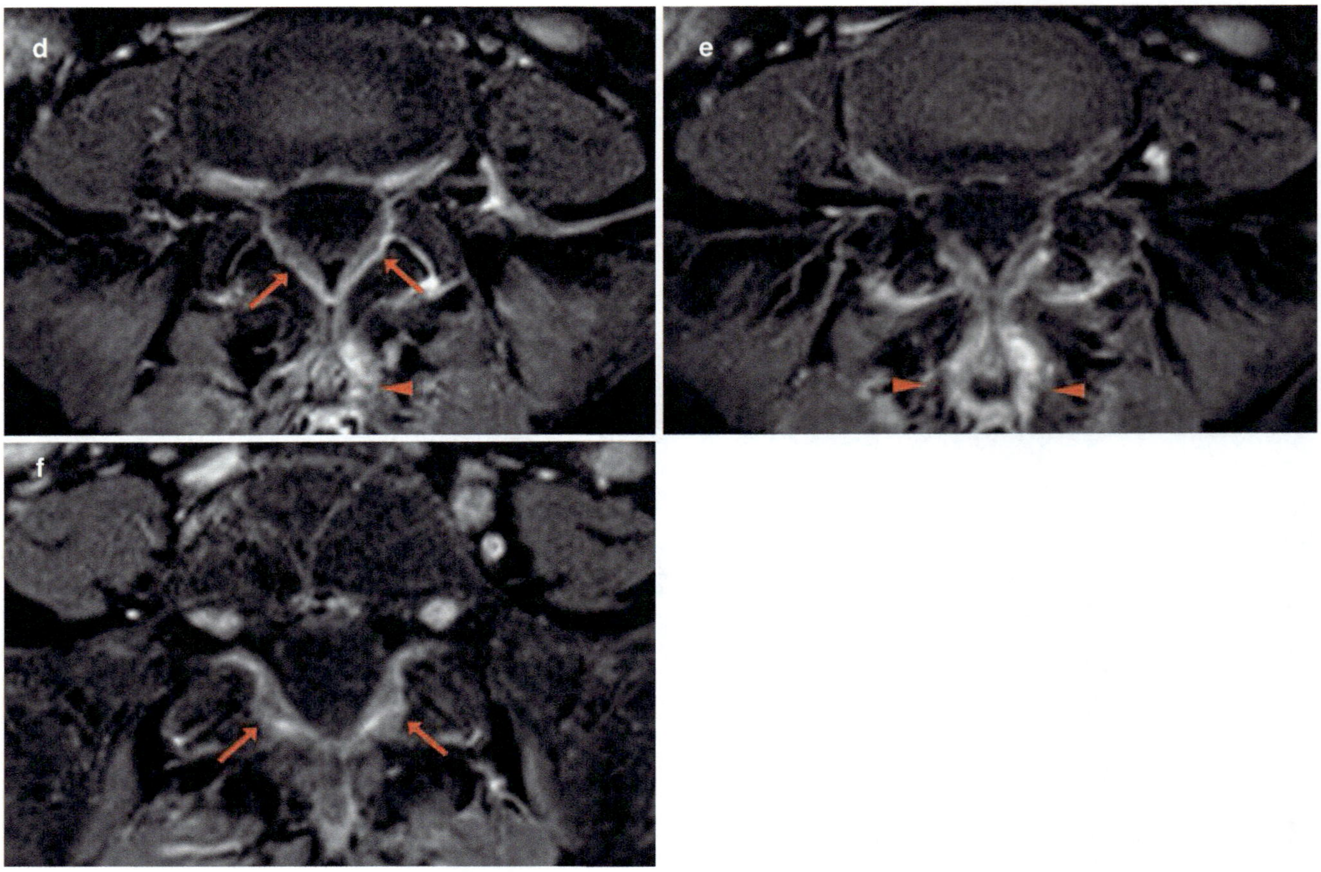

Fig. 2 (continued)

Case 47: Degeneration-Inflammation of Ligaments

- A 74-year-old man
- Patient with persistent low back pain
- Limited lumbar motion
- Exacerbation of pain by extension

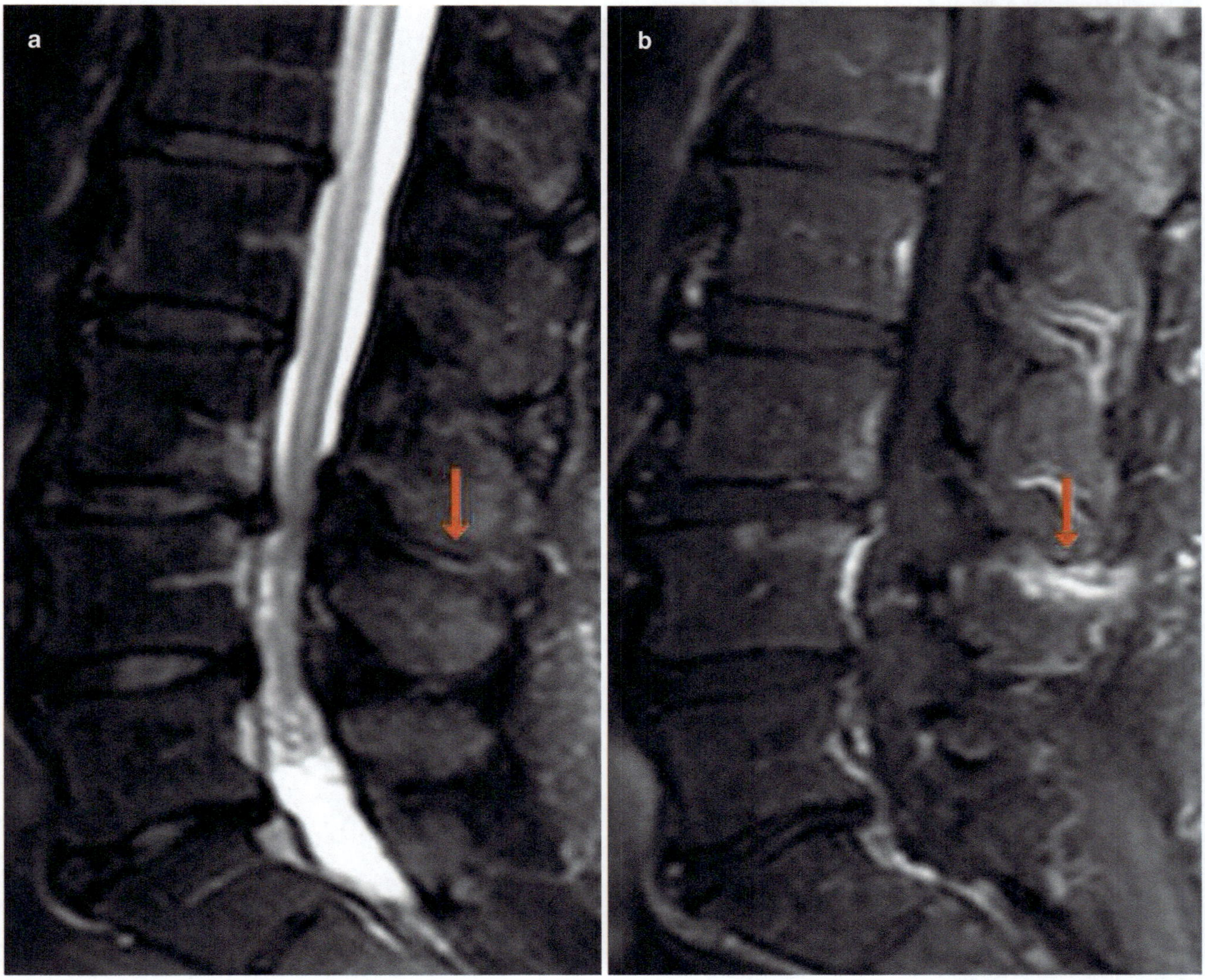

Fig. 3 Sagittal TSE T2-weighted image with fat saturation (**a**), sagittal and axial T1-weighted images with fat saturation following the administration of contrast medium (**b**, **c**). Mild retrolisthesis of L3 over L4, with posterior osteochondritis and bulging disc at the same level L3/L4 (**a**, **b**). Reduction in height of the L3/L4 interspinous space (**a**, *arrow*). Marked contrast enhancement of the L3/L4 interspinous ligament (**b**, **c**, *arrow*), indicating degenerative inflammatory ligamentous changes; these changes are presumably due to collision of the spinous processes and injury of the interposed ligament

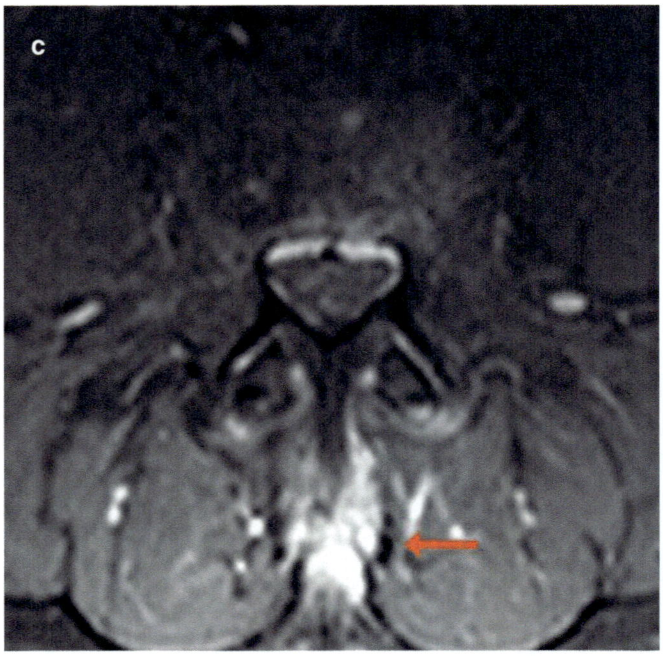

Fig. 3 (continued)

Case 48: Degeneration-Inflammation of Ligaments

- A 51-year-old woman
- Patient with cervical pain and tenderness to palpation of interspinous spaces
- No previous trauma
- No clinical or laboratory signs of spondyloarthritis

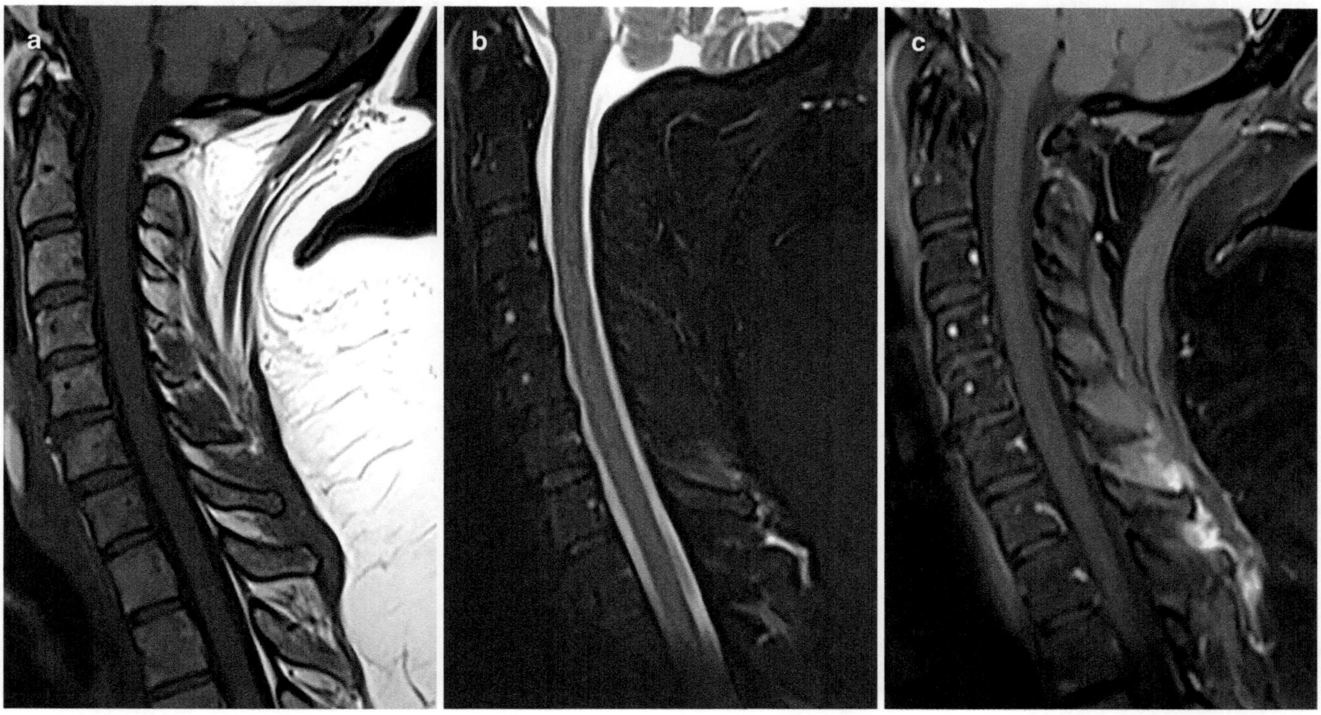

Fig. 4 (**a**–**f**) Sagittal TSE T1-weighted image (**a**), sagittal TSE T2-weighted image with fat saturation (**b**), sagittal and axial TSE T1-weighted images with fat saturation after administration of contrast medium (**c**–**f**). No signal changes in T1-weighted images (**a**). Mild hyperintensity of the interspinous space at C6/C7 in fat saturated T2-weighted image (**b**). The administration of contrast medium shows enhancement of the interspinous and supraspinous ligaments at C6/C7 and supraspinous ligament at C7/T1, indicating ligamentous degenerative inflammatory phenomena (**c**–**f**)

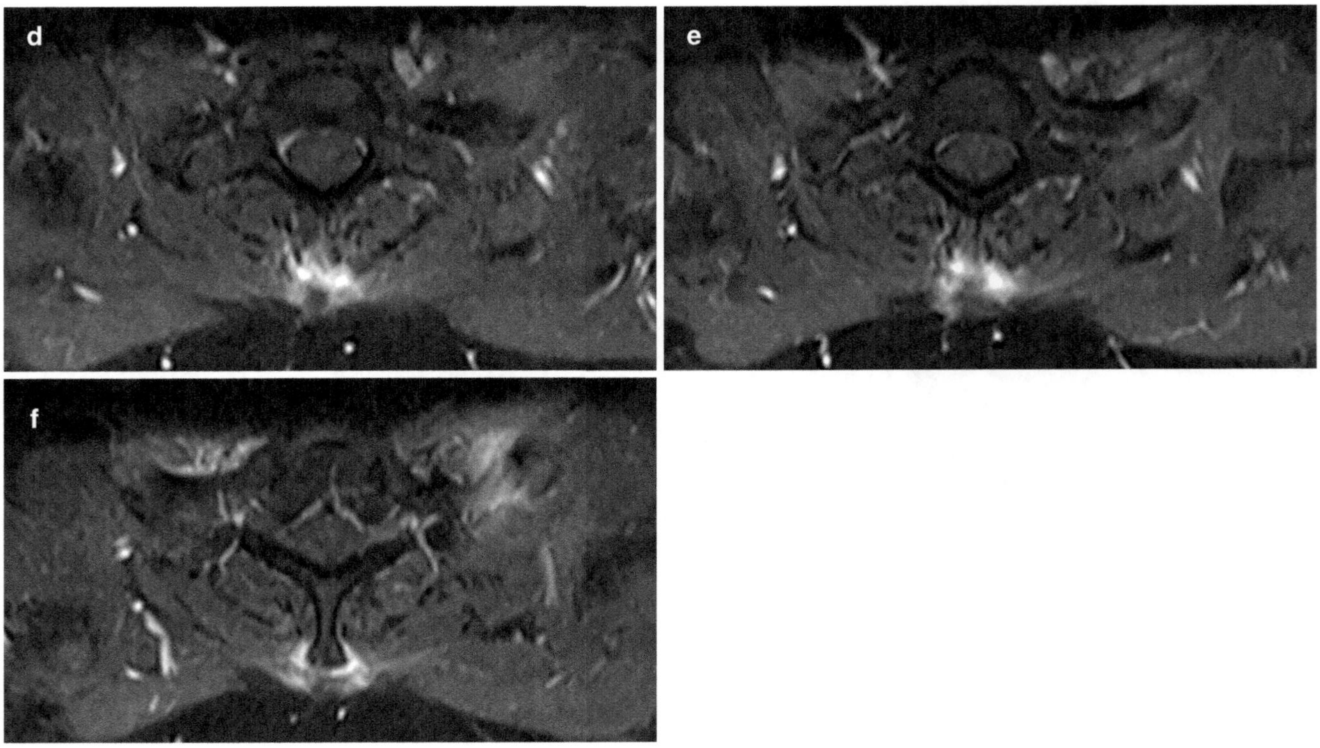

Fig. 4 (continued)

Case 49: Degeneration-Inflammation of Ligaments

- A 58-year-old woman
- Chronic low back pain more marked in flexion and weakness in the legs

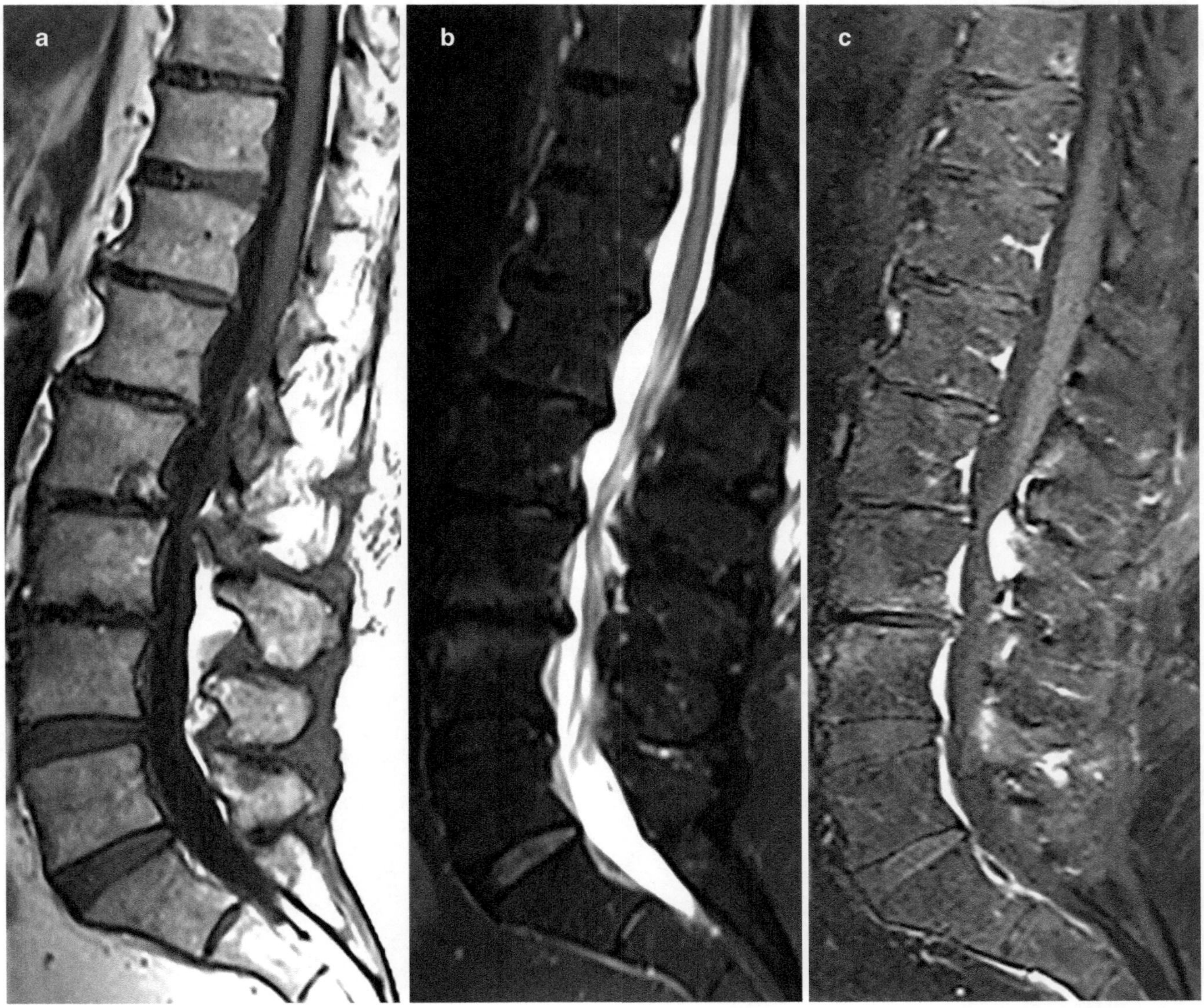

Fig. 5 (**a**–**e**) Sagittal TSE T1-weighted image (**a**), sagittal TSE T2-weighted image with fat saturation (**b**), sagittal and axial TSE T1-weighted images with fat saturation after administration of contrast medium (**c**–**e**). Mild anterolisthesis of L2 over L3 (**a**). Prominence of the anterior aspect of the interspinous ligament L2/L3 (**a**, **b**). Contrast enhancement of the same interspinous ligament L2/L3, prominent into the central vertebral canal, with stenosis of the central spinal canal (**c**–**e**). This finding indicates degenerative inflammatory phenomena of the interspinous ligament due to vertebral instability at the same level

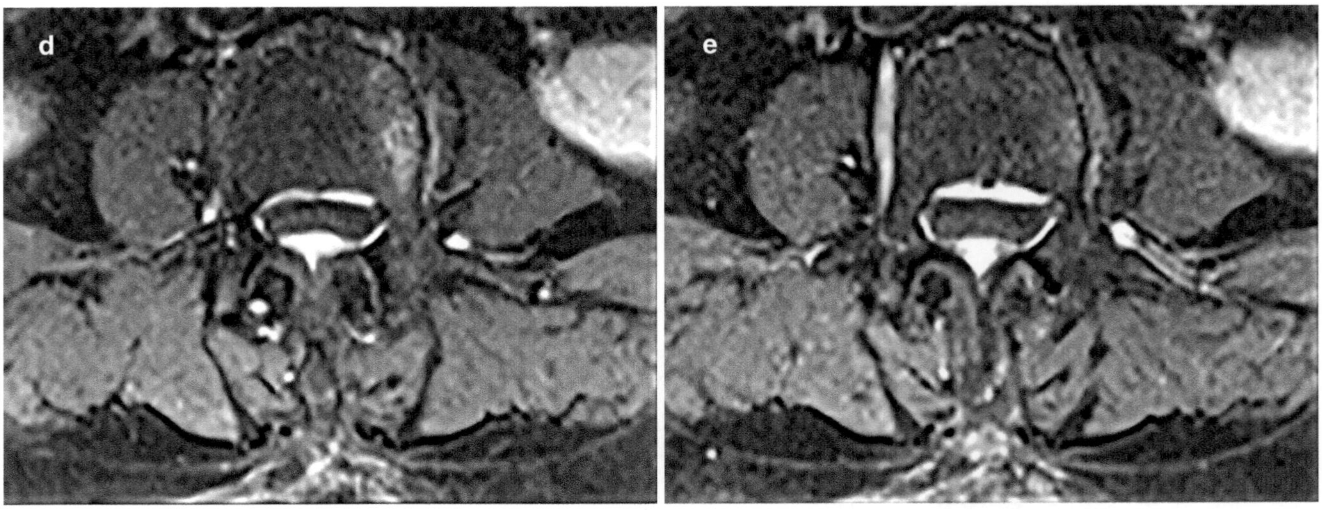

Fig. 5 (continued)

Case 50: Degeneration-Inflammation of Ligaments

- A 73-year-old man
- Patient with chronic low back pain
- Limited lumbar motion
- Exacerbation of pain by extension/flexion

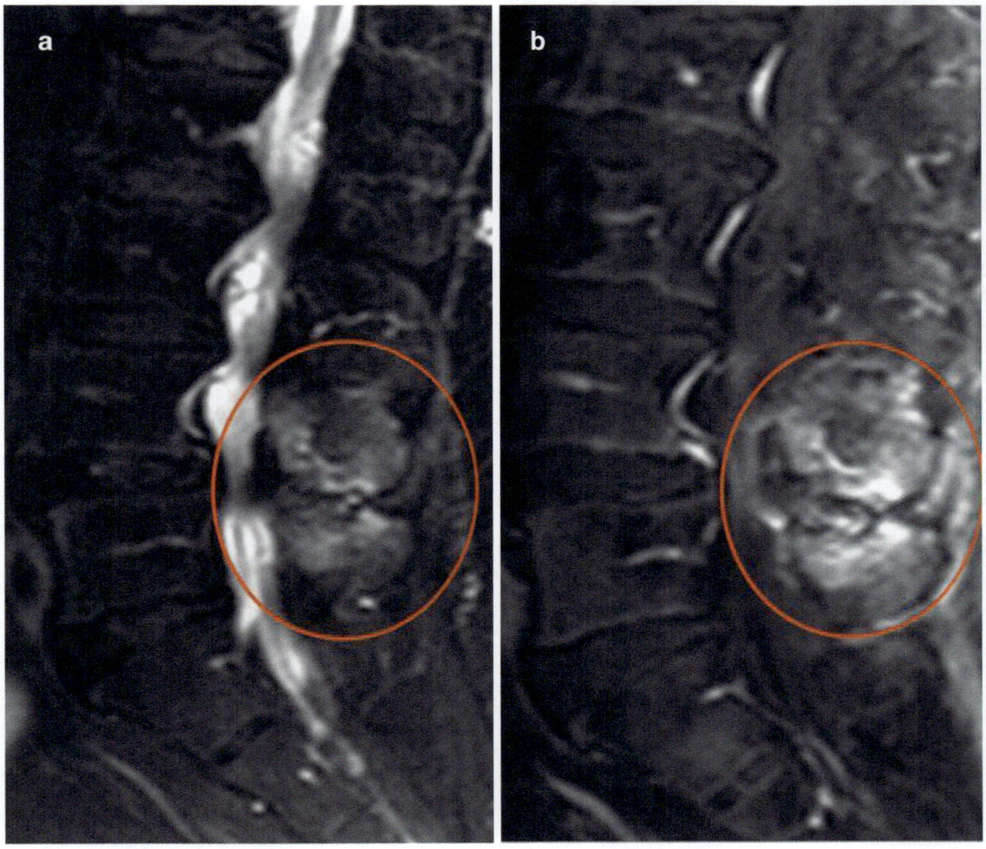

Fig. 6 Sagittal TSE T2-weighted image with fat saturation (**a**), sagittal and axial T1-weighted images with fat saturation following administration of contrast medium (**b**, **c**). Mild anterolisthesis of L4 over L5. High signal in T2 and contrast enhancement of the opposing L4/L5 spinous processes, due to bony collision and consequent stress-related reactive degenerative changes of the bone marrow (**a**, **b**, *circle*). The L4/L5 interspinous space is collapsed, and the corresponding interspinous ligament is degenerated. The axial image on L4/L5 shows also contrast enhancement of the perispinal muscles (e.g. interspinalis muscle) indicating degenerative inflammatory muscular changes and contrast enhancement of the facet joints, indicating bilateral osteoarthritis (**c**, *circle*)

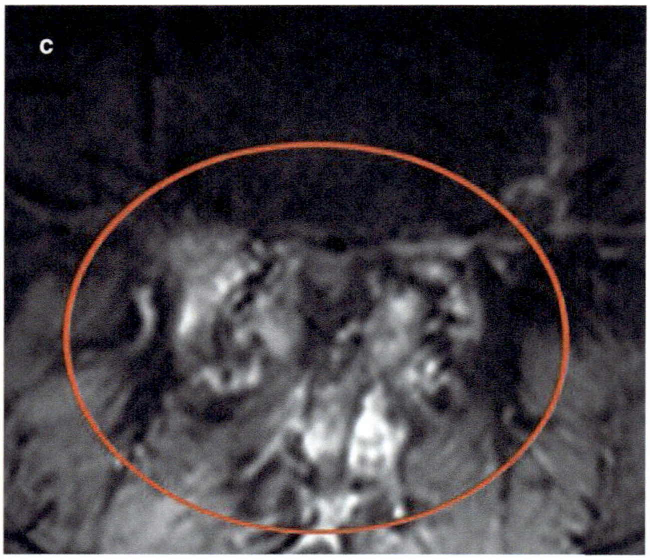

Fig. 6 (continued)

Case 51: Degeneration-Inflammation of Ligaments. Baastrup's Phenomenon

- A 52-year-old patient
- Persistent low back pain
- Limited lumbar motion
- Exacerbation of pain by hyperextension
- Tenderness on palpation of the interspinous spaces

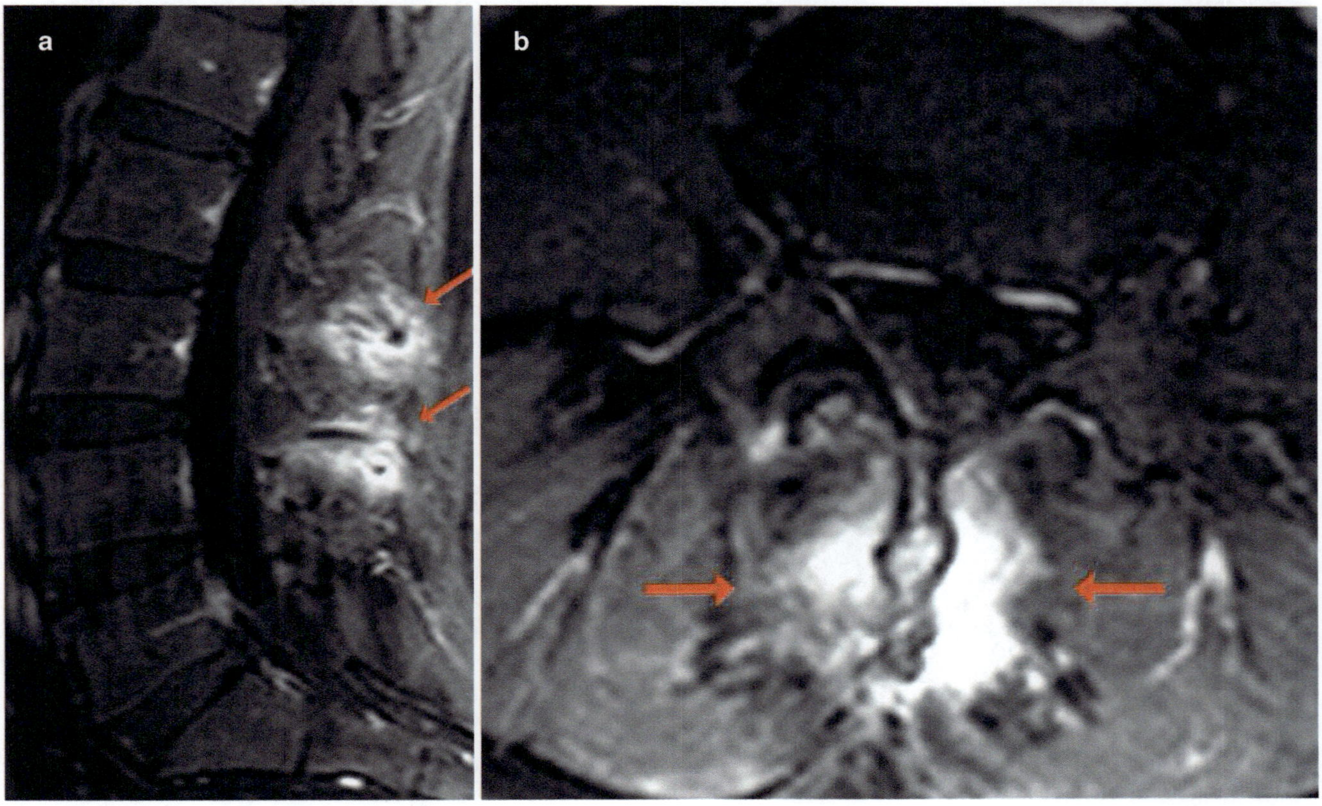

Fig. 7 Sagittal and axial SE T1-weighted images with fat saturation following the administration of contrast medium (**a**, **b**). Lumbar hyperlordosis is present, associated with collision of the spinous processes at L2-L3-L4 (i.e. Baastrup's phenomenon) (**a**). Contrast enhancement of the same opposing spinous processes, corresponding interspinous ligaments and interspinalis muscles (**a**, **b**, *arrows*). Bone marrow changes of the spinous processes represent stress-related bony reactive degenerative phenomena. Similarly, ligamentous and muscular changes represent stress-related degenerative inflammatory phenomena

Case 52: Degeneration-Inflammation of Ligaments. Baastrup's Phenomenon

- A 50-year-old woman
- Patient with persistent low back pain
- Limited lumbar motion

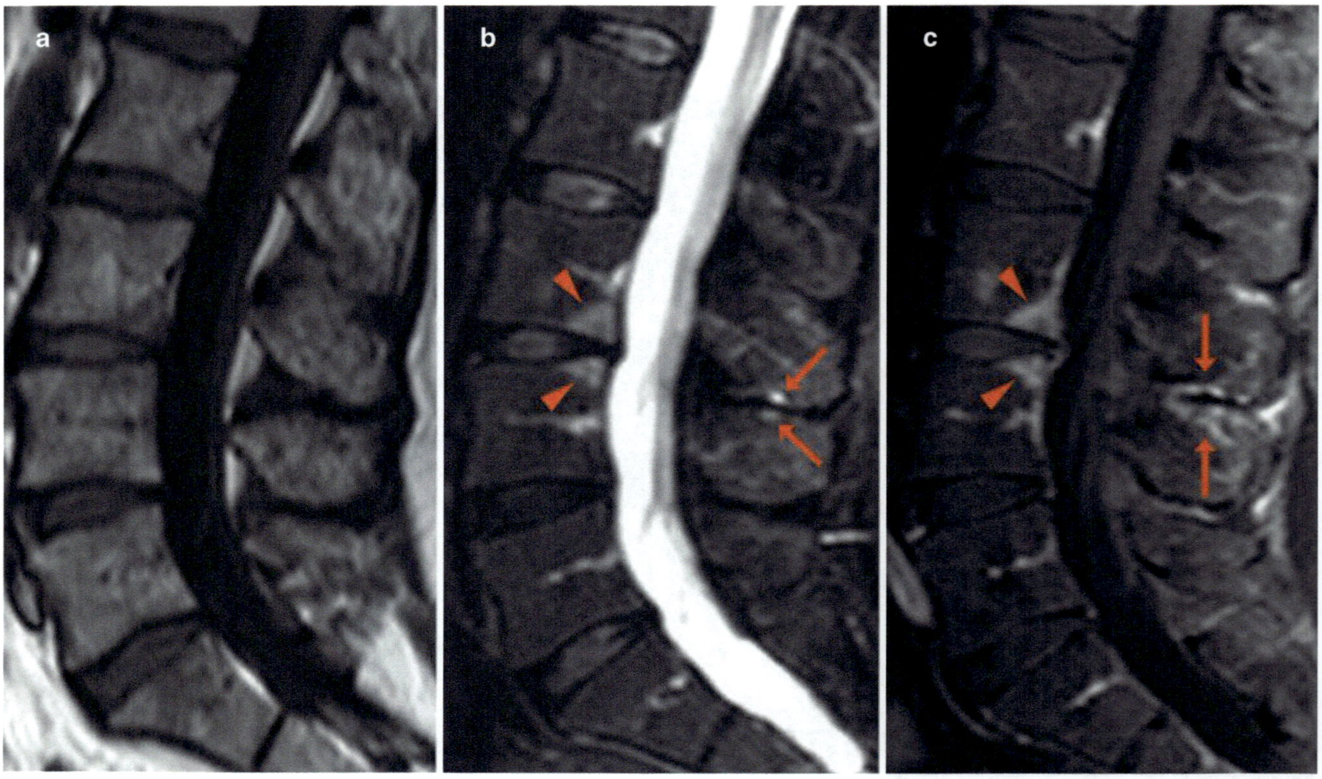

Fig. 8 Sagittal SE T1-weighted image (**a**), sagittal TSE T2-weighted image with fat saturation (**b**), sagittal and axial SE T1-weighted images with fat saturation after contrast medium administration (**c**, **d**). Lumbosacral hyperlordosis with collision of the spinous processes at L3/L4. Note small hyperintense areas in T2 (**b**, *arrows*) and contrast enhancement (**c**, *arrows*) in the same opposing spinous processes at L3/L4, due to stress-related bony reactive degenerative phenomena. Contrast enhancement of the interspinalis muscles at the same level (**d**, *arrows*), due to degenerative inflammatory phenomena. This patient presented also osteochondrosic changes at L3/L4, in active-inflammatory phase (**b**, **c**, *arrowheads*)

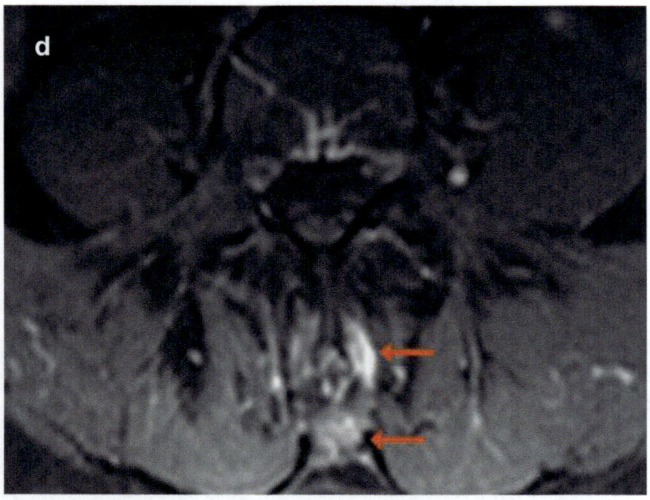

Fig. 8 (continued)

Case 53: Osteochondritis. Degeneration-Inflammation of Ligaments

- A 45-year-old man
- Patient with persistent low back pain that worsens with movement and prolonged upright position

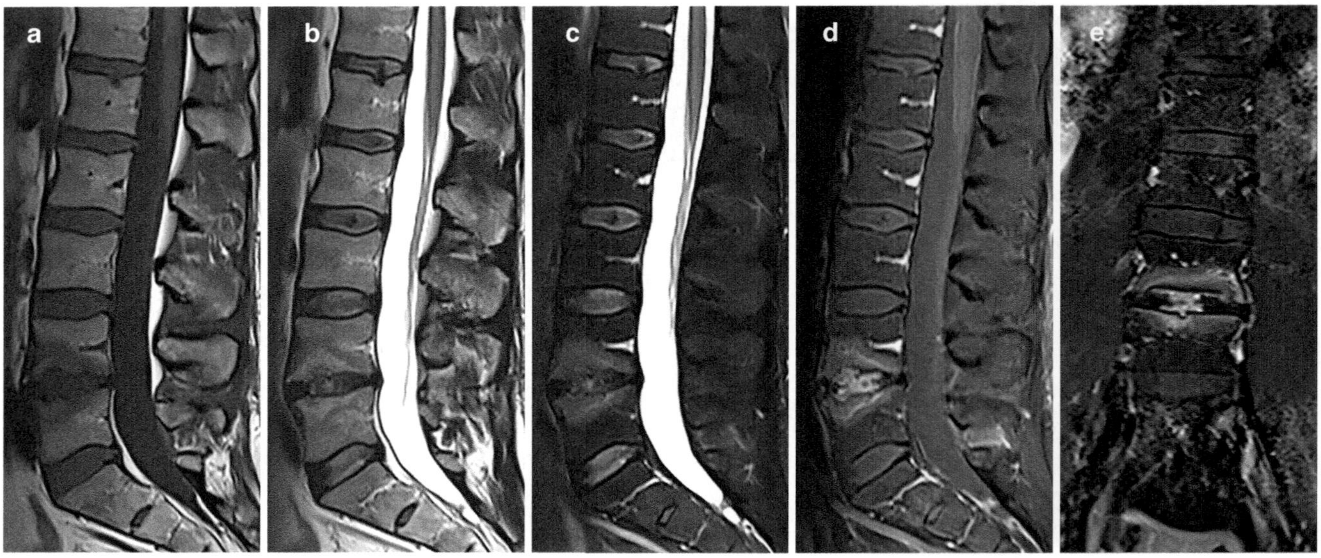

Fig. 9 (**a**–**h**) Sagittal TSE T1-weighted image (**a**), sagittal TSE T2-weighted image (**b**), sagittal TSE T2-weighted image with fat saturation (**c**), sagittal, coronal and axial TSE T1-weighted images with fat saturation after administration of contrast medium (**d**–**h**). The subchondral cancellous bone at L4/L5 shows marked signal changes, ipointense in T1 (**a**) and hyperintense in T2 (**b**, **c**), indicating oedematous pattern; note that oedema is more evident by using T2-weighted images with fat saturation (**c**) than standard T2-weighted images (**b**). The administration of contrast medium shows enhancement of the same subchondral cancellous bone and chondral surfaces at L4/L5, indicating osteochondritis in active inflammatory phase (**d**–**f**) other than enhancement of the interposed disc, indicating aseptic discitis (**d**–**g**). Diagnosis: osteochondritis in acute inflammatory phase with aseptic discitis. Note also contrast enhancement of the interspinous ligament at L5/S1, indicating ligamentous degeneration-inflammation (**d**, **h**)

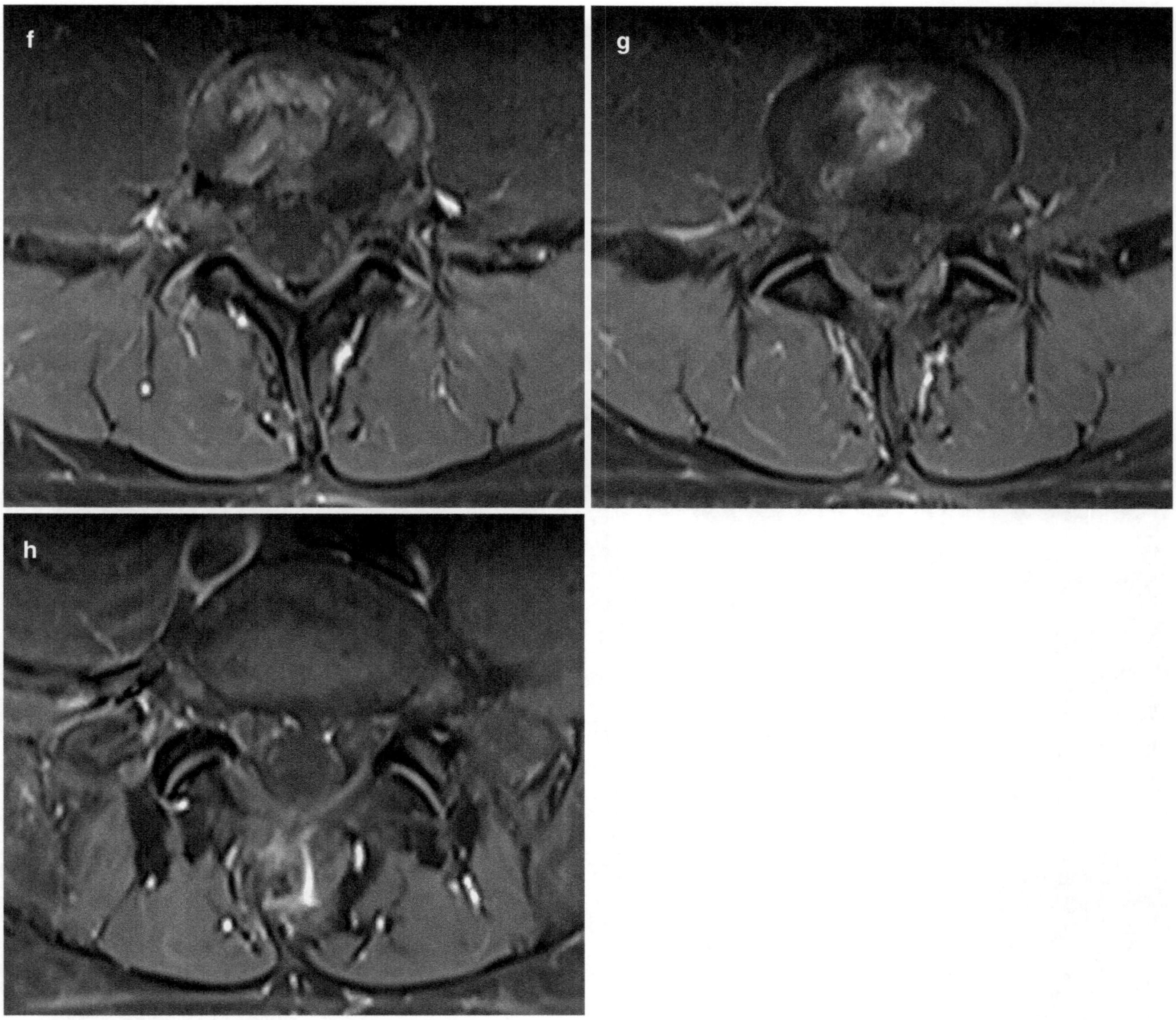

Fig. 9 (continued)

Case 54: Osteochondritis. Osteoarthritis. Muscular Inflammation

- A 58-year-old man
- Persistent low back pain
- Focal tenderness on the right side

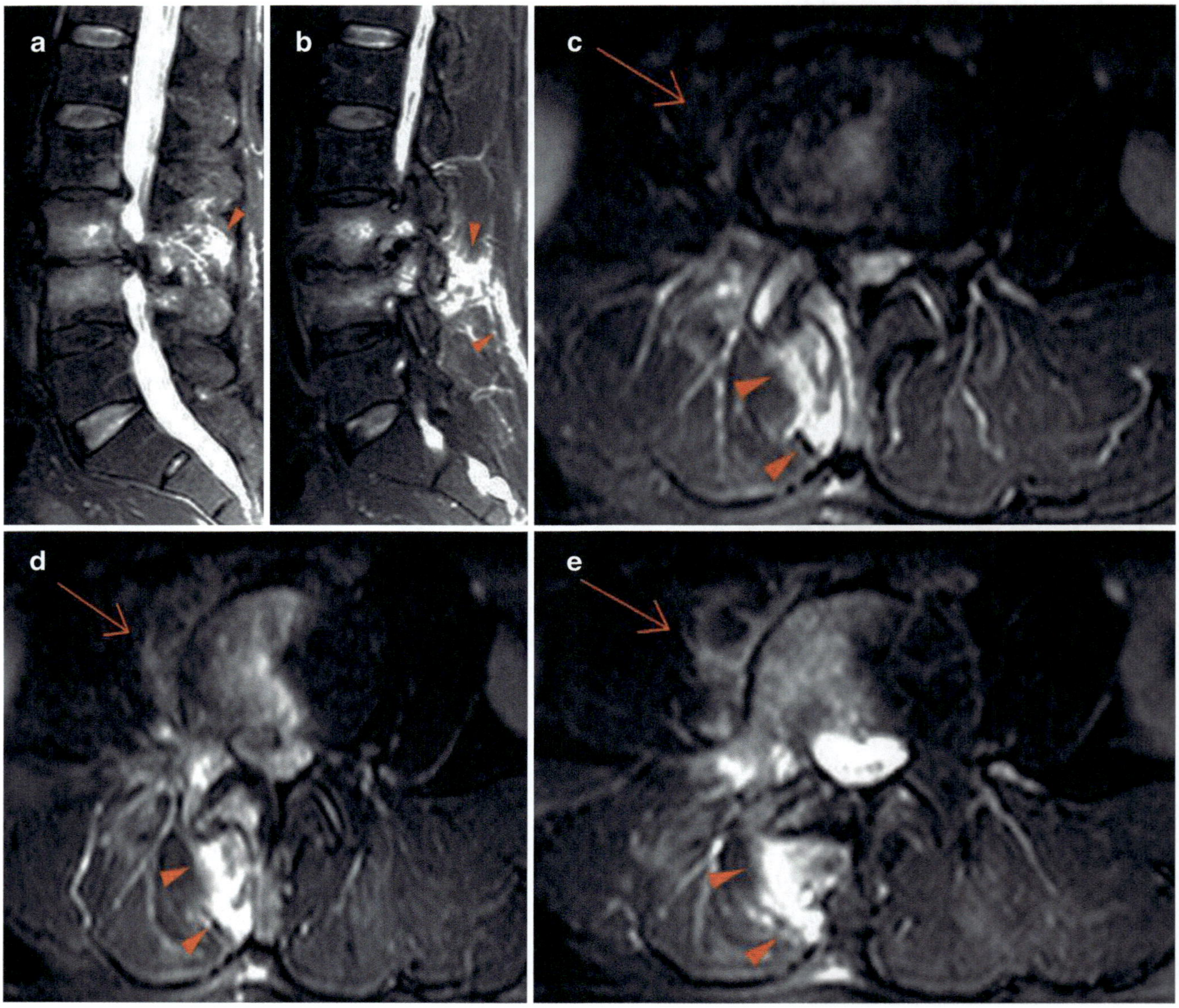

Fig. 10 Sagittal and axial TSE T2-weighted images with fat saturation (**a–e**), sagittal, coronal and axial SE T1-weighted images with fat saturation after the administration of contrast medium (**f–m**). Osteochondritis at L3/L4, in active inflammatory phase, with peridiscal inflammation involving the adjacent psoas muscle (**a–m**, *thin arrow*). Right facet joint osteoarthritis al the same level L3/L4 (**c–e**, **j–m**). Degeneration-inflammation on the right multifidus muscle that shows hyperintensity in T2 and contrast enhancement (**a–m**, *arrowheads*). Left-convex scoliosis (**h**). All the above-mentioned changes, i.e. osteochondritis, osteoarthritis and muscular changes, are presumably due to scoliosis with consequent biomechanical deterioration of the spine and perispinal muscles

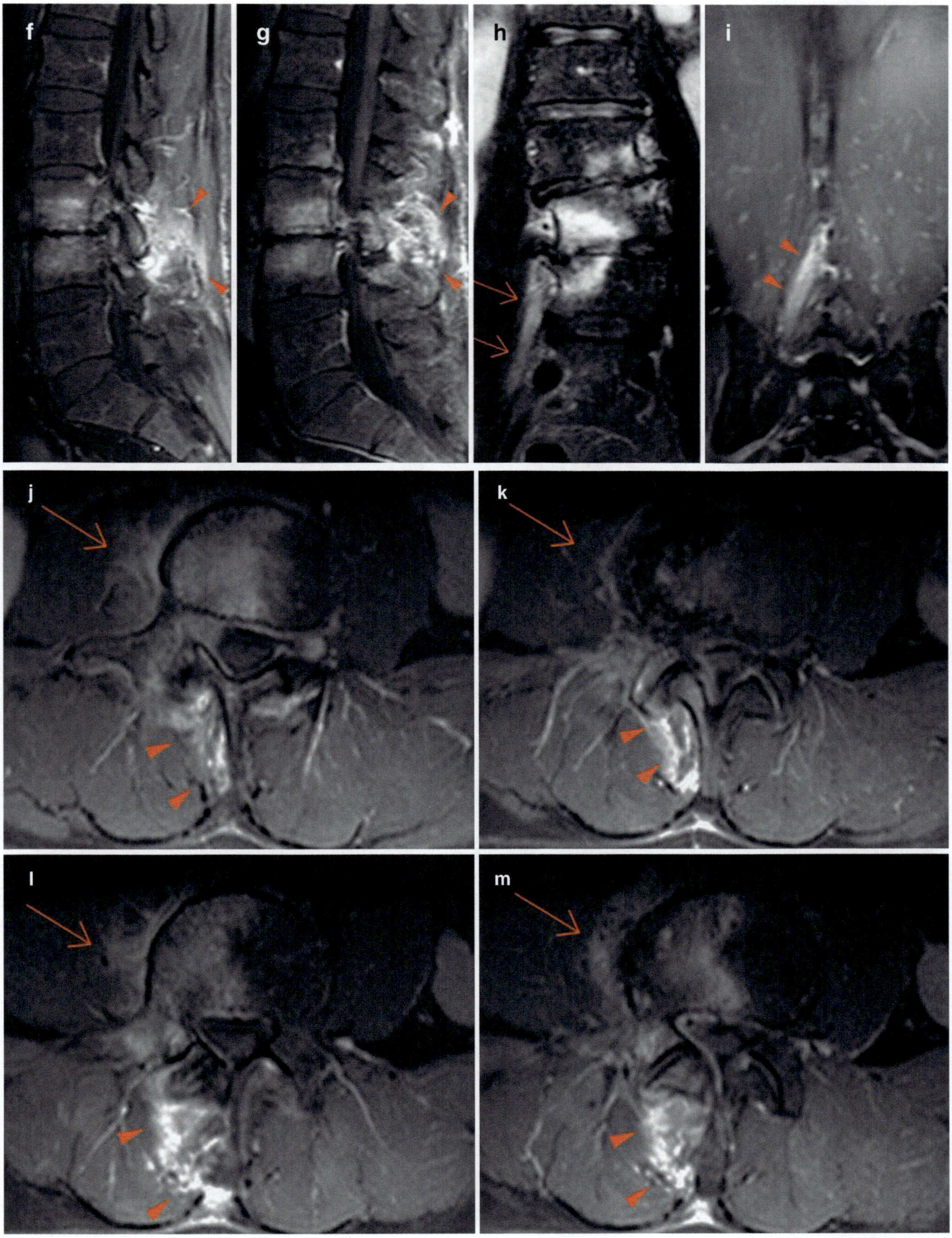

Fig. 10 (continued)

Case 55: Degeneration-Inflammation of Ligaments. Ligamentous Cyst. Facet Joint Osteoarthritis. Synovitis

- A 68-year-old woman
- Low back pain
- Weakness in the legs
- Focal tenderness on palpation of the interspinous space at L4/L5

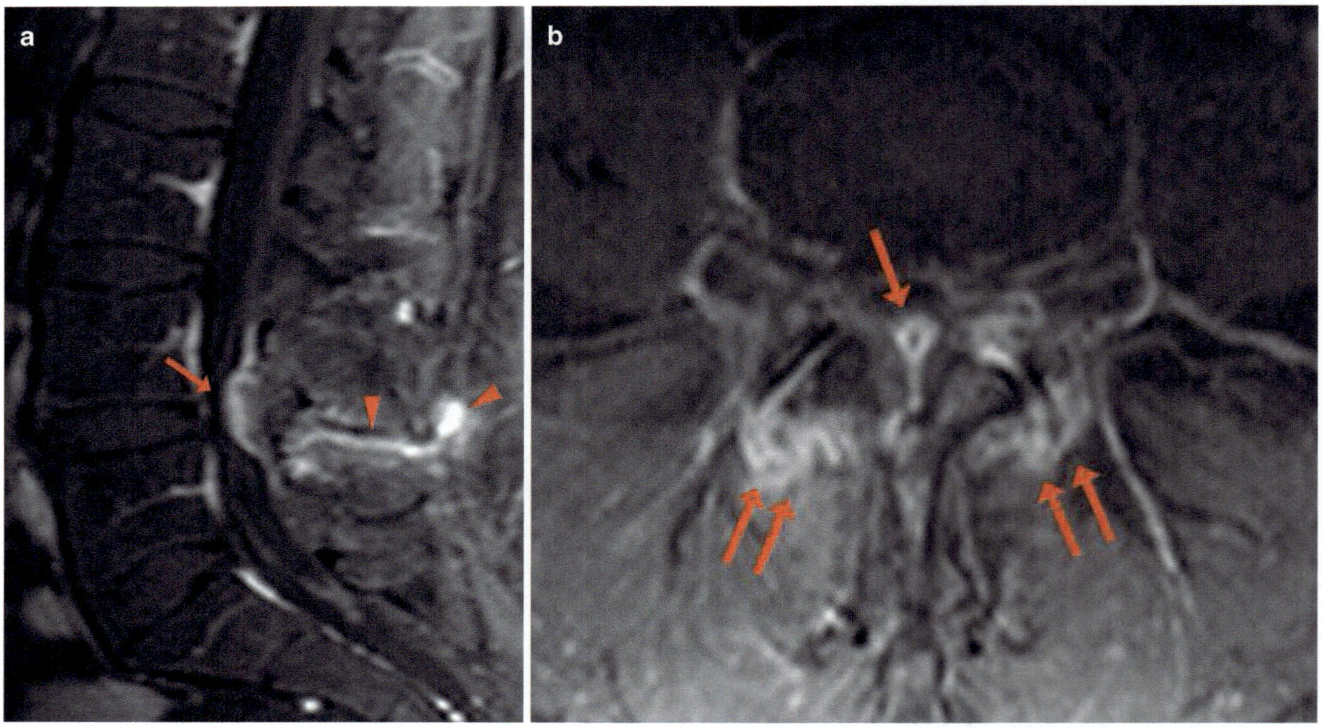

Fig. 11 Sagittal and axial SE T1-weighted images with fat saturation following the administration of contrast medium (**a–c**). Mild anterolisthesis of L4 over L5. Contrast enhancement of the interspinous and supraspinous ligaments at L4/L5, indicating ligamentous degeneration-inflammation (**a–c**, *arrowheads*). Note the anterior neo-/pseudocyst with peripheral contrast enhancement, in the epidural space of the posterior aspect of the central spinal canal at L4/L5 in the midline (**a**, **b**, *arrow*). The cyst arises from the collision of the corresponding spinous processes and progressive degeneration of the interspinous ligament, with pseudocyst formation. The same cyst contributes to the stenosis of the central spinal canal at the same level. Bilateral osteoarthritis with synovitis-synovial hypertrophy at L4/L5 (**b**, **c**, *double arrows*)

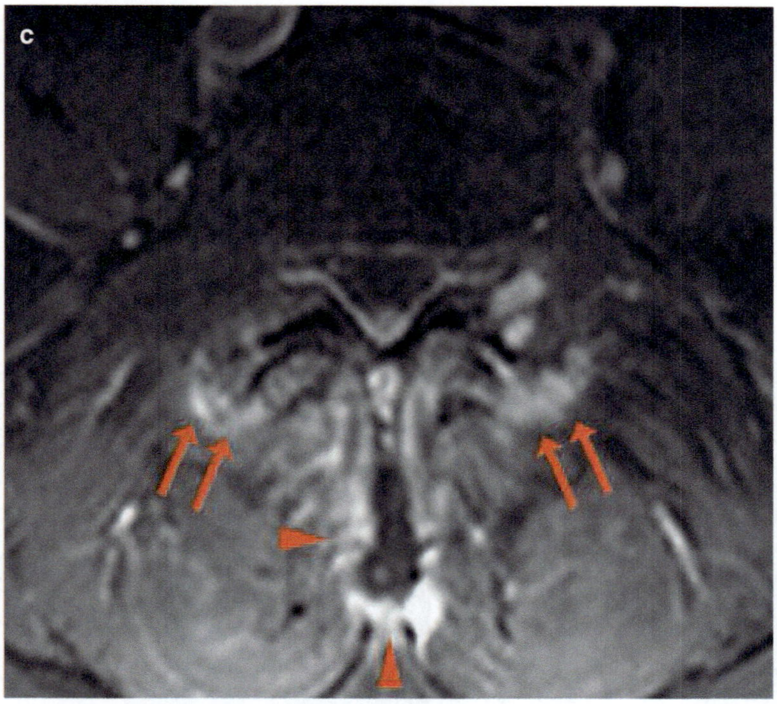

Fig. 11 (continued)

Case 56: Degeneration-Inflammation of Ligaments and Paravertebral Muscles

- A 66-year-old man
- Chronic low back pain
- Pain on palpation of the lumbar interspinous spaces and posterior paravertebral muscles on the left side

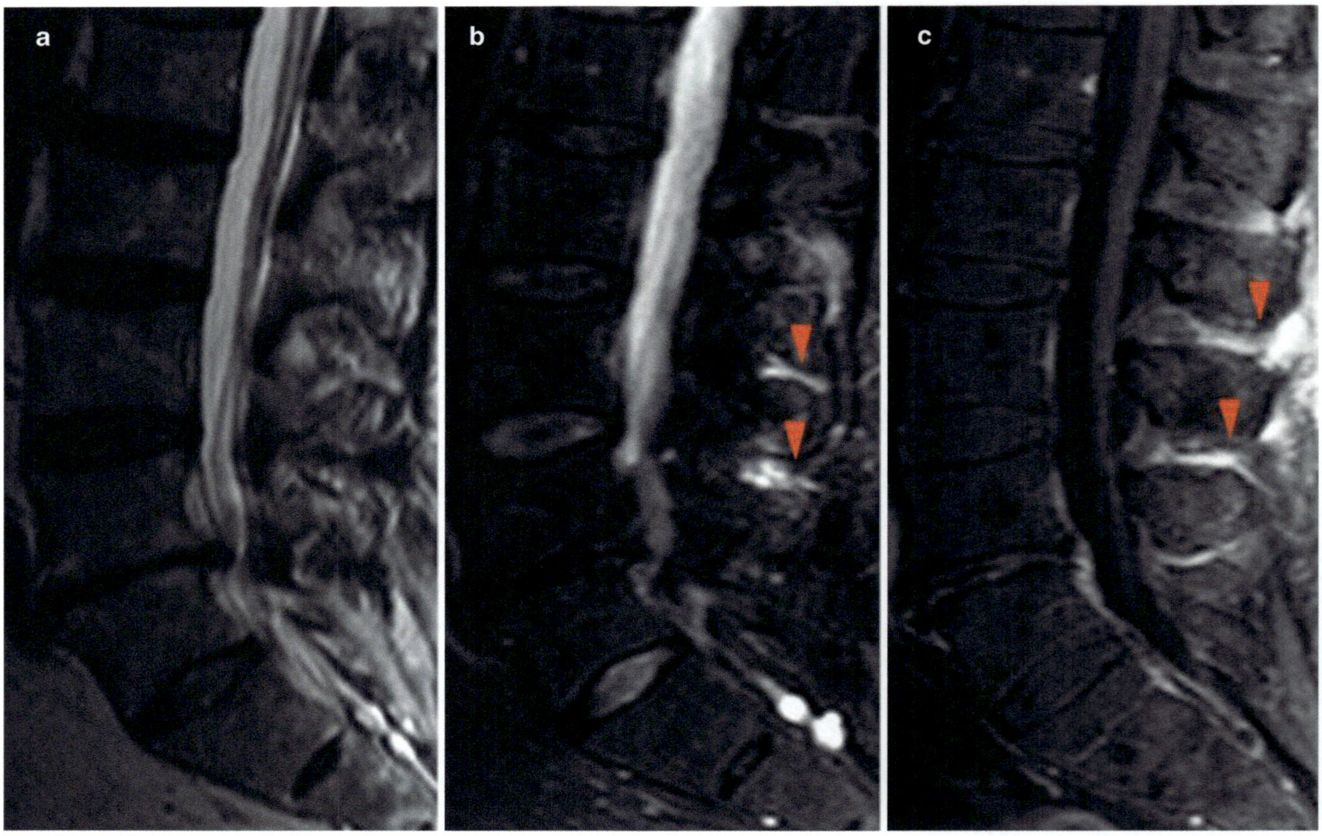

Fig. 12 Sagittal SE T2-weighted image (**a**), sagittal and axial TSE T2-weighted images with fat saturation (**b**, **d**, **e**), sagittal and axial SE T1-weighted images with fat saturation following administration of contrast medium (**c**, **f**, **g**). Osteochondrosis at L4-L5. T2 hyperintensity and contrast enhancement of the interspinous and/or supraspinous ligaments from L1 to L5, indicating degeneration-inflammation of the same ligaments (**b**, **c**, *arrowhead*). The same patient presented T2 hyperintensity and contrast enhancement of the interspinalis muscles (**e–g**, *arrowhead*) and left multifidus muscle (**d–g**, *arrow*), referable to degeneration-inflammation of the same muscles

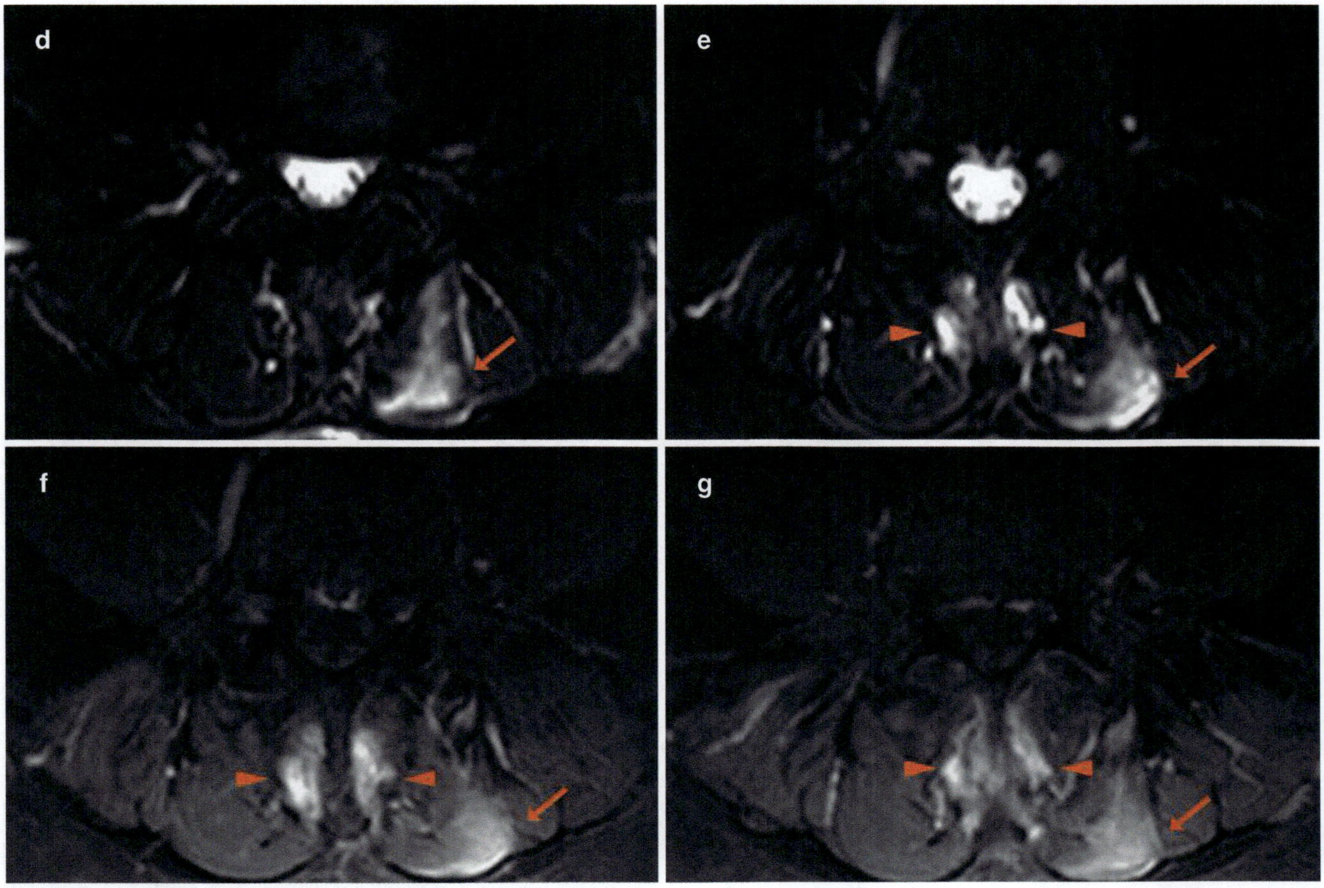

Fig. 12 (continued)

Case 57: Muscular Inflammation

- A 31-year-old woman
- Low back pain
- Focal tenderness on palpation of the lumbar perispinal muscles

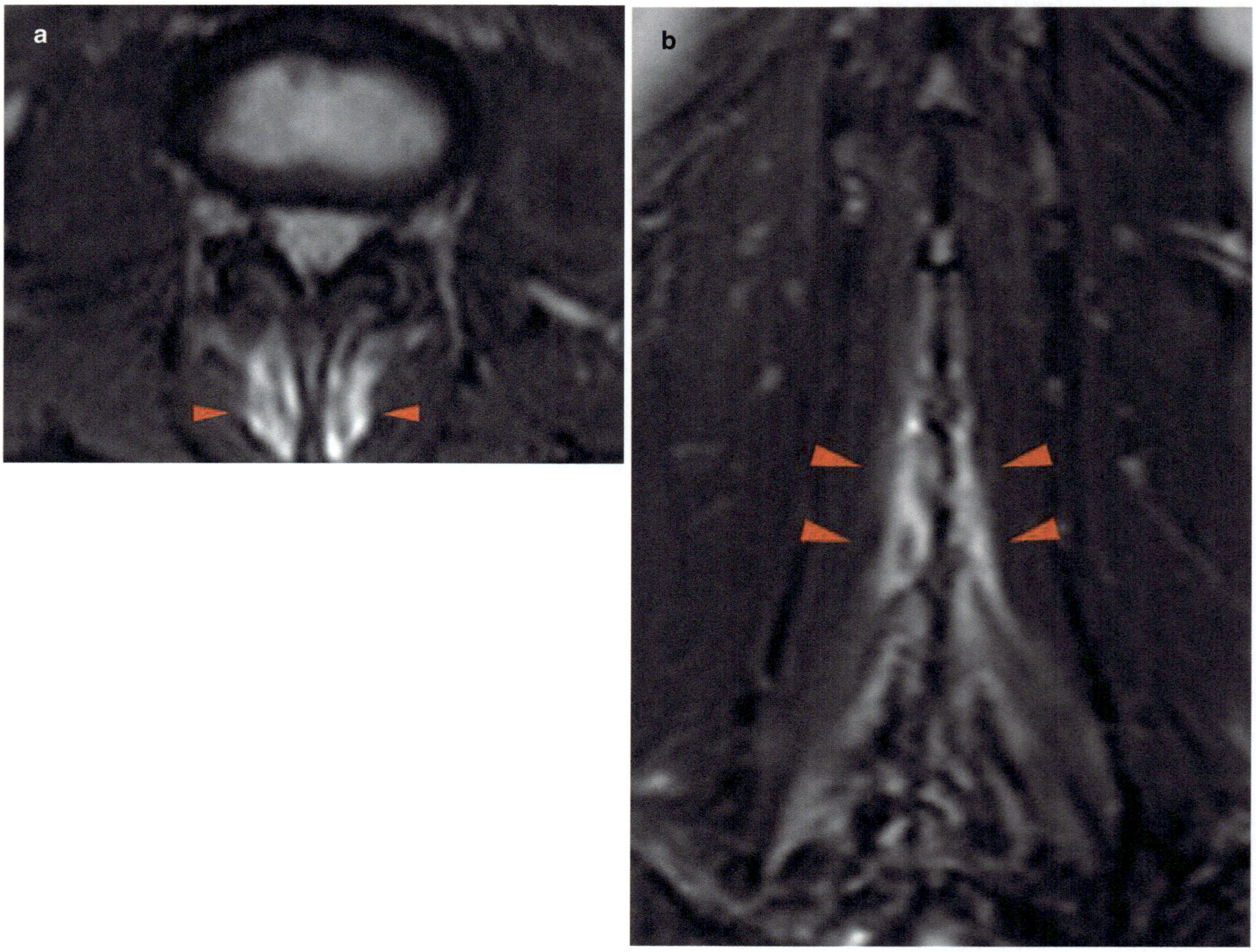

Fig. 13 Axial and coronal TSE T2-weighted images with fat saturation image (**a**, **b**). T2 hyperintensity of the interspinalis muscles, due to oedema (**a**, **b**, *arrowheads*). This patient had a trauma 10 days before MR examination

Case 58: Muscular Inflammation

- A 66-year-old man
- Right-sided low back pain
- Focal tenderness

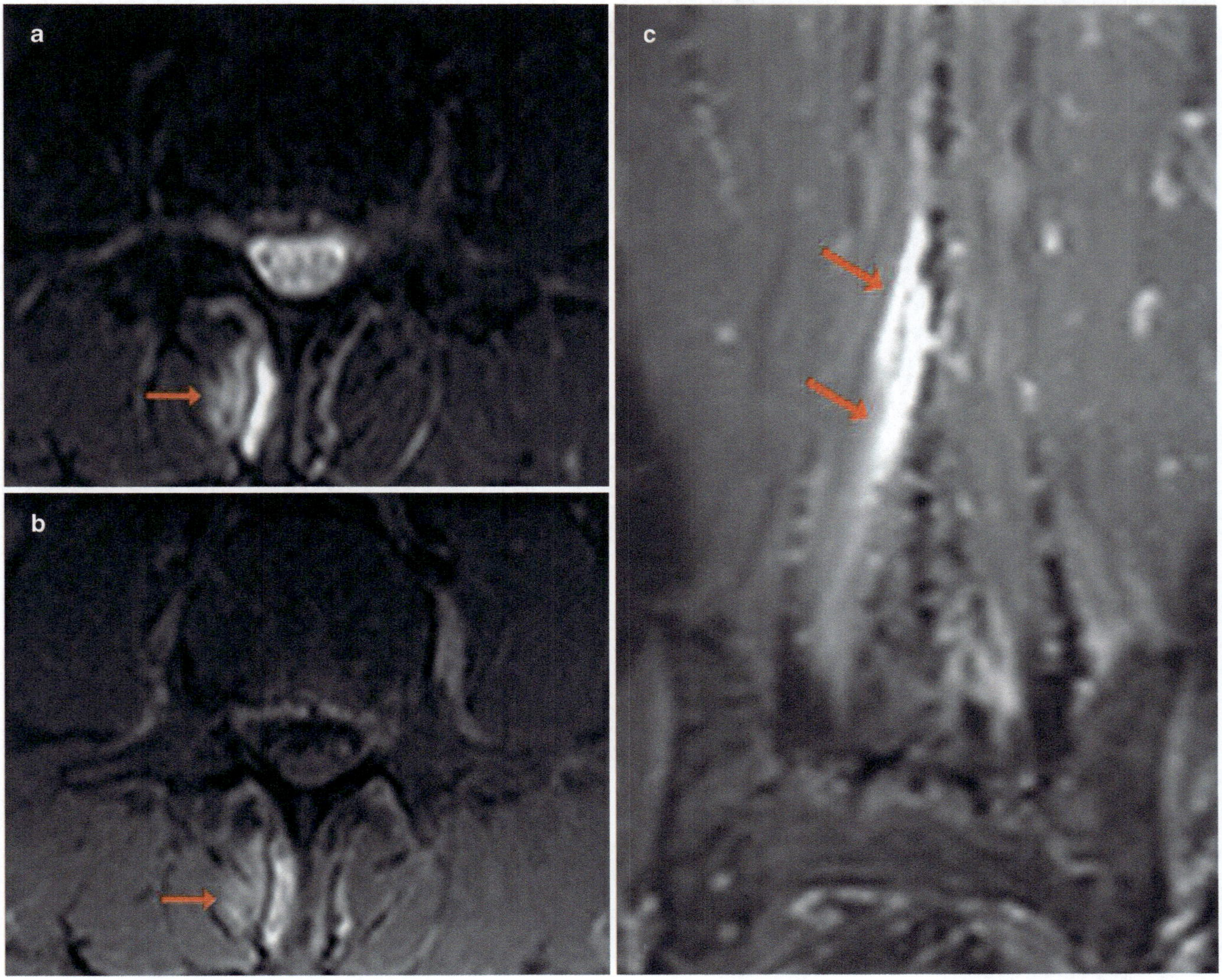

Fig. 14 Axial TSE T2-weighted image with fat saturation (**a**), axial and coronal SE T1-weighted images with fat saturation after contrast medium administration (**b**, **c**). T2 hyperintensity of the perispinal muscles (e.g. interspinalis muscle and multifidus muscle) on the right side (**a**, *arrow*). Contrast enhancement of the same muscles (**b**, **c**, *arrows*). These finding indicate degenerative oedematous muscular changes

Case 59: Muscular Inflammation

- A 27-year-old man
- Right back pain after physical exercise

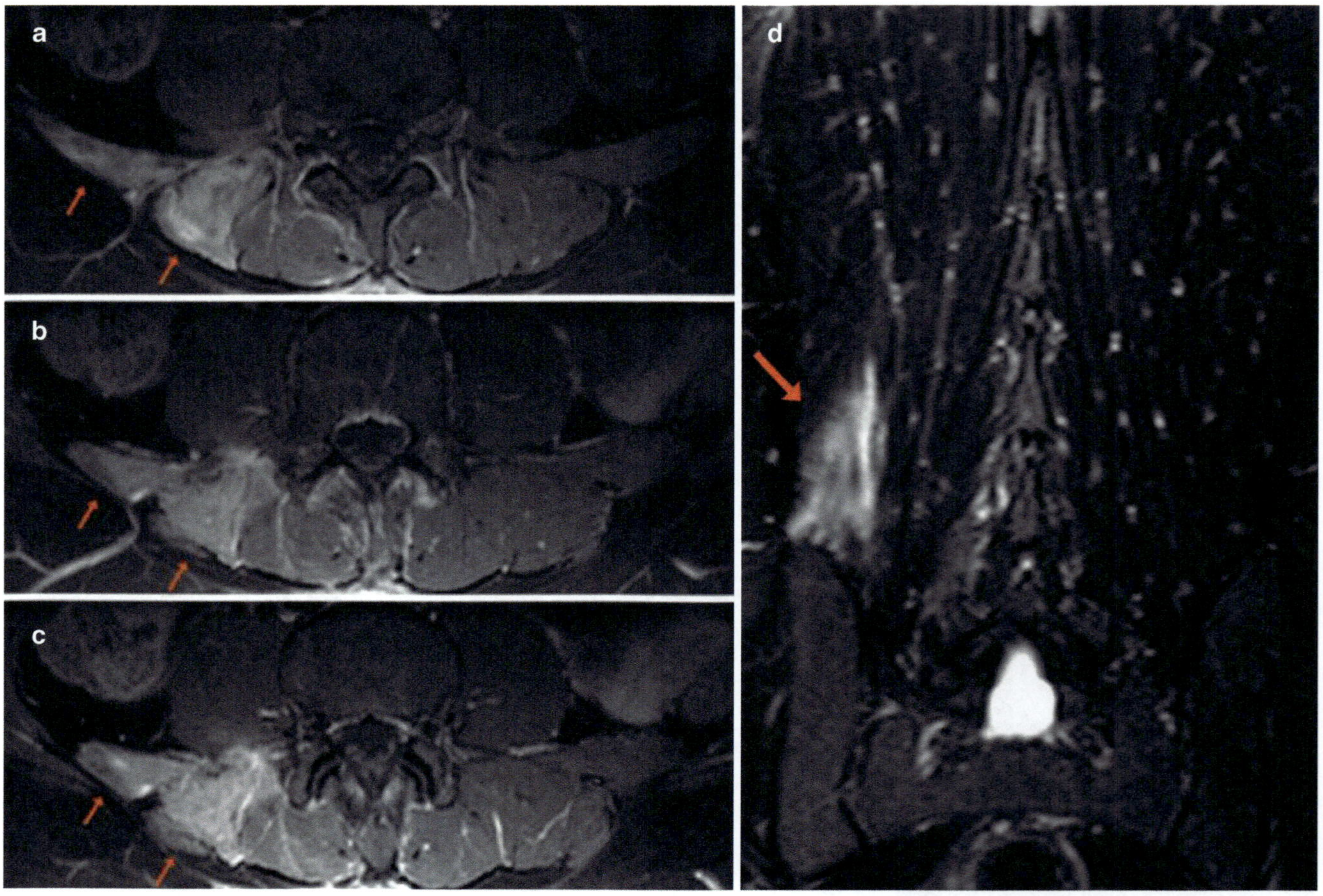

Fig. 15 Axial SE T1-weighted images with fat saturation following administration of contrast medium (**a–c**), coronal TSE T2-weighted with fat saturation (**d**). Signal changes of the posterior paravertebral muscles on the right side. In particular, the iliocostalis and quadratus lumborum muscles show contrast enhancement (**a–c**, *arrows*) and high signal in T2 (**d**, *arrow*). These findings indicate inflammatory muscular changes. There was precise correlation between MRI findings and the patient's focus of pain

Case 60: Muscular Inflammation

- A 30-year-old patient
- Lumbar radiculopathy on the right side
- Limited motion
- Focal tenderness corresponding to lumbar perispinal muscles on the right side

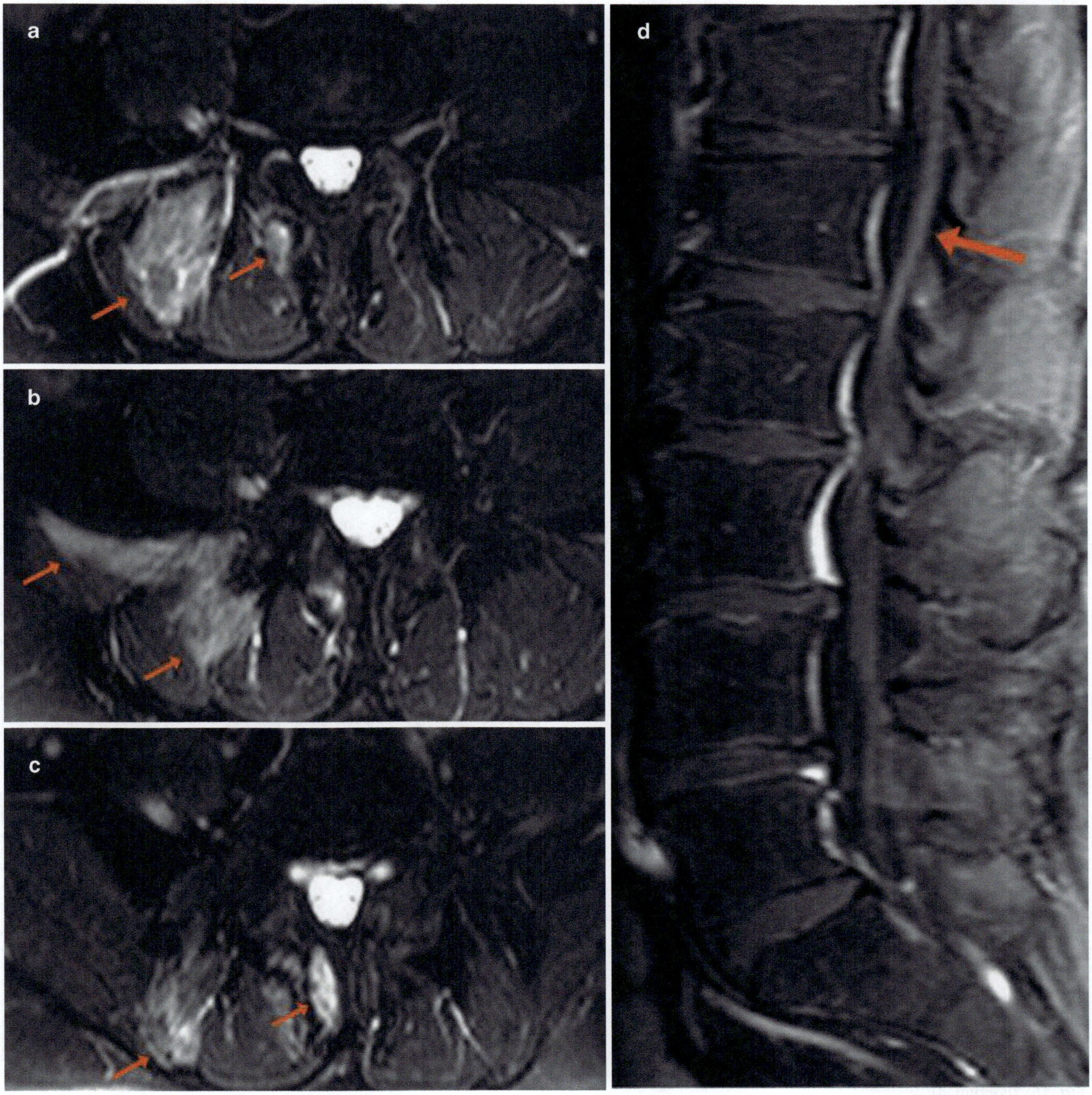

Fig. 16 Axial TSE T2-weighted images with fat saturation (**a–c**), sagittal, axial and coronal SE T1-weighted images with fat saturation following administration of contrast medium (**d–m**). Signal changes of the lumbar perispinal muscles on the right side, e.g. interspinalis, multifidus, thoracocostalis, longissimus, quadratus lumborum (**a–c**, **e–g**, **j**, **k**, *arrows*). These muscles exhibit high signal in T2-weighted images (**a–c**), with marked contrast enhancement (**e–g**, **j**, **k**, *arrows*). The same patient presented contrast enhancement of a nerve root on the right side (**d**, **h**, **i**, *arrow*), indicating sterile radiculitis

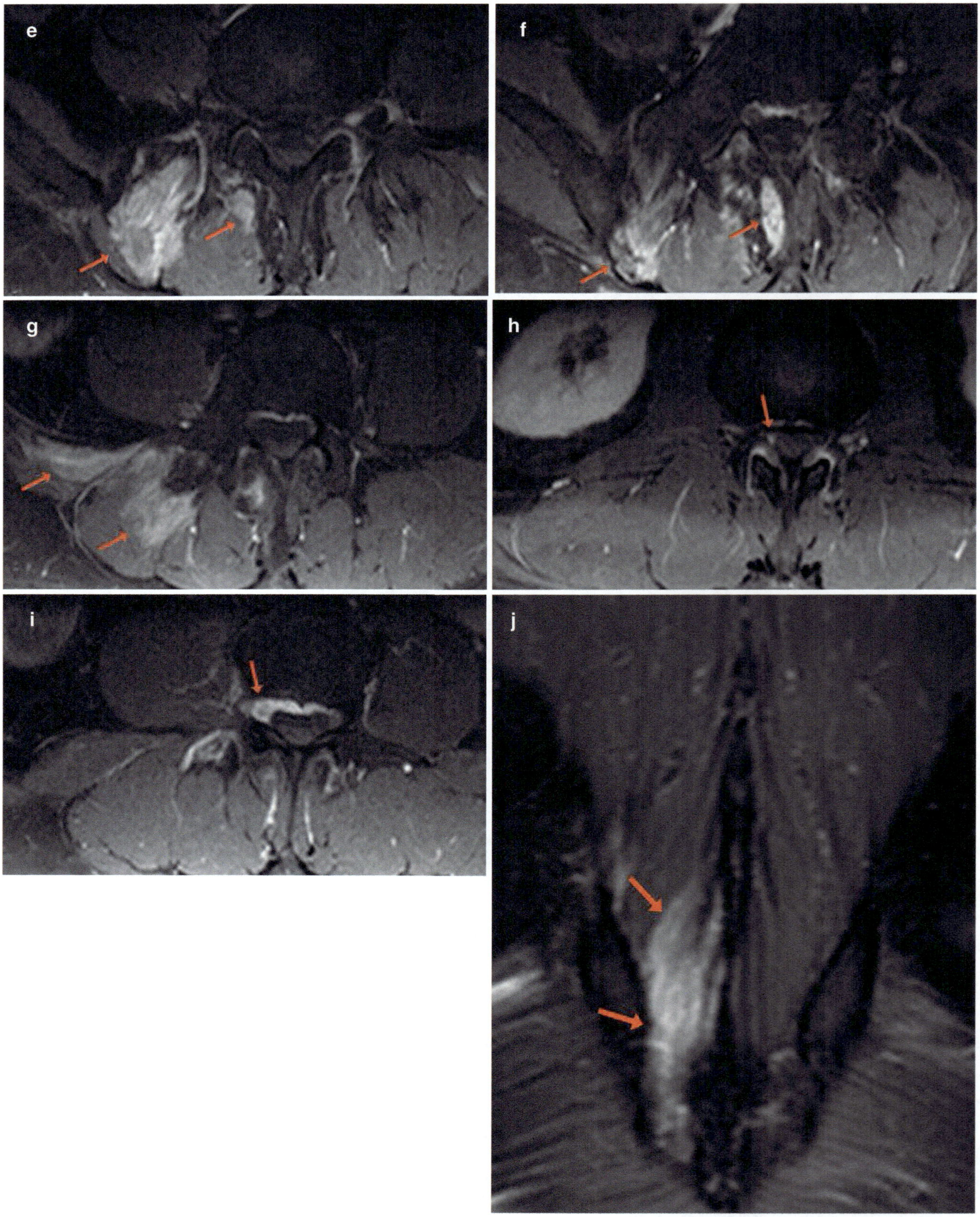

Fig. 16 (continued)

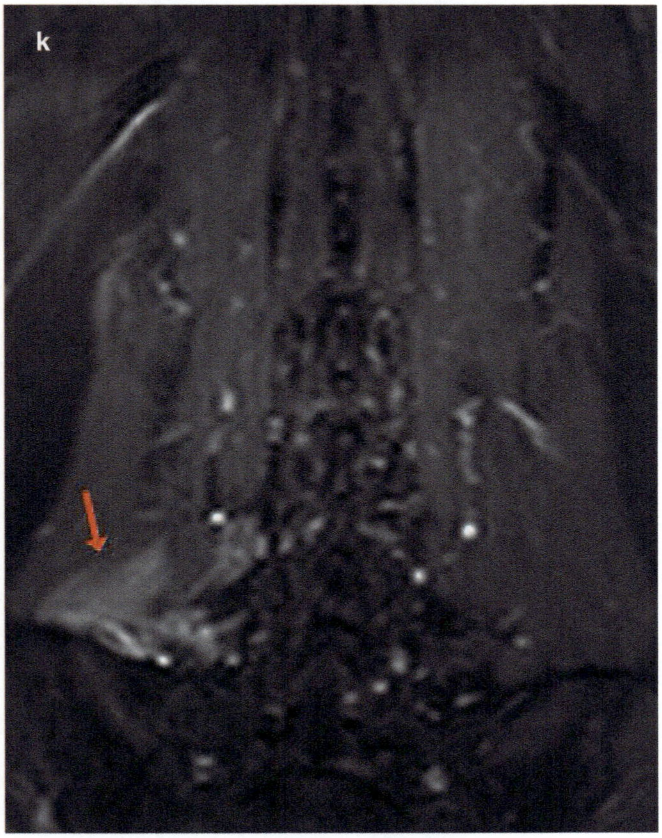

Fig. 16 (continued)

Unusual Cases

8

Case 61: Unusual Case. Herniated Disc in Unusual Location

- A 58-year-old woman
- Sudden onset of back pain and right anterior thigh pain following physical exercise

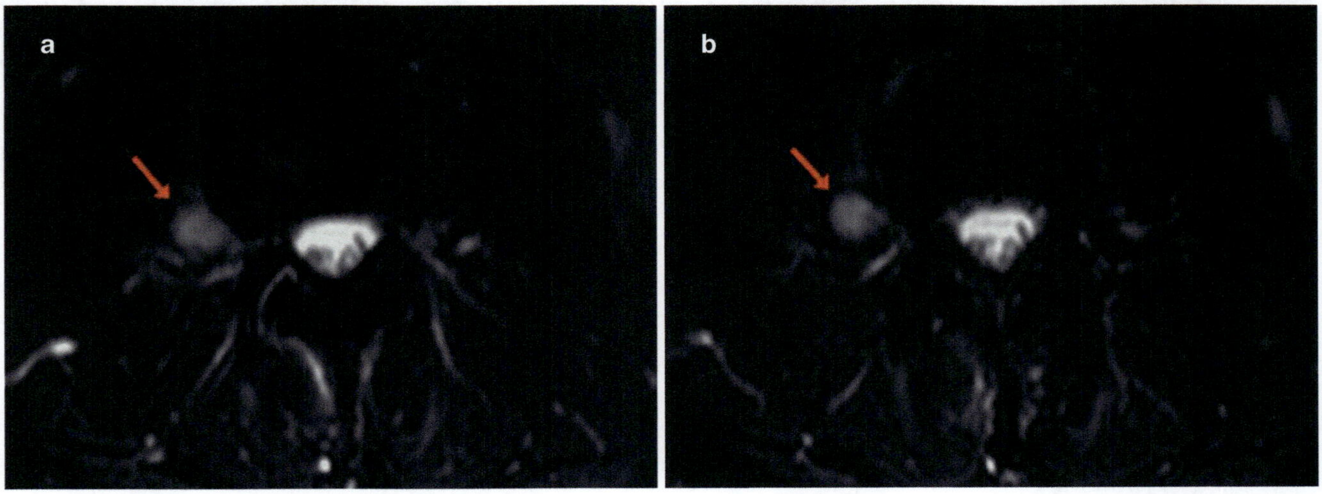

Fig. 1 Axial TSE T2-weighted images with fat saturation (**a**, **b**), axial and coronal SE T1-weighted images with fat saturation following administration of contrast medium (**c**–**f**). Small rounded mass lateral to the right L1/L2 neural foramen and adjacent to the ipsilateral psoas. The mass shows high signal on T2-weighted images (**a**, **b**, *arrow*), probably caused by associated oedema and has an enhancing rim on contrast-enhanced T1-weighted studies (**c**–**f**, *arrow*). This is an extraforaminal disc fragment (so-called far lateral herniation), well delineated by peripheral contrast enhancement due to peridiscal inflammatory reaction

P. D'Aprile, A. Tarantino, *MRI of Degenerative Disease of the Spine*, https://doi.org/10.1007/978-3-030-73707-8_8

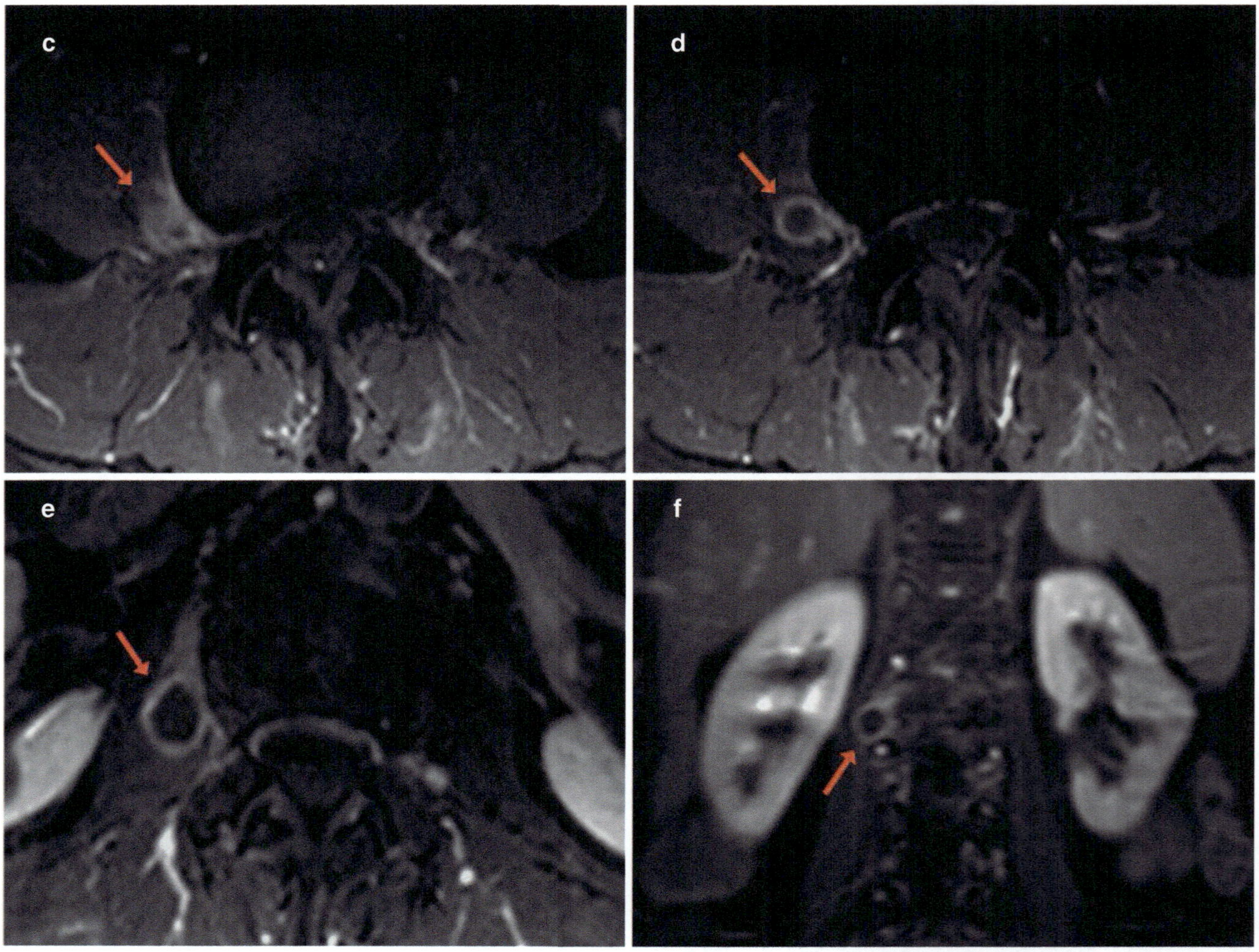

Fig. 1 (continued)

Case 62: Unusual Case. Herniated Disc in Unusual Location

- A 55-year-old man
- Persistent low back pain
- Limited lumbar motion

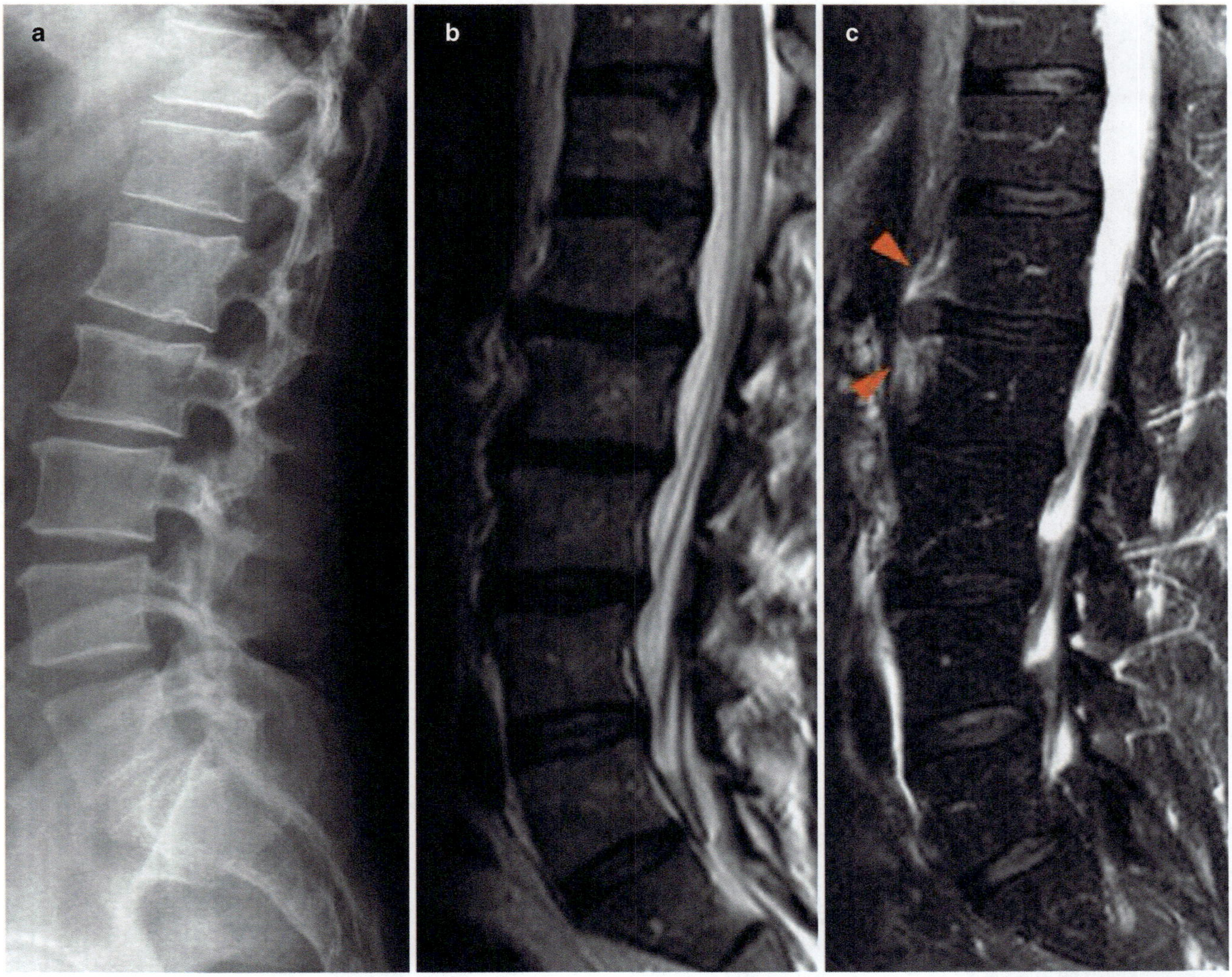

Fig. 2 Lateral lumbosacral X-ray (**a**), sagittal TSE T2-weighted image (**b**), sagittal and axial TSE T2-weighted images with fat saturation (**c**, **e**), axial SE T1-weighted image (**d**), sagittal and axial SE T1-weighted images with fat saturation after contrast medium administration (**f**, **g**). X-ray does not show spine changes (**a**). MRI shows an anterior herniated disc at L1/L2 (**b**–**f**, *arrowheads*). Note that T2-weighted images with fat saturation (**c**) reveal peridiscal oedema that is not evident in the "standard" T2-weighted images without fat saturation (**b**). Note also peridiscal contrast enhancement indicating peridiscal inflammatory reaction (**f**, **g**, *arrowheads*)

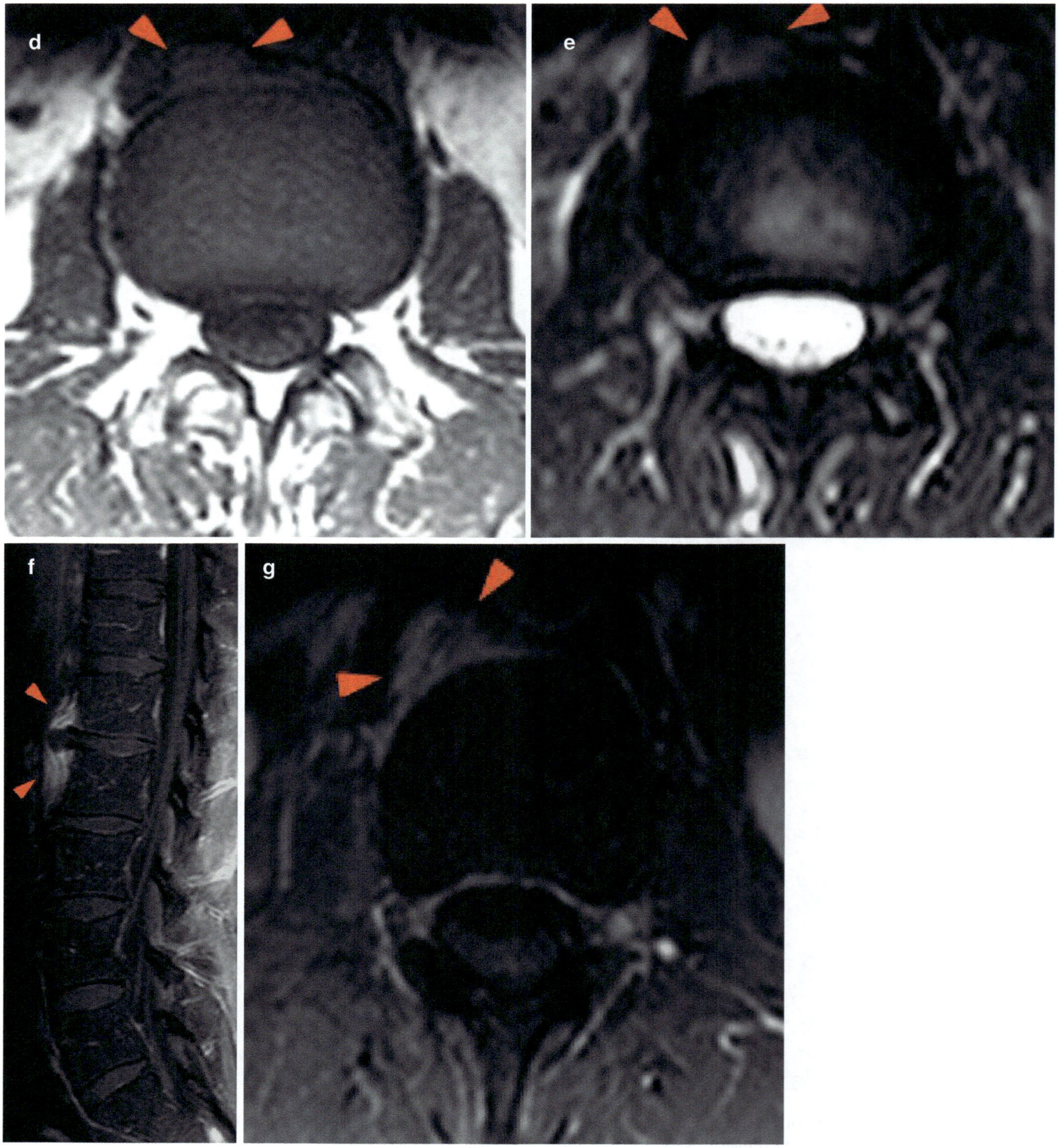

Fig. 2 (continued)

Case 63: Unusual Case. Giant Schmorl Hernia

- A 30-year-old man
- Low back pain

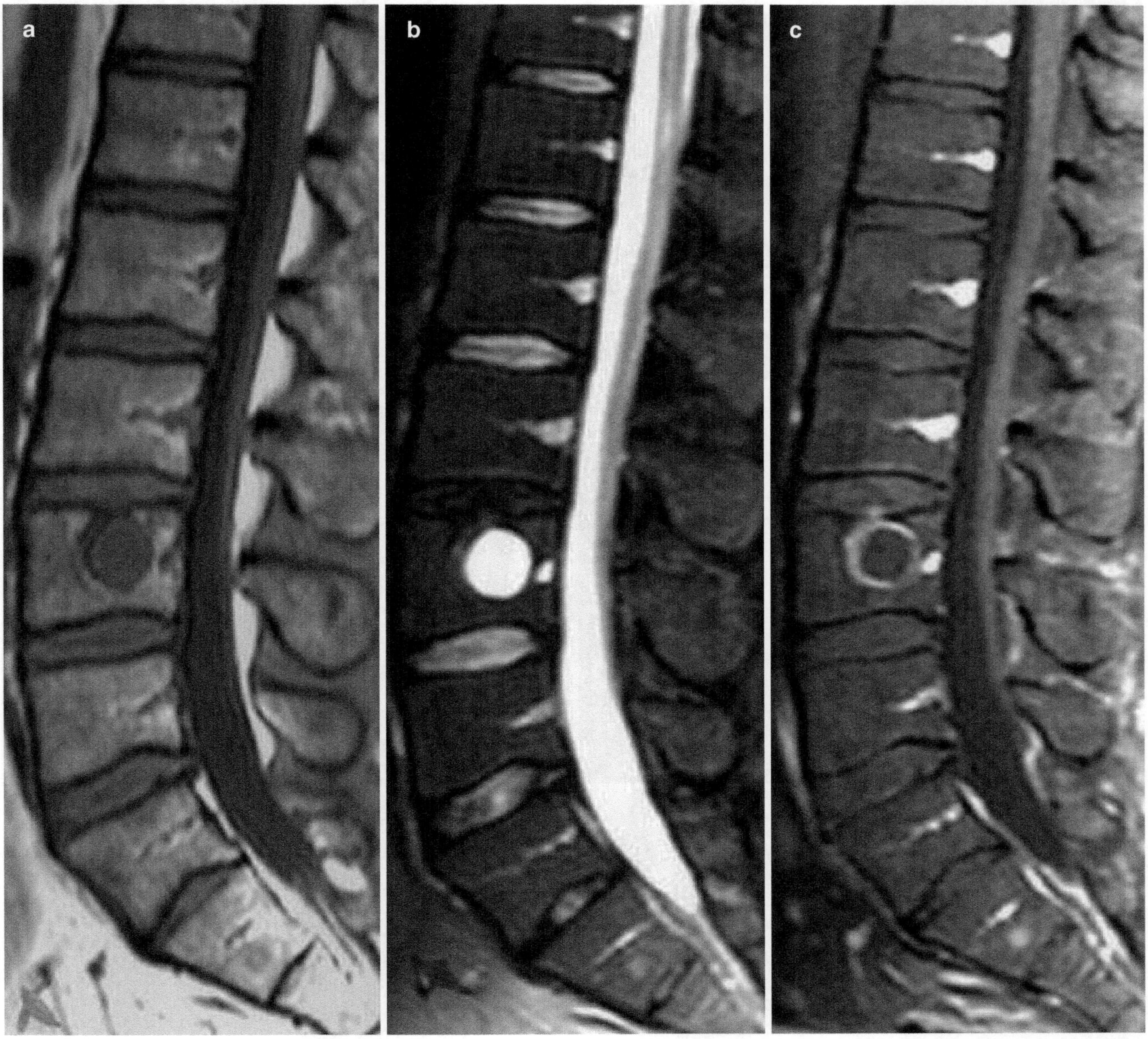

Fig. 3 Sagittal SE T1-weighted images (**a**), sagittal TSE T2-weighted image with fat saturation (**b**, **d**), sagittal and axial SE T1-weighted images with fat saturation following administration of contrast medium (**c**, **e**), CT scan with coronal and sagittal reconstruction (MRP) (**f**–**h**). Presence of round lesion in the vertebral body of L4. The lesion shows a cystic appearance, hypointense in T1 (**a**), hyperintense in T2 (**b**, **d**), with peripheral contrast enhancement (**c**, **e**). There is a small interruption of the adjacent vertebral endplate. CT images show a thin osteosclerotic margin of the lesion and confirm the interruption of the upper adjacent vertebral end-plate. Diagnosis: giant Schmorl hernia with cystic-degenerative phenomena

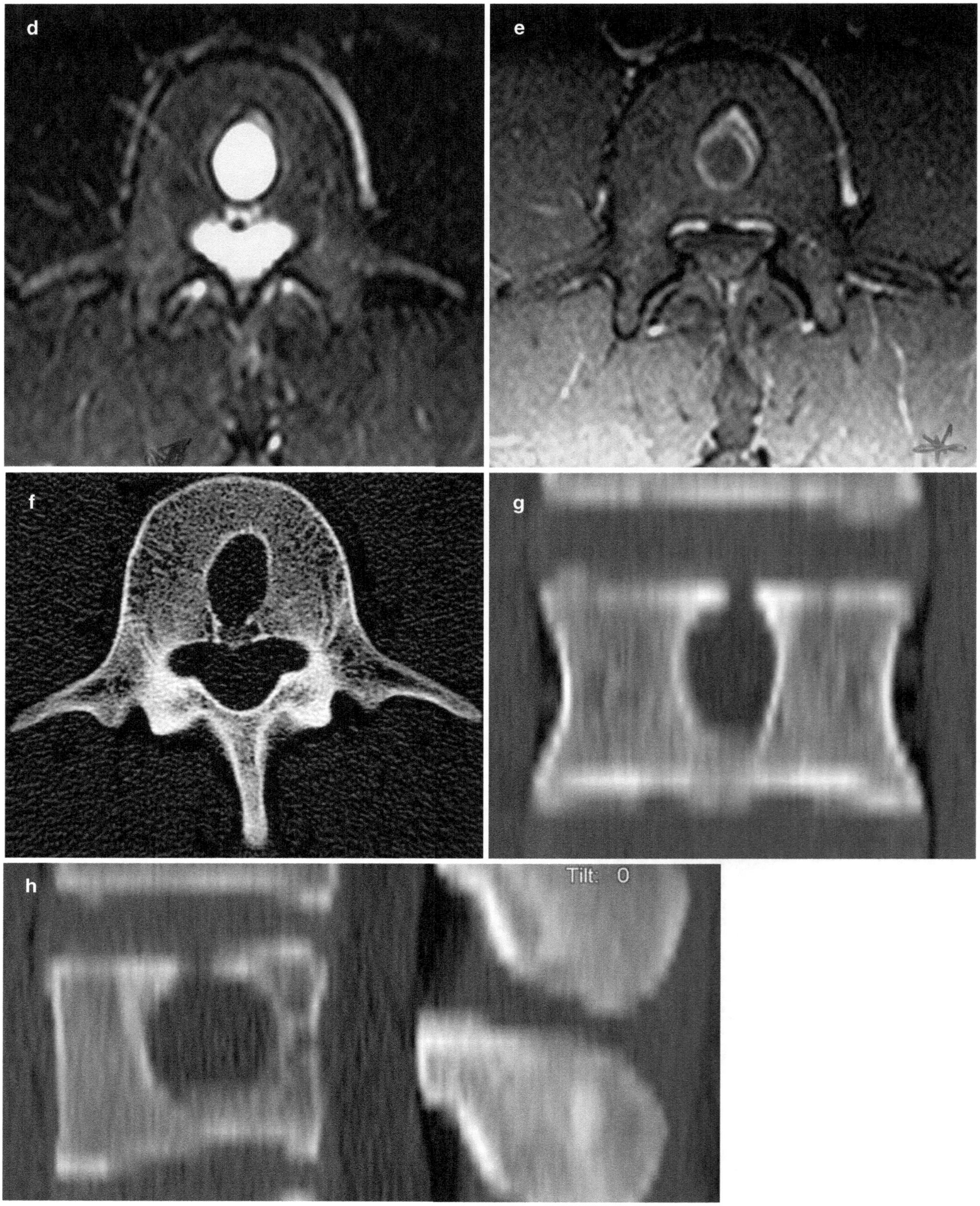

Fig. 3 (continued)

Case 64: Unusual Case. Ganglion Cyst

- An 18-year-old boy
- Low back pain with sciatica on the left side

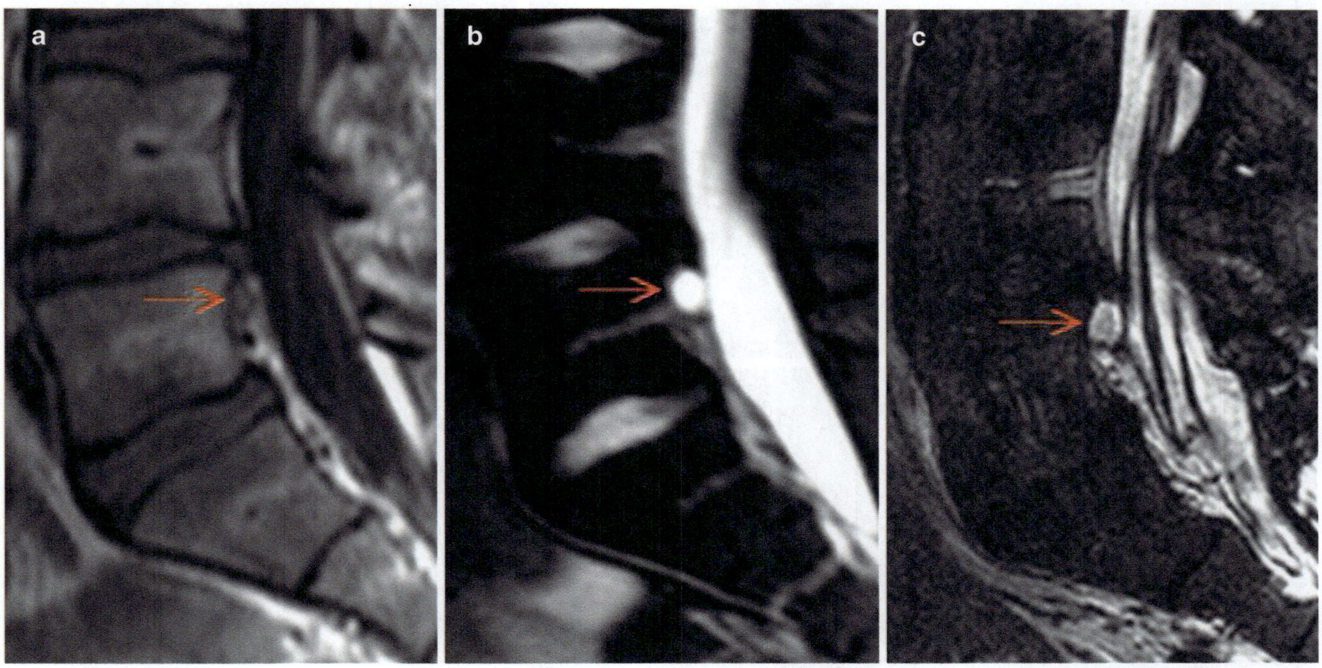

Fig. 4 Sagittal SE T1-weighted image (**a**), sagittal TSE T2-weighted image with fat saturation (**b**), sagittal and axial CISS images (**c**, **d**), SE T1-weighted images with fat saturation following administration of contrast medium (**e**, **f**). Cystic lesion in the anterior epidural space, on the left side (**a**–**f**, *arrows*). The cyst content resembles the CSF in all pulse sequences (**a**–**d**) and shows peripheral contrast enhancement. This is a so-called ganglion cyst, arising from the posterior longitudinal ligament. Epidural cysts, either synovial or ganglion, are an unusual case of radicular compression

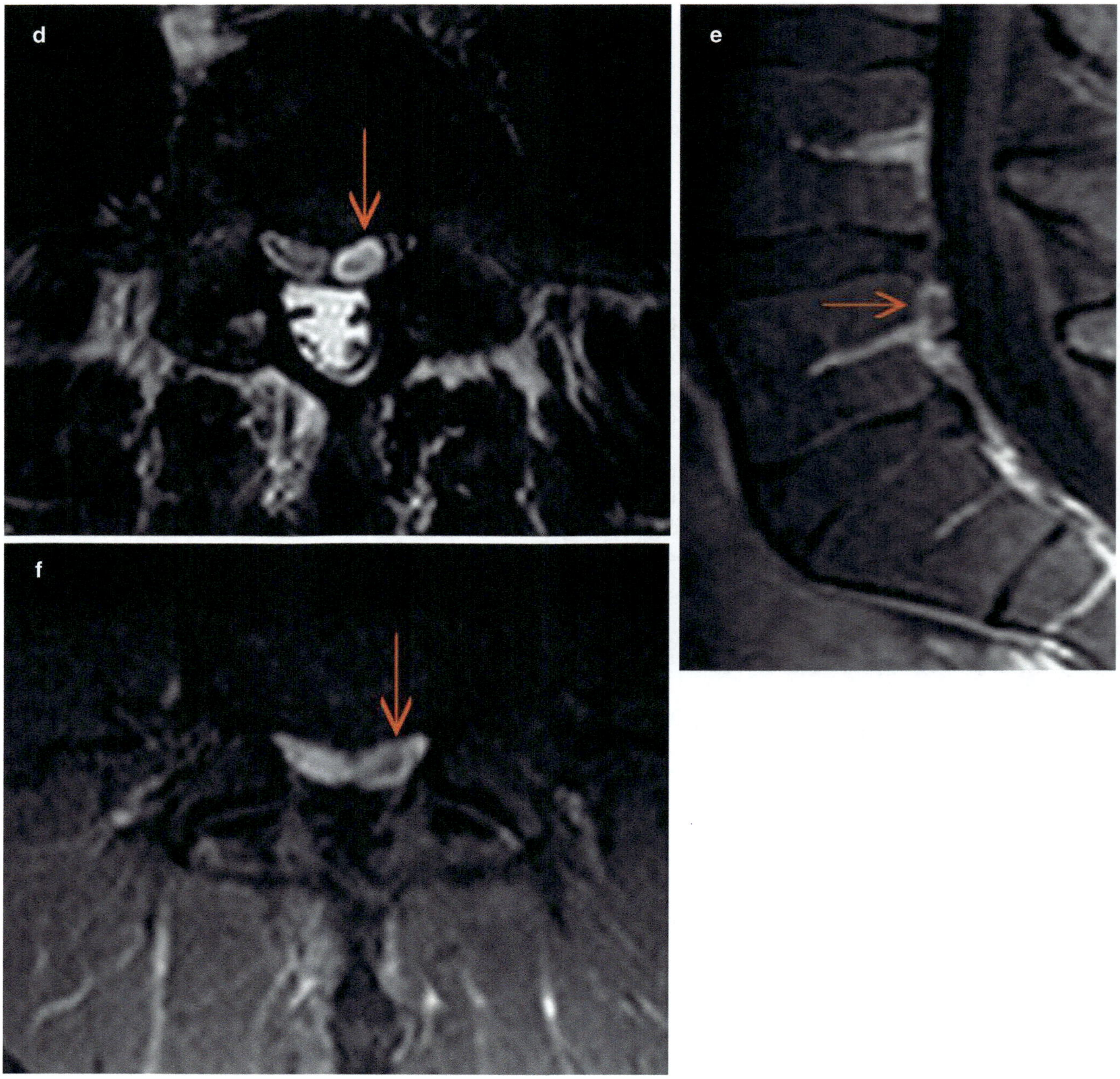

Fig. 4 (continued)

Case 65: Unusual Case. Periradicular Cyst

- A 54-year-old woman
- Left sciatica

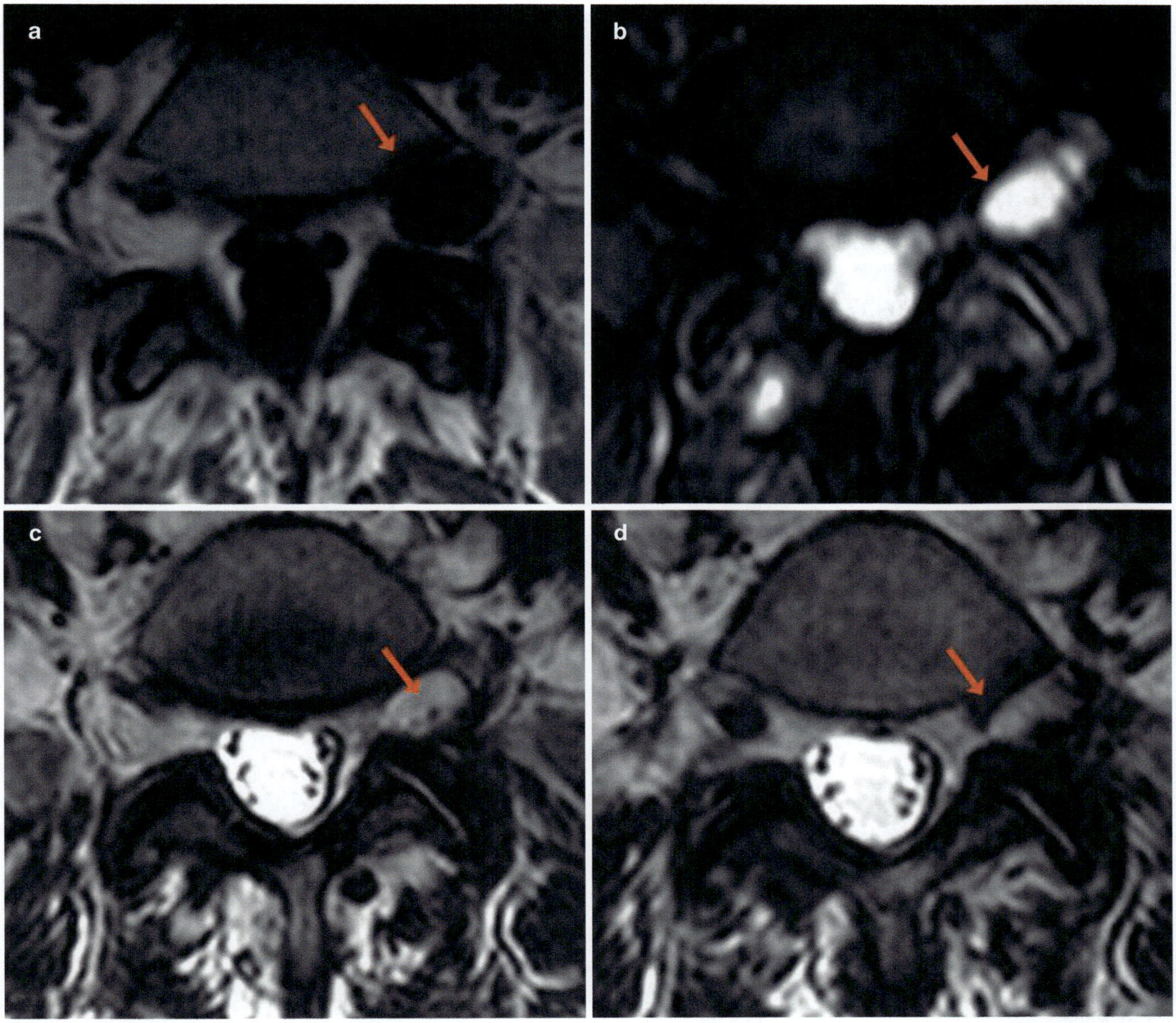

Fig. 5 Axial SE T1-weighted image (**a**), axial TSE T2-weighted image with fat saturation (**b**), axial CISS images (**c**, **d**). Intraforaminal periradicular cyst at L5/S1 on the left side (**a–c**, *arrow*). The cyst compresses and displaces the adjacent nerve root (**d**, *arrow*)

Case 66: Unusual Case. Perigangliar Cyst

- A 44-year-old woman
- Right sciatica

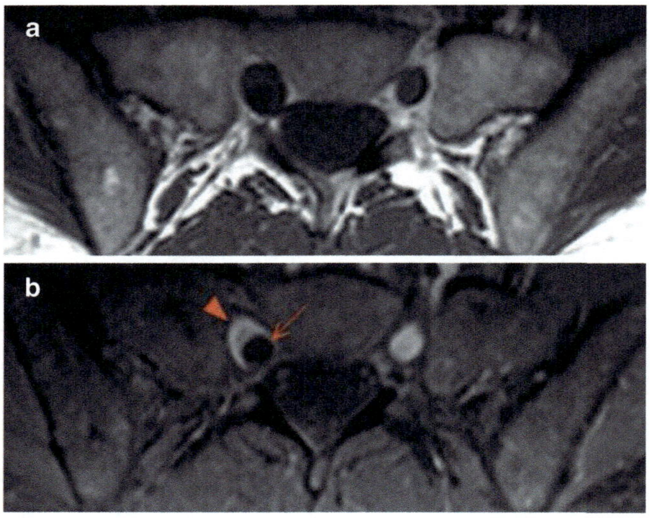

Fig. 6 Axial SE T1-weighted image (**a**), axial SE T1-weighted image with fat saturation after contrast medium administration (**b**). Periradicular perigangliar cyst at S1. The cyst (**b**, *arrow*) compresses and displaces the corresponding ganglion (**b**, *arrowhead*)

Case 67: Unusual Case. Pigmented Villonodular Synovitis

- A 35-year-old man
- 3 weeks history of left-sided low back pain

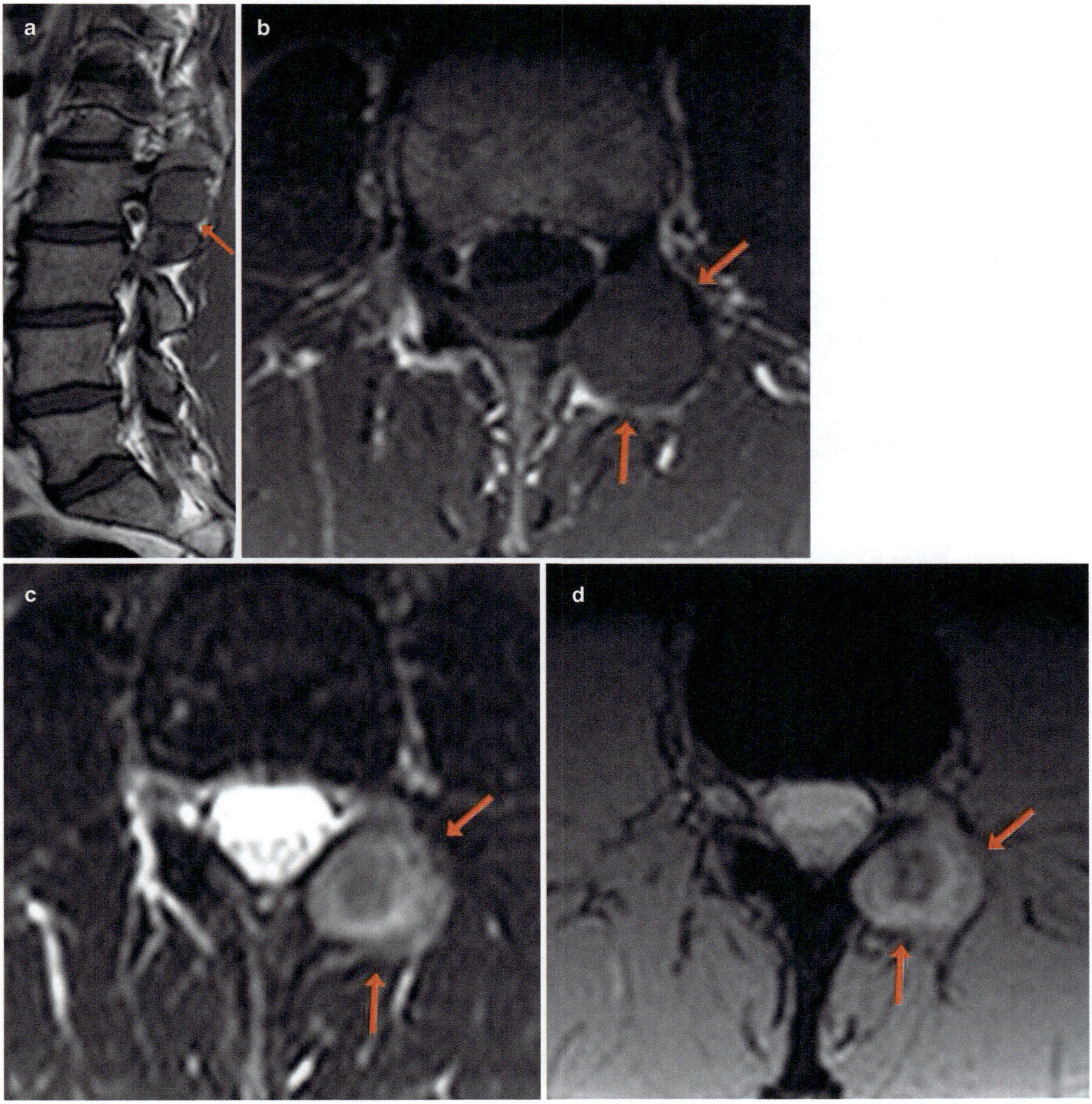

Fig. 7 Sagittal and axial SE T1-weighted image (**a**, **b**), axial TSE T2-weighted image with fat saturation (**c**), axial GE T2*-weighted image (**d**), sagittal and axial SE T1-weighted images with fat saturation following administration of contrast medium (**e**, **f**), axial CT scan (**g**). Extradural mass arising from the left facet joint at L2/L3 (*arrow*). The lesion shows intermediate-low signal intensity in T1 (**a**, **b**) and hyperintensity in T2 (**c**, **d**), with marked contrast enhancement (**e**, **f**). CT scan shows osteolysis of the same facet joint (**g**, *arrows*). The patient underwent a biopsy of the lesion, with histological diagnosis of pigmented villonodular synovitis (PVNS) [1]. PVNS is a locally aggressive proliferative disorder affecting synovium lined joints. The anatomopathological findings of PVNS are constituted by synovial cells lined by villous fronds containing mononuclear cells, multinucleated giant cells, fibroblasts and macrophages

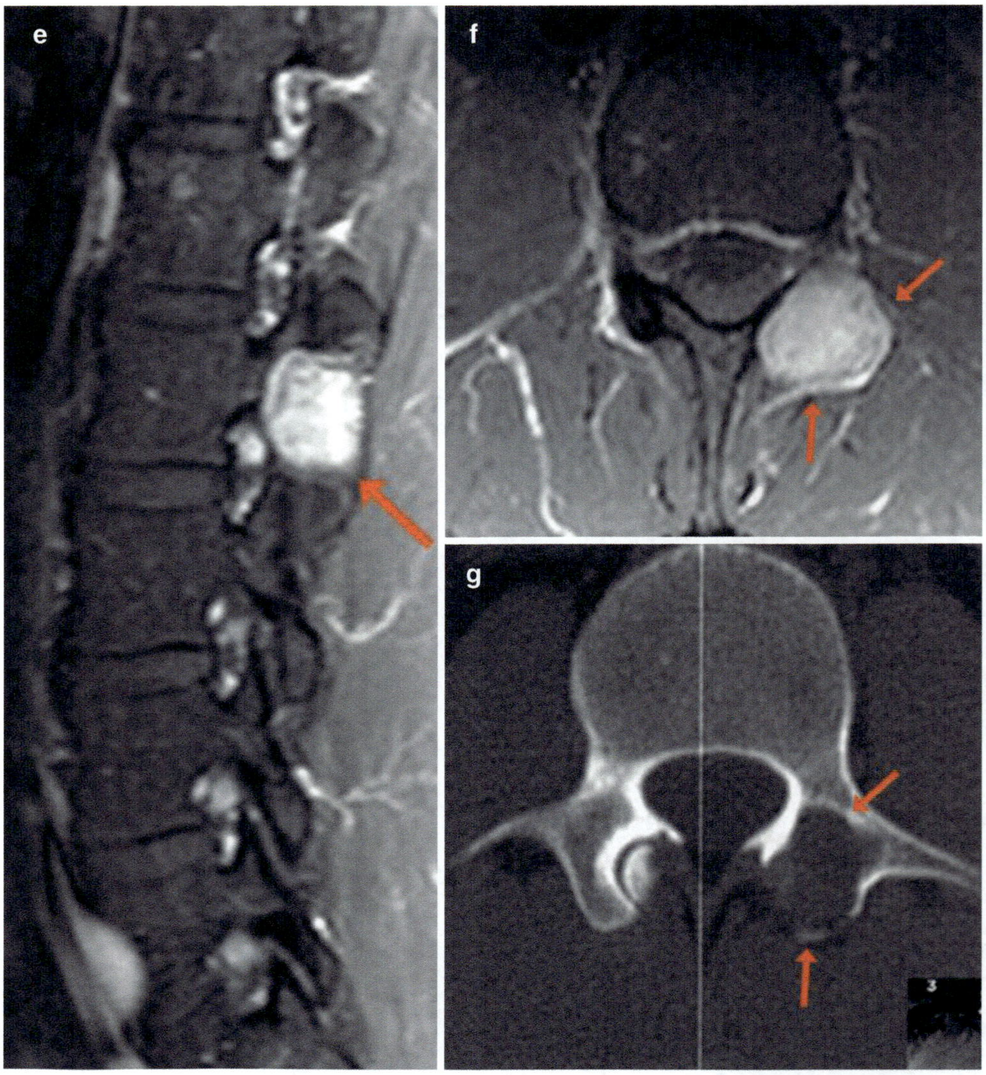

Fig. 7 (continued)

Reference

1. Oreste D, Tarantino A, D'Aprile P (2009) MRI of pigmented villonodular synovitis of the lumbar spine. Euro Rad. (online, case 7520). http://www.eurorad.org/case.php?id=7520

Radiculitis/Neuritis

9

Case 68: Radiculitis

- A 43-year-old woman
- Right low back pain with radiculopathy

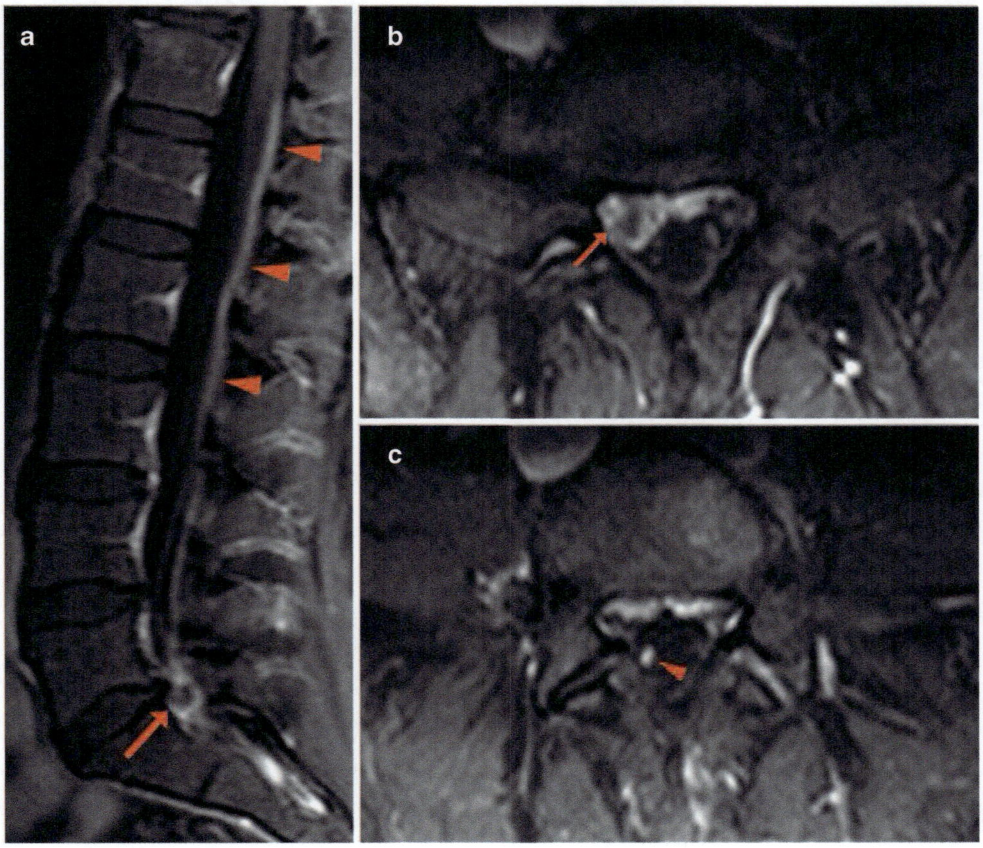

Fig. 1 Sagittal and axial SE T1-weighted images with fat saturation after contrast medium administration (**a–c**). Herniated disc fragment at L5/S1, with reactive peripheral contrast enhancement (**a**, **b**, *arrow*). Diffuse intradural contrast enhancement of the compressed nerve root (**a**, **c**, *arrowhead*), referable to sterile, benign radiculitis. In some cases of lateral recess stenosis, the compressed nerve root enhances after contrast medium administration as a result of a breakdown of the blood–nerve barrier and/or intravascular enhancement of radicular veins

P. D'Aprile, A. Tarantino, *MRI of Degenerative Disease of the Spine*, https://doi.org/10.1007/978-3-030-73707-8_9

Case 69: Radiculitis

- A 65-year-old woman
- Low back pain with radiculopathy

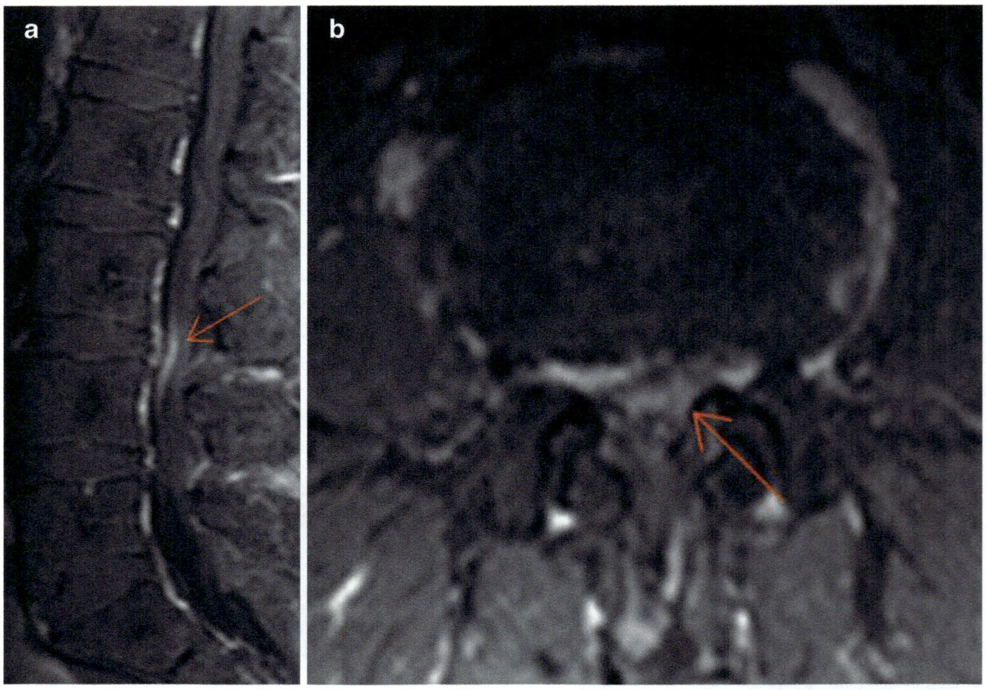

Fig. 2 Sagittal and axial T1-weighted images with fat saturation following administration of contrast medium (**a**, **b**). Contrast enhancement of nerve roots at L3/L4 (**a**, **b**, *arrow*), in correspondence of a canal stenosis. This finding is referable to aseptic radiculitis caused by compression of nerve roots

Case 70: Radiculitis

- A 48-year-old man
- Low back pain with radiculopathy

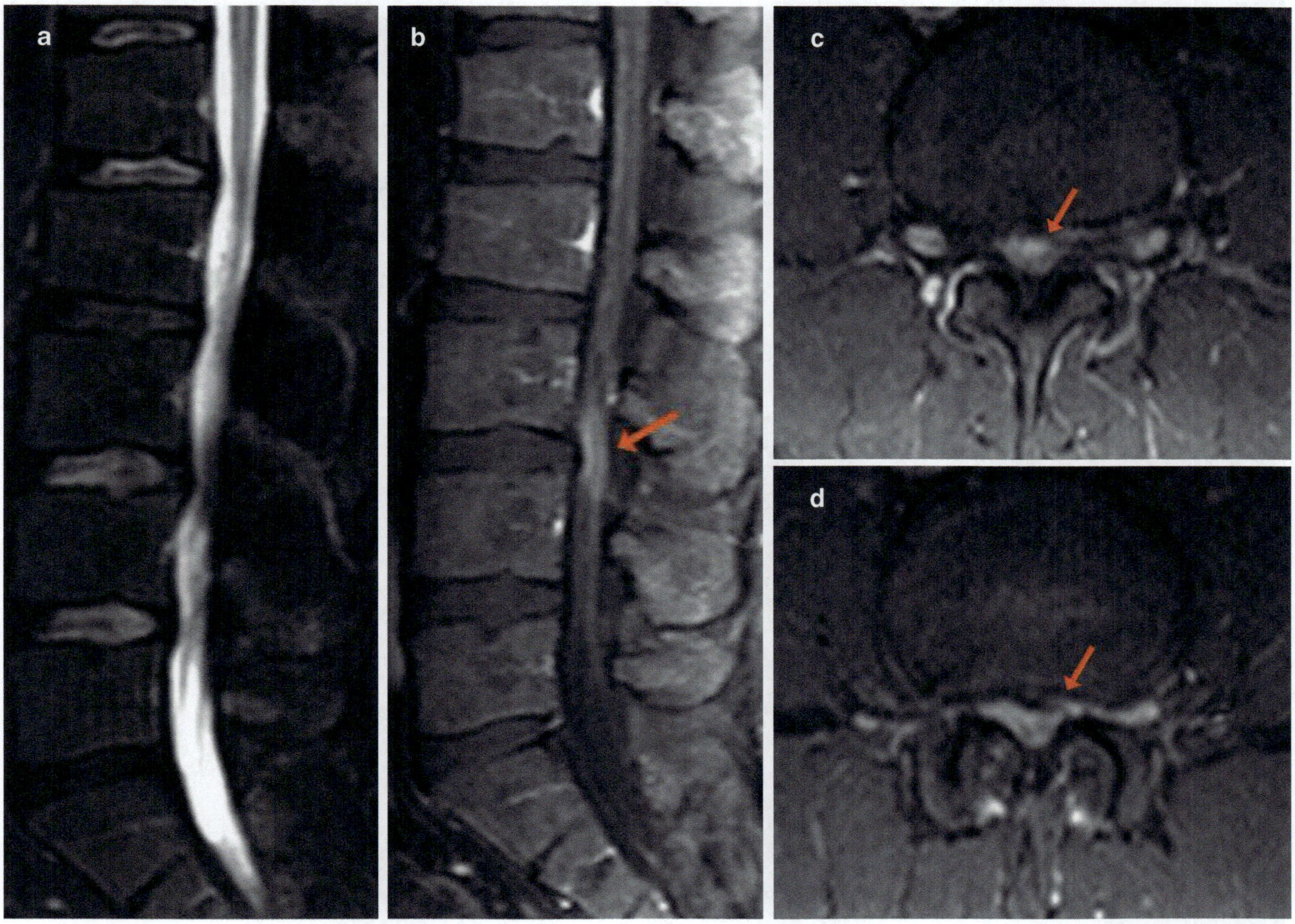

Fig. 3 Sagittal TSE T2-weighted image with fat saturation (**a**), sagittal and axial SE T1-weighted images with fat saturation following administration of contrast medium (**b–d**). Herniated disc and canal stenosis at L3/L4. At the same level, there is contrast enhancement of nerve roots (**b–d**, *arrow*). Diagnosis: radiculitis due to compression of nerve roots

Case 71: Radiculitis

- A 73-year-old woman
- Left low back pain with radiculopathy

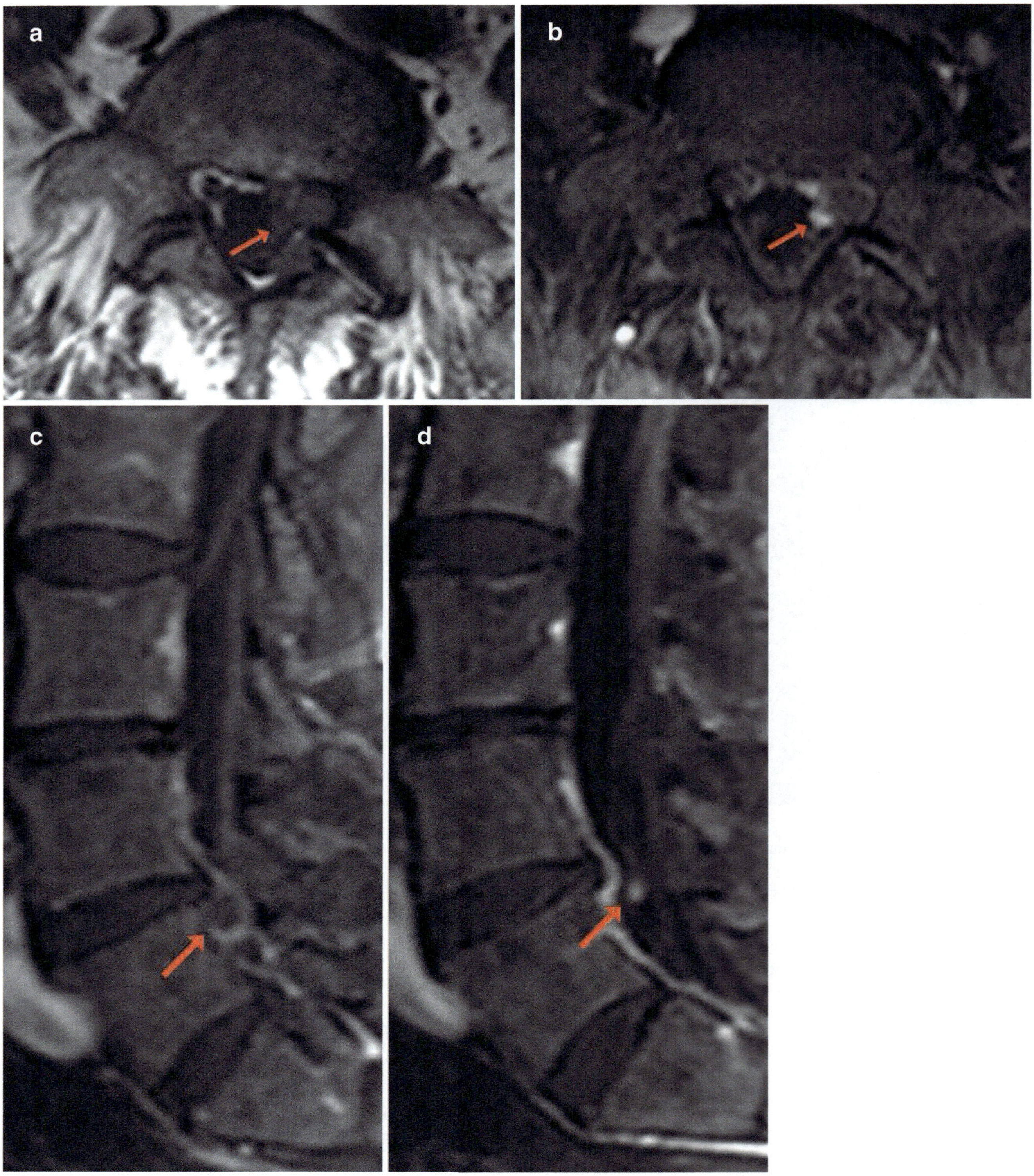

Fig. 4 Axial SE T1-weighted image (**a**), sagittal and axial SE T1-weighted images with fat saturation following contrast medium administration (**b–d**). Herniated disc with inferior migratory fragment behind the L5 vertebral body on the left side (**a**, **c**, *arrows*). It coexists with contrast enhancement of the adjacent intradural nerve root (**b**, **d**, *arrows*), indicating sterile radiculitis

Case 72: Radiculitis

- A 78-year-old man
- Low back pain with bilateral radiculopathy

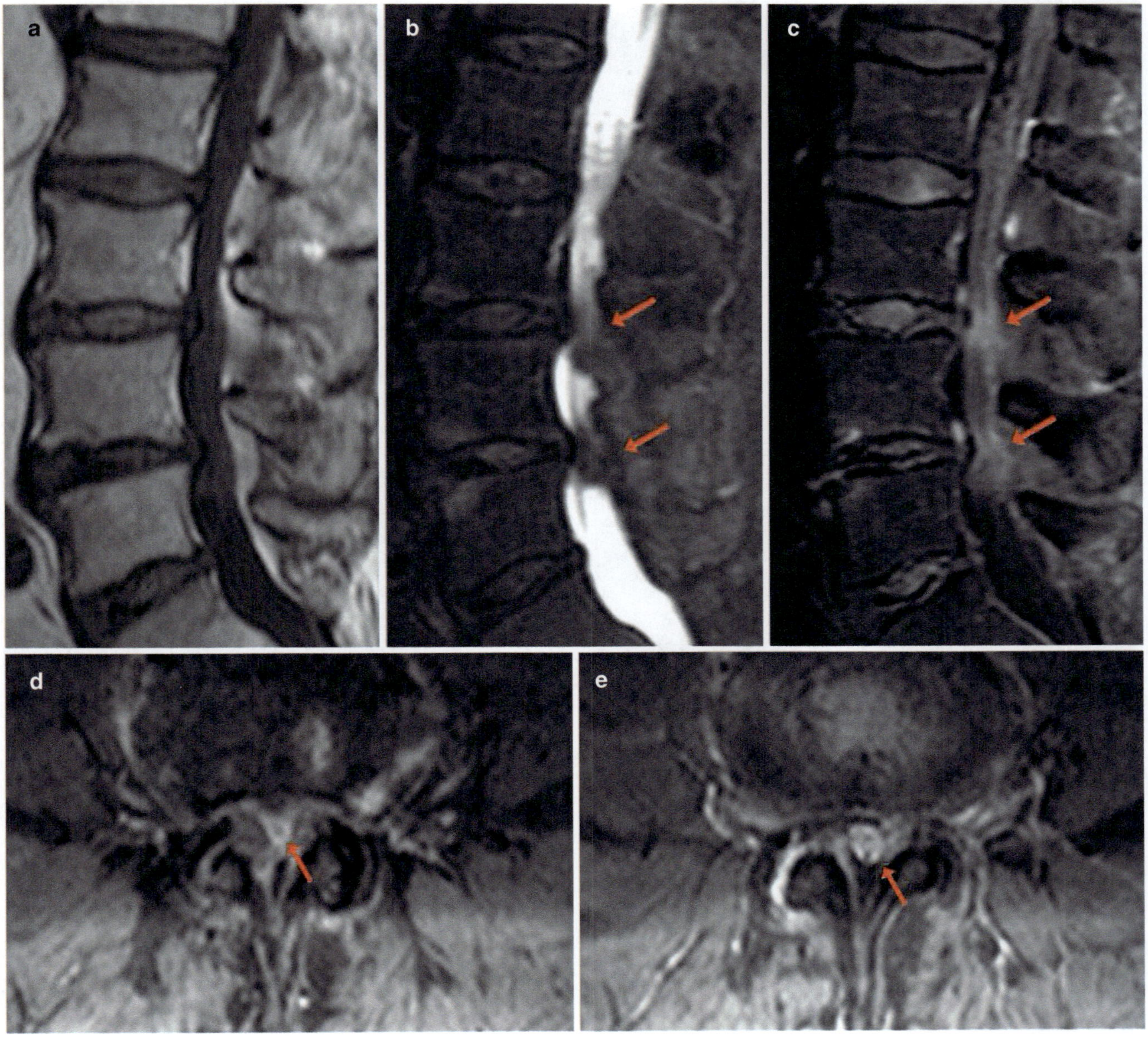

Fig. 5 Sagittal SE T1-weighted image (**a**), sagittal TSE T2-weighted image with fat saturation (**b**), sagittal and axial SE T1-weighted images with fat saturation after administration of contrast medium (**c–e**). Disc herniation/protrusion and canal stenosis at L3/L4 and L4/L5 (**a**, **b**, *arrows*). Contrast enhancement of the nerve roots at the same levels (**c–e**, *arrow*), indicating sterile, benign radiculitis due to radicular compression

Case 73: Neuritis

- A 35-year-old man
- Low back pain on the right side

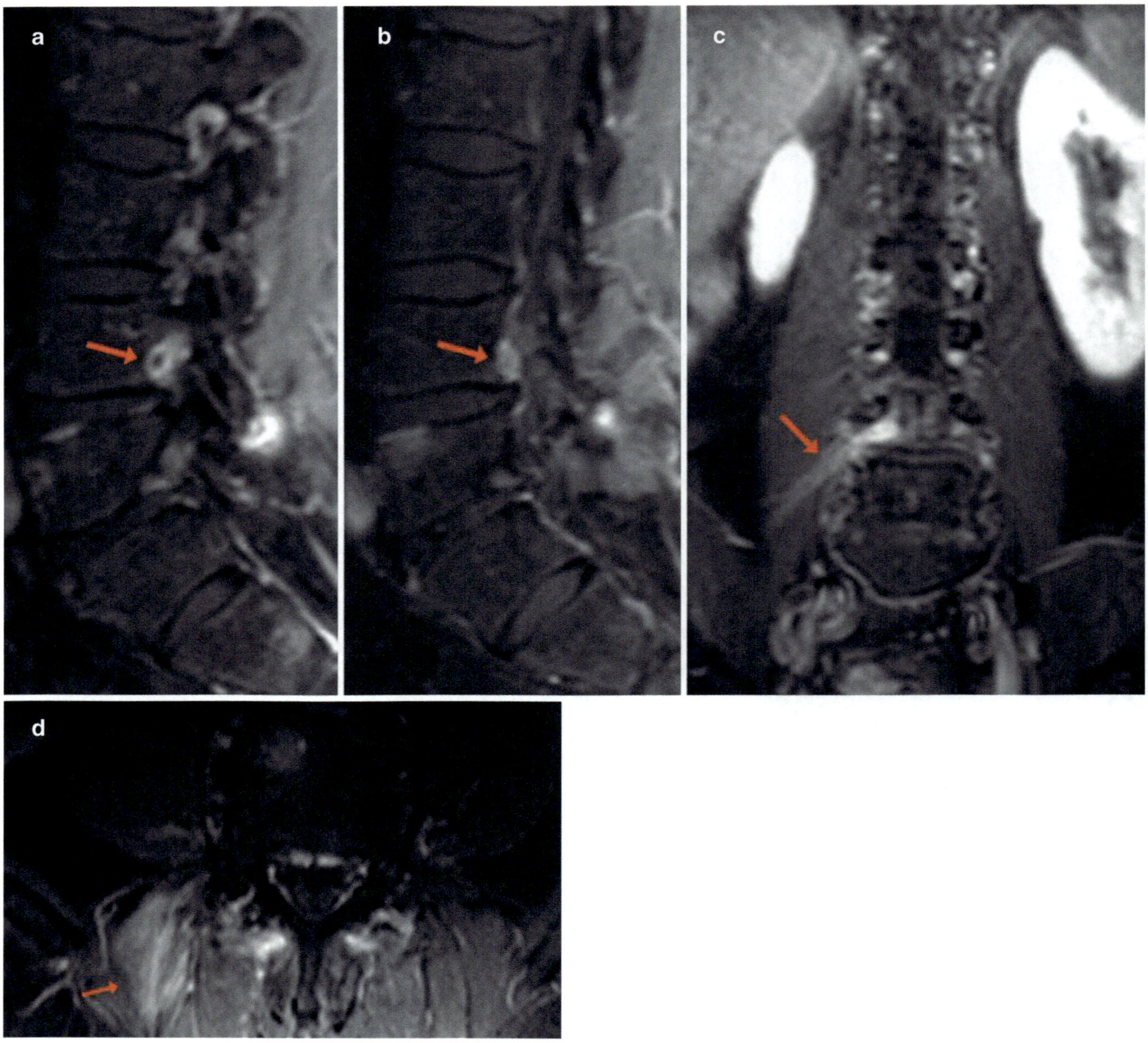

Fig. 6 Sagittal, coronal and axial SE T1-weighted images with fat saturation following administration of contrast medium (**a**–**d**). Herniated disc with superior migratory fragment within the right L4/L5 neural foramen and behind the L4 vertebral body (**a**, **b**, *arrow*). The same disc fragment shows peripheral enhancement after contrast medium administration, due to peridiscal reactive inflammation. It coexists with contrast enhancement of the corresponding nerve passing through the fibers of the psoas muscle (**c**, *arrow*), indicating sterile neuritis. Note also contrast enhancement of the corresponding posterior perispinal muscle, e.g. thoracocostalis muscle (**d**, *arrow*)

10 Postoperative Spine

Case 74: Discectomy. Recurrent Herniated Disc

- A 60-year-old man
- Right persistent low back pain in L5/S1 herniated disc treated by discectomy, laminectomy and removal of facet joint.
- MR early postoperative follow-up.

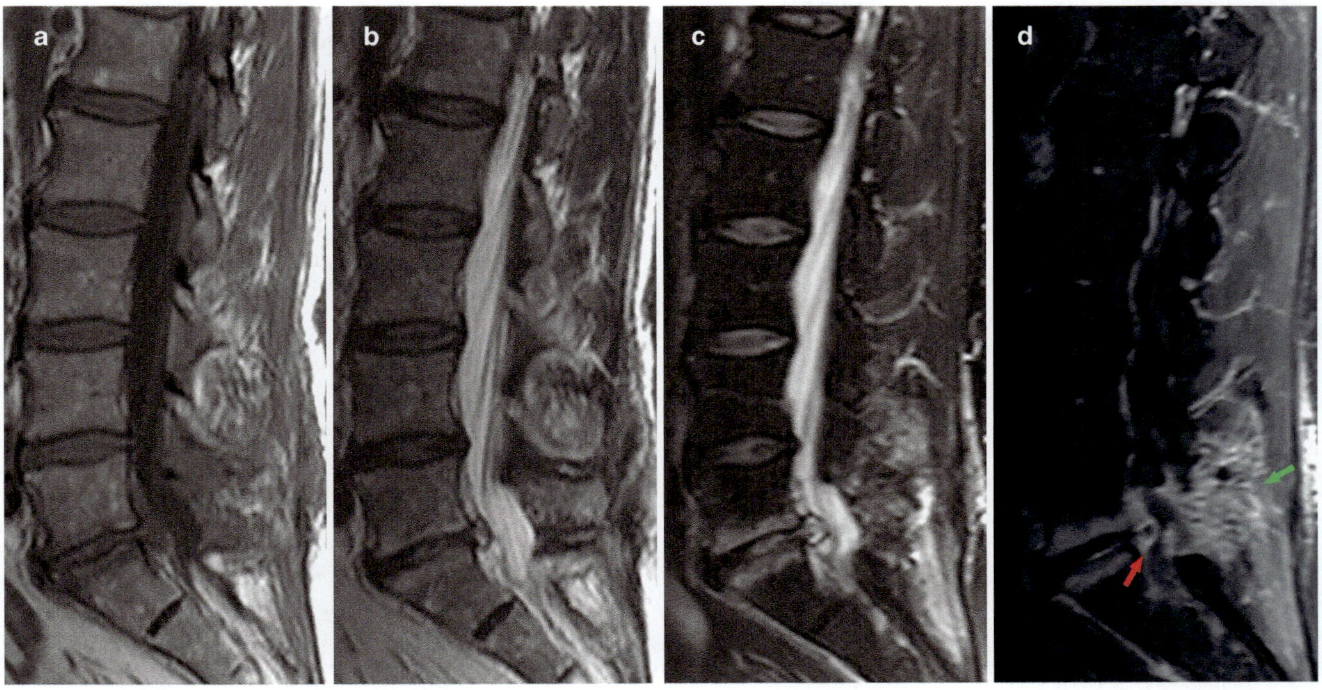

Fig. 1 (**a–g**) Sagittal TSE T1-weighted image (**a**), sagittal TSE T2-weighted image (**b**), sagittal TSE T2-weighted image with fat saturation (**c**), sagittal and axial TSE T1-weighted images with fat saturation following administration of contrast medium (**d–g**). Right L5/S1 recurrent hernia (**a–c**) surrounded by contrast enhanced granulation tissue (**d**, **f**, *red arrow*). Marked contrast enhancement along the surgical breach due to reactive scarring phenomena (**e–g**, *green arrow*). Both nerve roots at lower level are clearly visualized (**g**)

P. D'Aprile, A. Tarantino, *MRI of Degenerative Disease of the Spine*, https://doi.org/10.1007/978-3-030-73707-8_10

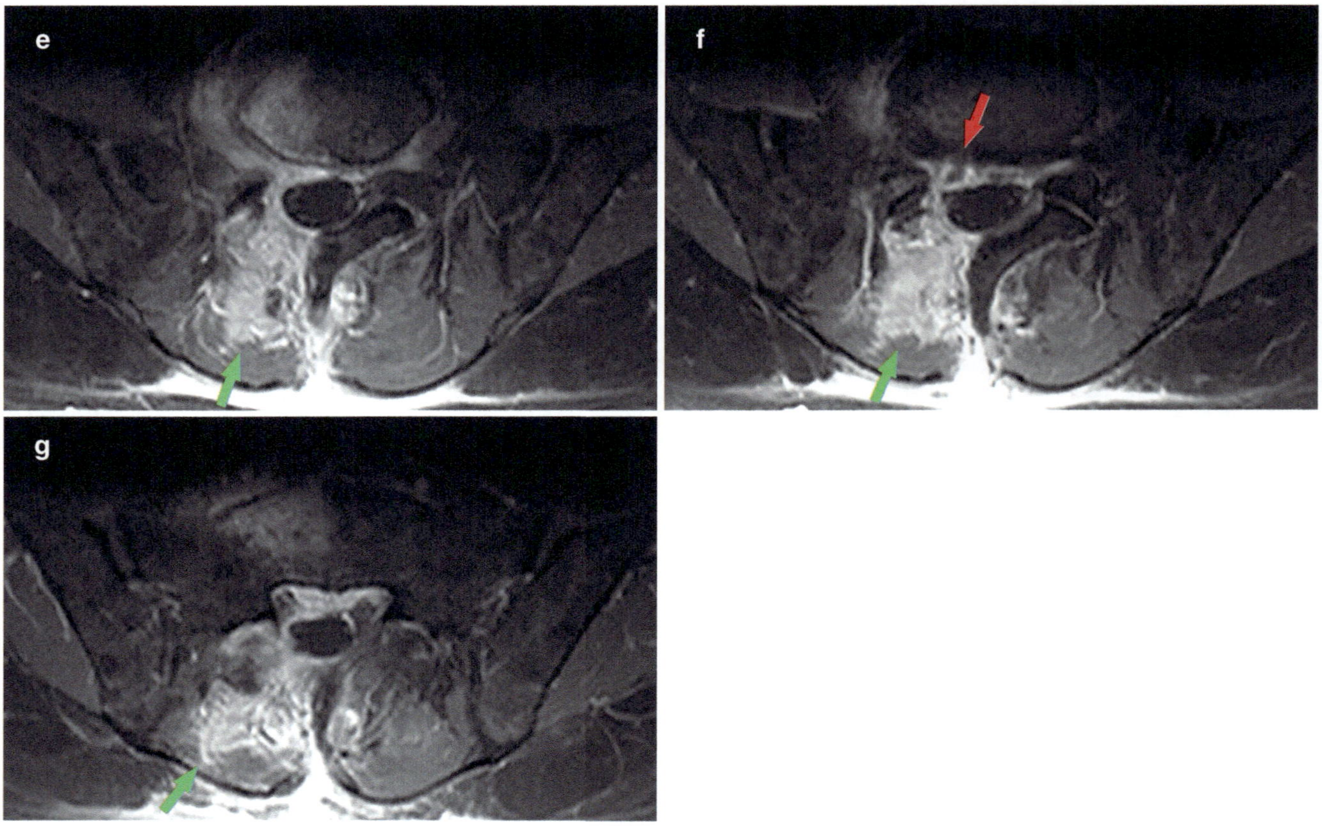

Fig. 1 (continued)

Case 75: Discectomy. Recurrent Herniated Disc. Fibrous Scar

- A 33-year-old man
- Persisting left low back pain in L4/L5 herniated disc treated by discectomy and laminectomy
- MR postoperative follow-up

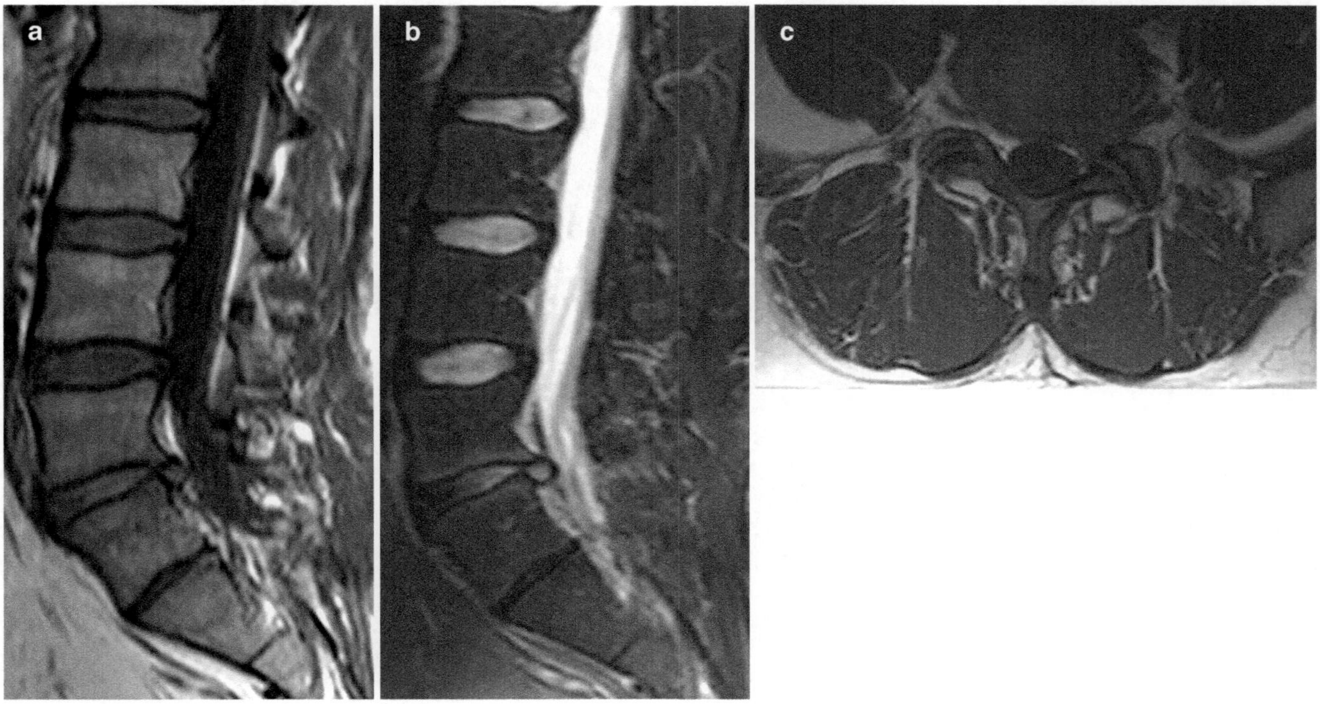

Fig. 2 (**a–g**) Sagittal TSE T1-weighted image (**a**, **c**, **d**), sagittal TSE T2-weighted image with fat saturation (**b**), sagittal and axial TSE T1-weighted images with fat saturation after administration of contrast medium (**e–g**). Small recurrent hernia at L4/L5 (**a–d**), with peripheral contrast enhancement (**e**, **g**, *red arrow*). It coexists contrast enhancement of the fibrous scar in site of laminectomy and left lateral spine recess (**f**, **g**). The axial images before contrast medium administration do not allow to clearly delimit hernia from scar (**c**, **d**), whereas contrast-enhanced imaging allows an accurate diagnosis (**e–g**)

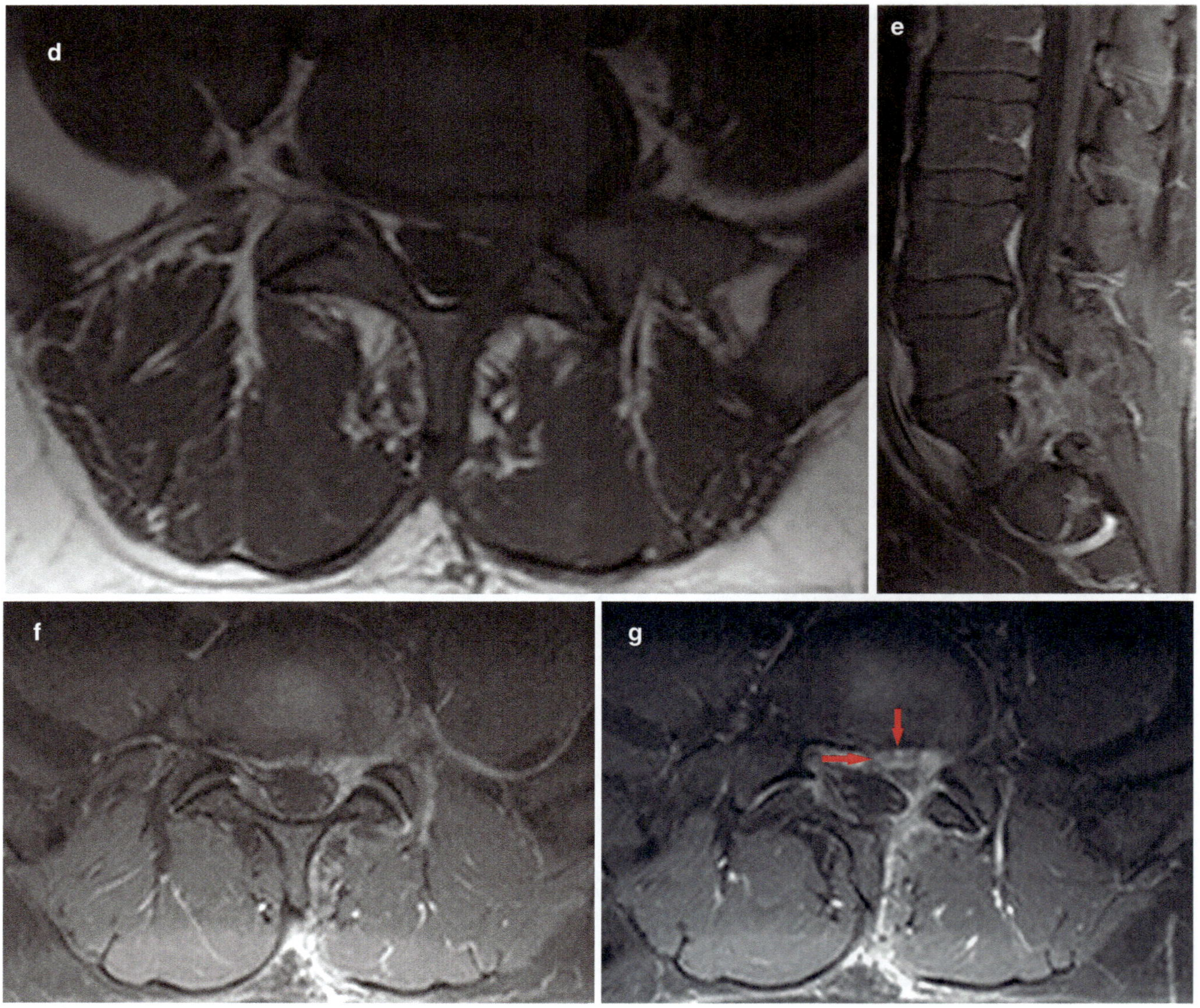

Fig. 2 (continued)

Case 76: Discectomy. Fibrous Scar

- A 38-year-old woman
- Patient with persistent right low back pain in L5/S1 herniated disc treated by discectomy and laminectomy
- Late MR postoperative follow-up

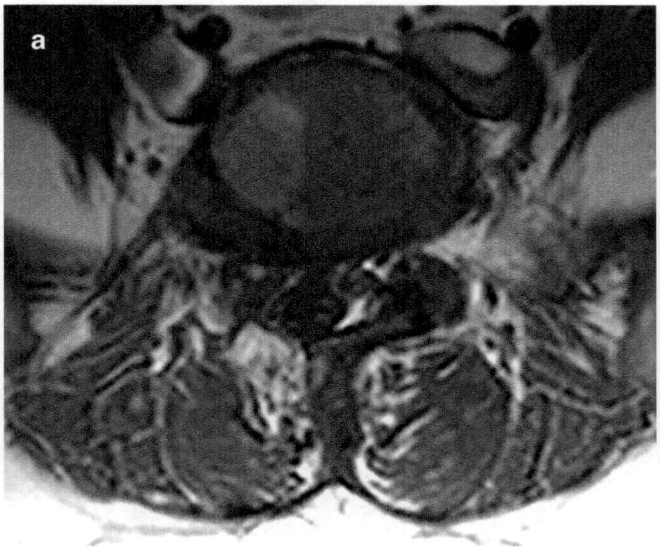

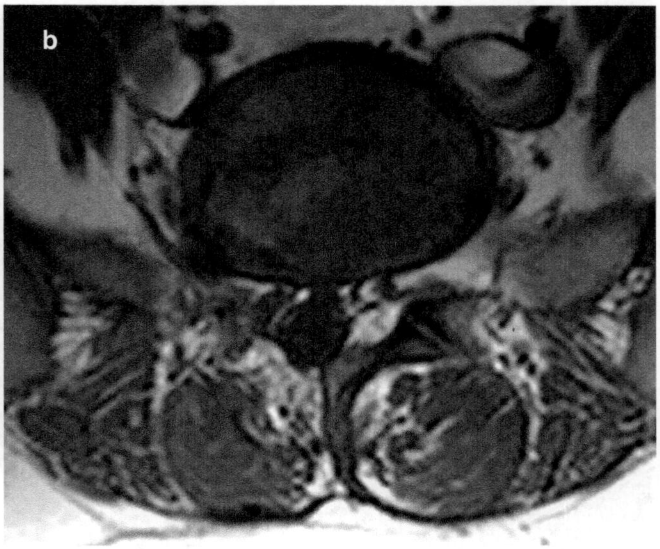

Fig. 3 (**a**–**f**) Axial TSE T1-weighted images (**a**, **b**), axial TSE T1-weighted images with fat saturation after administration of contrast medium (**c**–**f**). Right laminectomy at L5/S1 (**a**, **b**). Right peridural and periradicular contrast enhancement at the same level L5/S1 indicating exuberant postoperative fibrous scar (**c**–**f**)

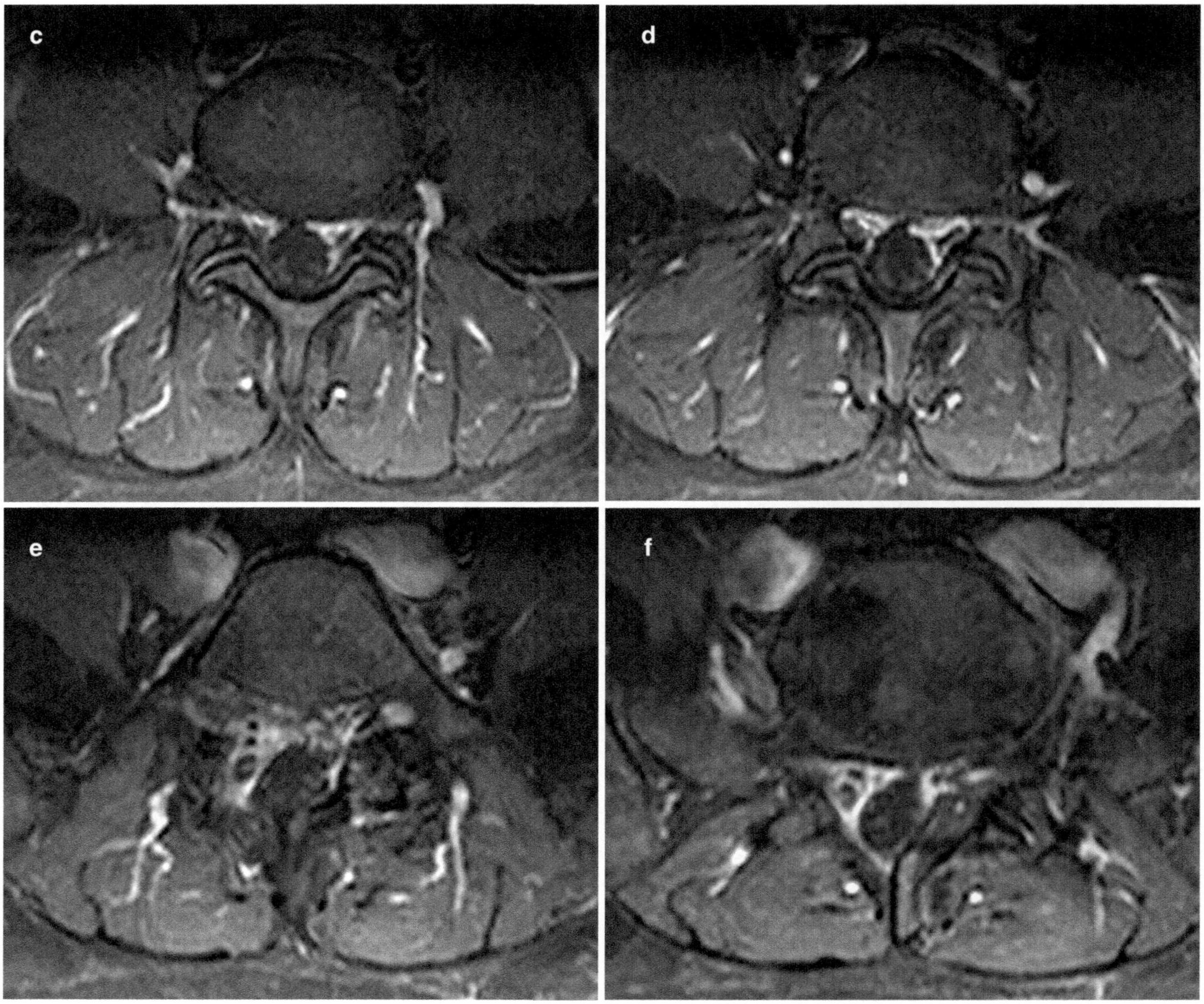

Fig. 3 (continued)

Case 77: Discectomy. Recurrent Herniated Disc. Fibrous Scar. Radiculitis

- A 53-year-old man
- Right persistent low back pain in L5/S1 herniated disc treated by discectomy
- Late MR postoperative follow-up (6 months)

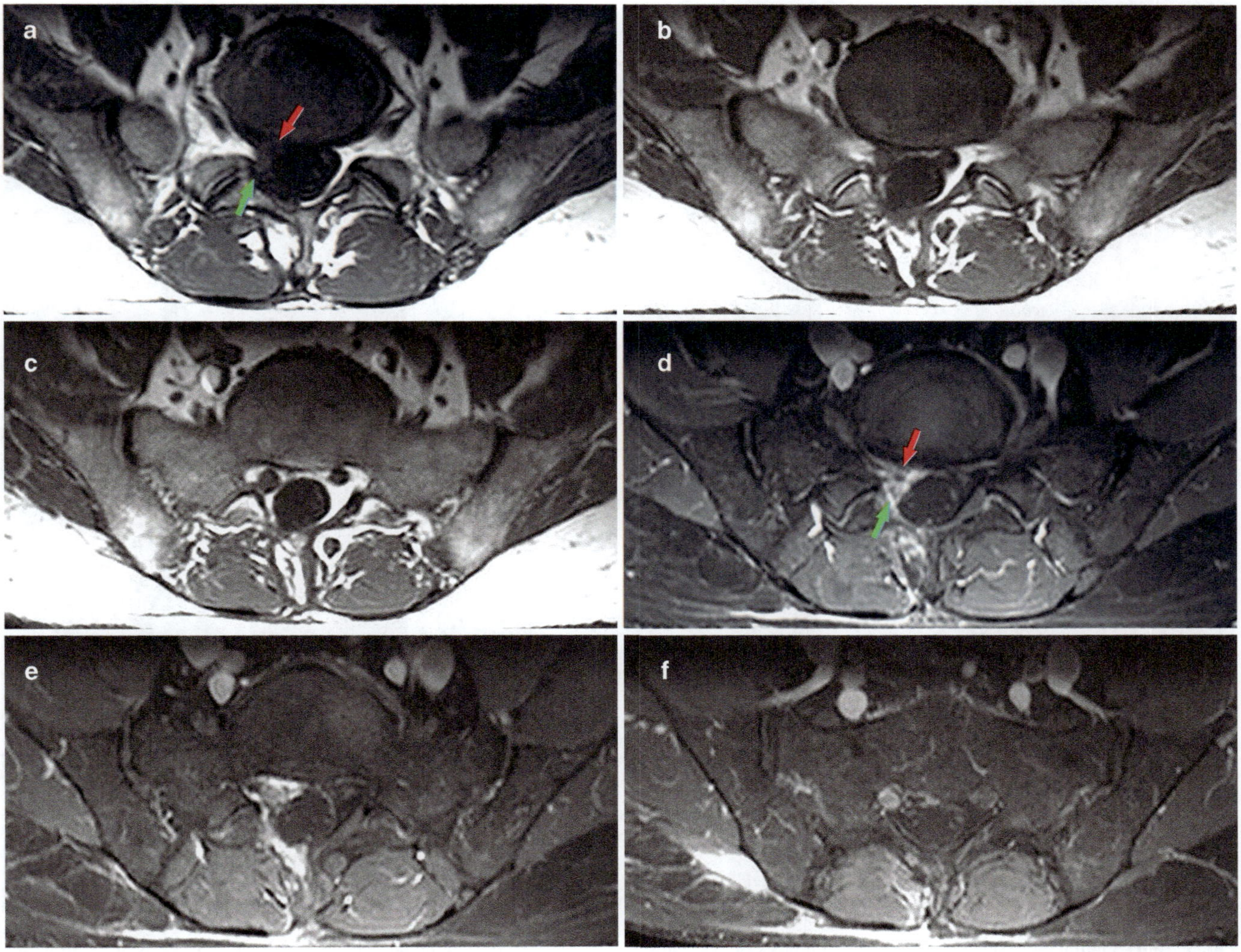

Fig. 4 (**a–f**) Axial TSE T1-weighted images (**a–c**), axial TSE T1-weighted images with fat saturation following administration of contrast medium (**d–f**). Small recurrent hernia (**a**, *red arrow*) that compresses the adjacent nerve root (**a**, *green arrow*). Contrast enhancement surrounding both the recurrent hernia (**d**, *red arrow*) due to granulation tissue, and the nerve root (**d**, *green arrow*) due to fibrous scar (**d**, **e**). Contrast enhancement of the right nerve root sheath, indicating radiculitis (**f**)

Case 78: Discectomy, Stabilization. Vertebral Instability. Herniated Disc

- A 70-year-old woman
- Patient surgically treated 4 years earlier for anterolisthesis of L4 over L5 and corresponding spinal canal stenosis, with laminectomy L4/L5, microdiscectomy, insertion of interbody cage and bone graft, posterior stabilization through metallic pedicular screws
- Chronic low back pain and left sciatica for 2 months

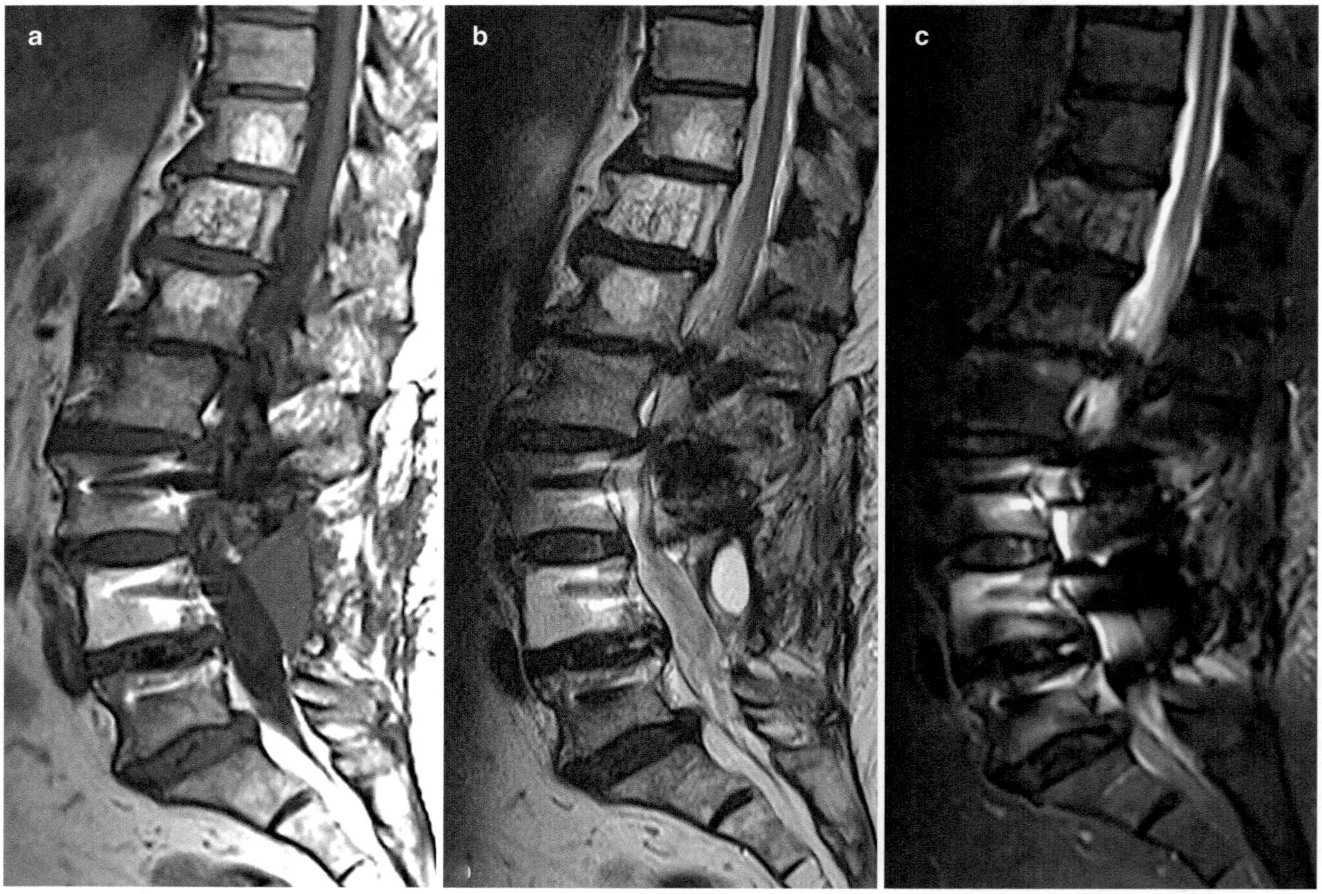

Fig. 5 (**a–f**) Sagittal and axial TSE T1-weighted images (**a**, **d**), sagittal and axial TSE T2-weighted images (**b**, **e**, **f**), sagittal TSE T2-weighted image with fat saturation (**c**). Mild anterolisthesis of L3 over L4 and L4 over L5, site of stabilization (**a–c**). It coexists mild retrolisthesis of L1 over L2 and L2 over L3, with corresponding disc pseudobulges (**a–c**). Fluid collection in the laminectomy side (**a**, **b**, **d**, **e**). New small hernia at lower level (L5/S1) on the left side (**f**). Note artifacts due to metallic devices that reduce image quality. These artifacts are more marked on fat-saturated images (**c**) and less evident on standard TSE T2-weighted images (**b**, **e**)

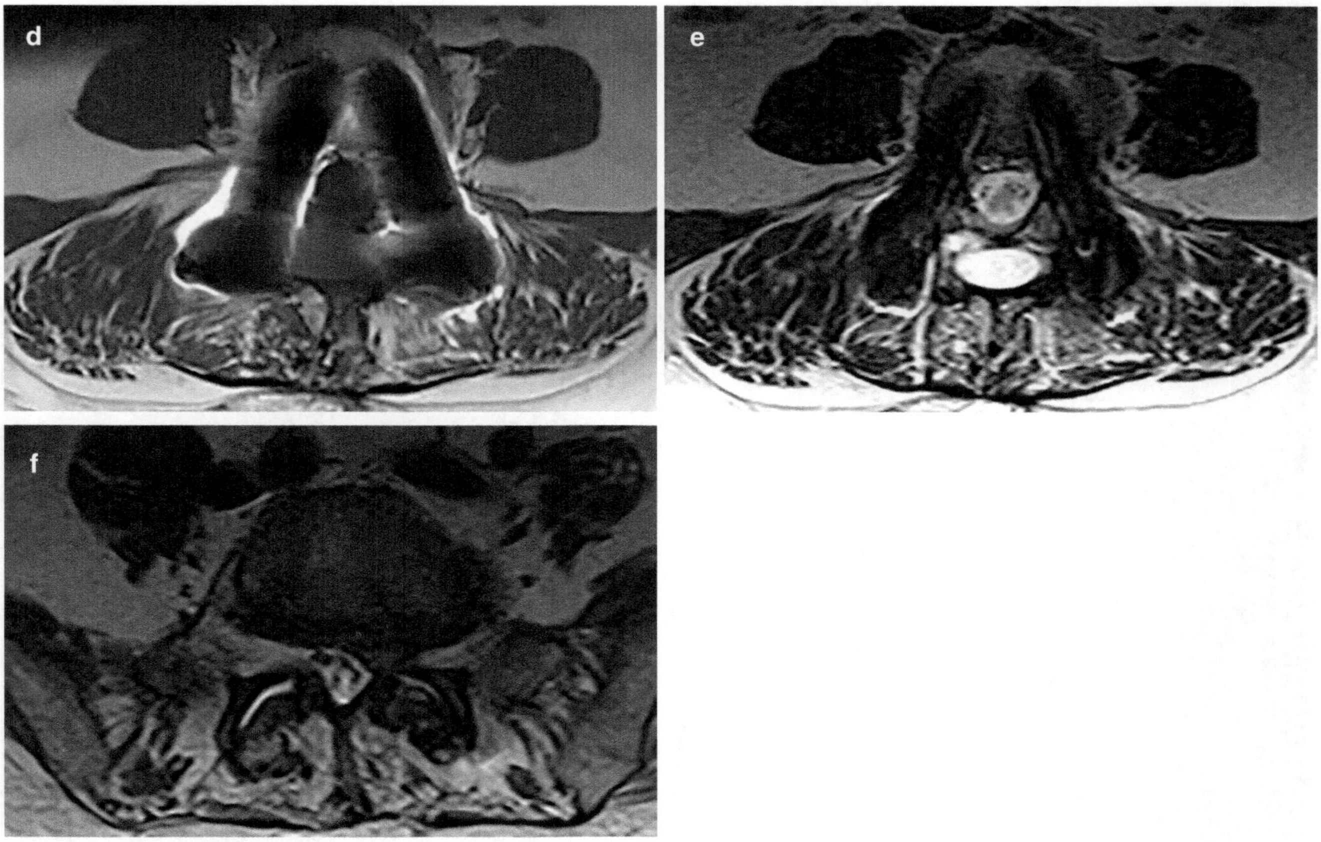

Fig. 5 (continued)

Case 79: Stabilization. Osteochondrosis. Aseptic Discitis

- An 80-year-old man
- Patient previously subjected to vertebral stabilization
- Persistent back pain, more marked on the right side

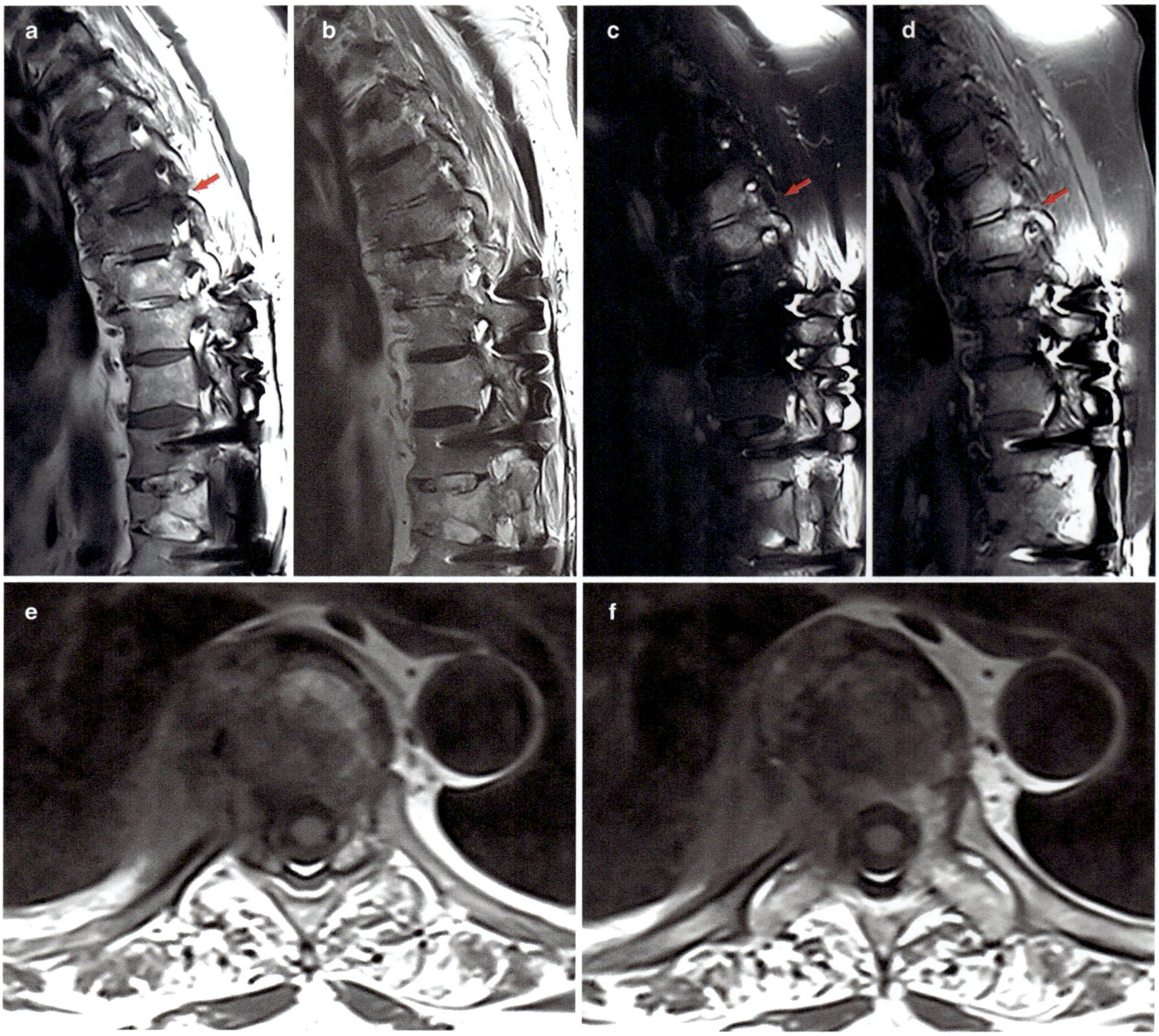

Fig. 6 (**a–p**) Sagittal and axial TSE T1-weighted image (**a**, **e–g**), sagittal TSE T2-weighted image (**b**), sagittal and axial TSE T2-weighted images with fat saturation (**c**, **h–j**), sagittal, axial and coronal TSE T1-weighted images with fat saturation after administration of contrast medium (**d**, **k–p**). Conspicuous artifacts due to metal devices (**a–d**), more marked in fat-saturated imaging (**c**, **d**). Signal changes in the right part of the vertebral bodies D7/D8, hypointense in T1 (**a**, **e–g**), hyperintense in T2 (**b**, **c**, **h–j**), with contrast enhancement (**d**, **k–p**). Note that the oedematous component is best seen by utilizing fat-saturated T2-weighted images (**c**), whereas it is poorly appreciated with standard T2-weighted images (**b**). It coexists contrast enhancement of the disc D7/D8 (**d**, **n–p**) and oedematous changes with contrast enhancement of the rib homolaterally (**h–m**). Note also lateral osteophytosis on the right side and pathologic tissue with contrast enhancement surrounding the same vertebral bodies at D7/D8 (**k–p**). These findings raised the suspicion of infection or, secondly, tumour. The patient underwent biopsy that showed inflammatory tissue. Diagnosis: osteochondrosis in active inflammatory phase, with aseptic discitis and perivertebral inflammatory soft tissue

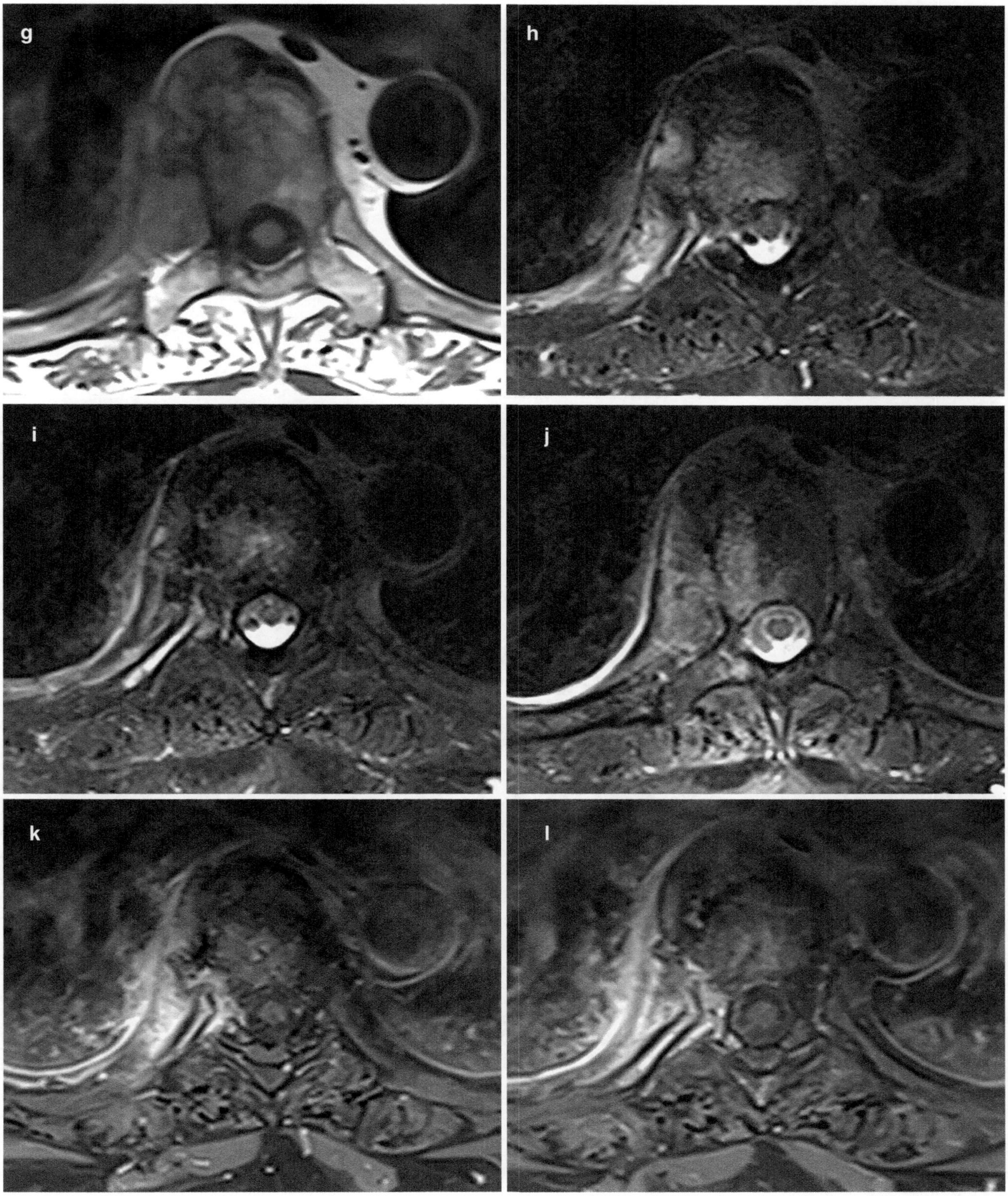

Fig. 6 (continued)

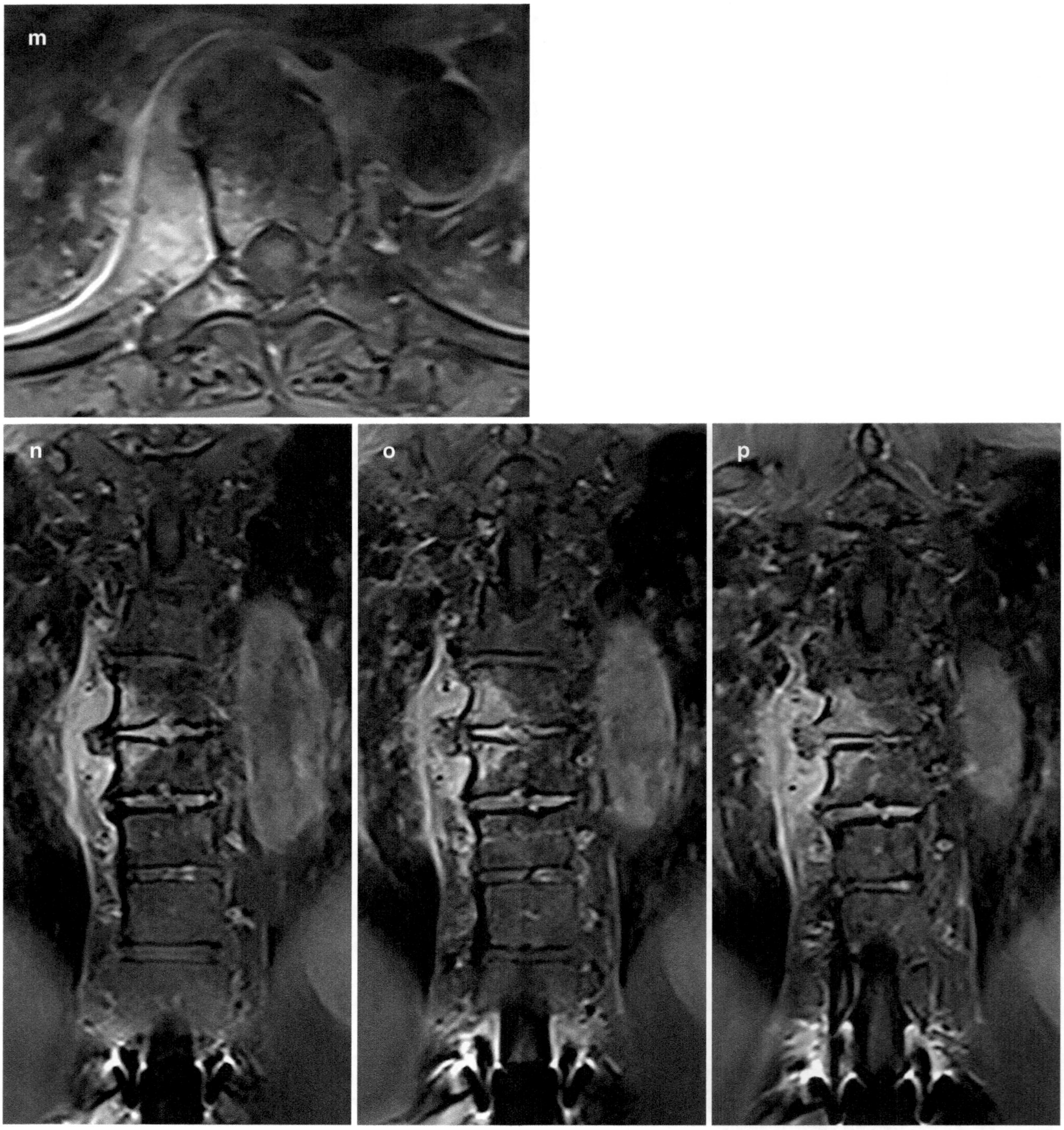

Fig. 6 (continued)

Case 80: Stabilization. Osteochondrosis. Muscular Inflammation

- A 58-year-old woman
- Spinal stabilization
- Chronic back pain and low back pain
- Worsening of symptoms in prolonged upright position
- Improvement of symptoms with rest
- MR postoperative follow-up

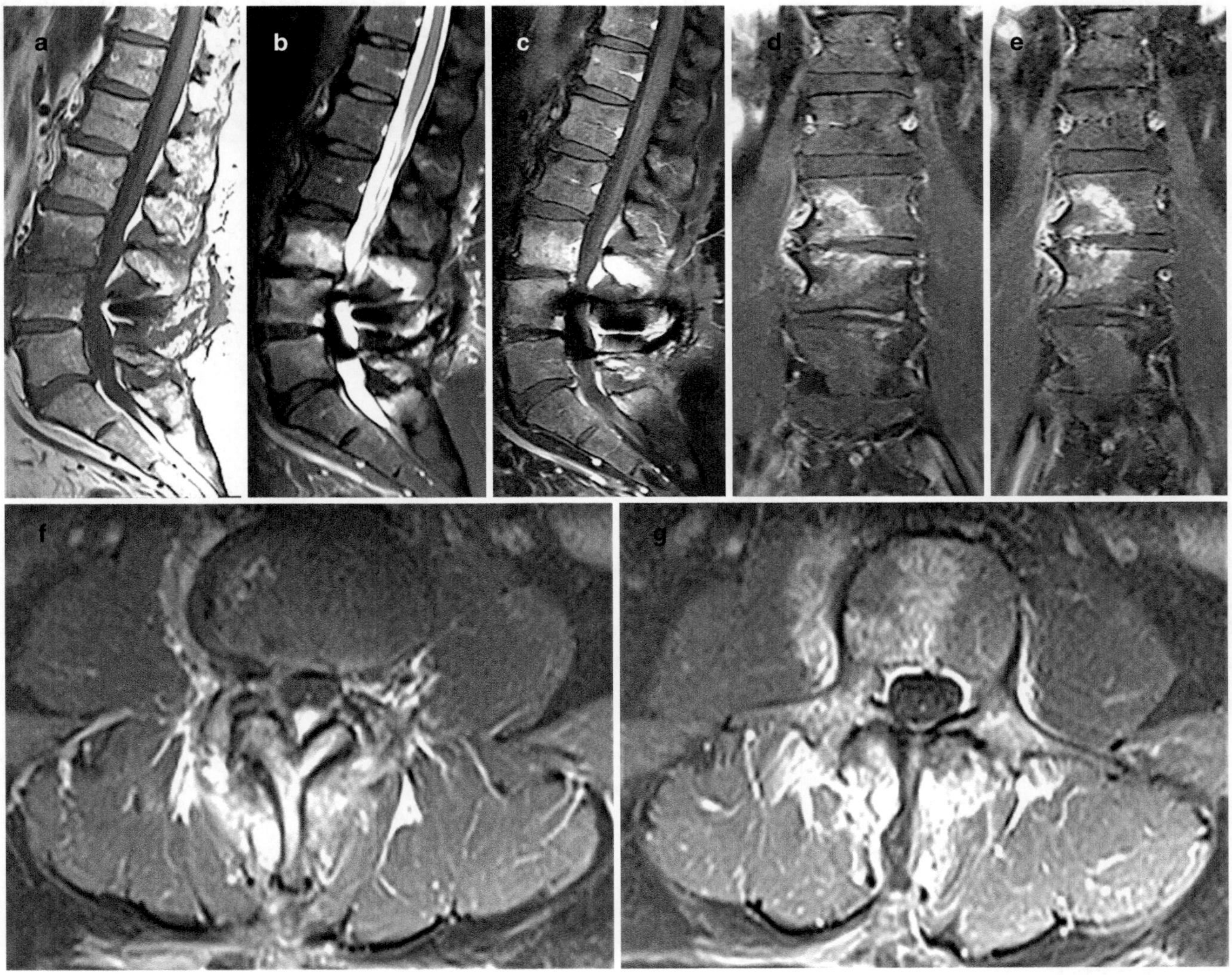

Fig. 7 (**a**–**j**) Sagittal TSE T1-weighted image (**a**), sagittal TSE T2-weighted image with fat saturation (**b**), sagittal, coronal, and axial TSE T1-weighted images with fat saturation after administration of contrast medium (**c**–**j**). Posterior stabilization at L4/L5, with consequent metal artifacts (**a**–**c**). Mild retrolisthesis of L3 over L4 (**a**–**c**). Marked osteochondritis at the same level L3/L4 on the right side (**a**–**e**), in active inflammatory phase, with peridiscal inflammation homolaterally (**d**–**h**). Note also contrast enhancement of the posterior perispinal soft tissues bilaterally (**f**–**h**), indicating periapophyseal inflammation and degeneration-inflammation of the perispinal muscles (e.g. interspinalis and multifidus muscles). The same patient presented mild dorsal hyperkyphosis and marked osteochondritis at D7/D9, in active inflammatory phase (**i**, **j**). Note that the lesions develop at the apex of the kyphosis, in the point of maximum load

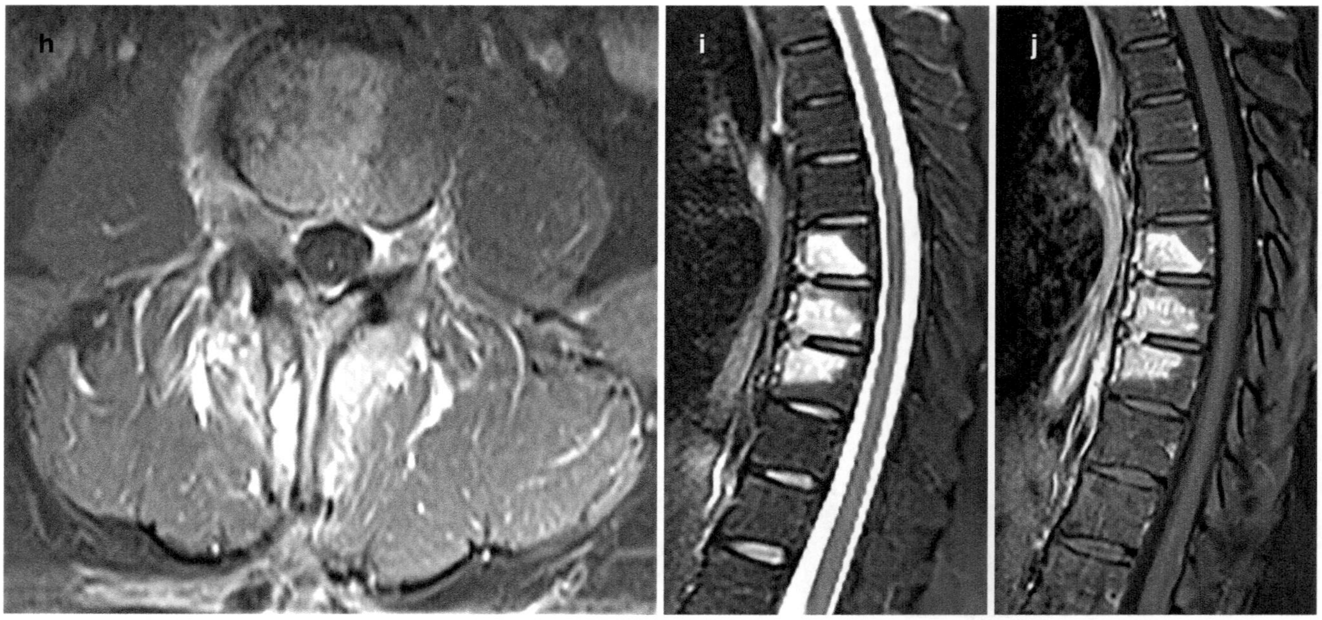

Fig. 7 (continued)

Case 81: Discectomy. Spondylodiscitis

- A 54-year-old man
- Right low back pain and high-level flogosis markers following L4/L5 discectomy
- MR postoperative follow-up with PWI

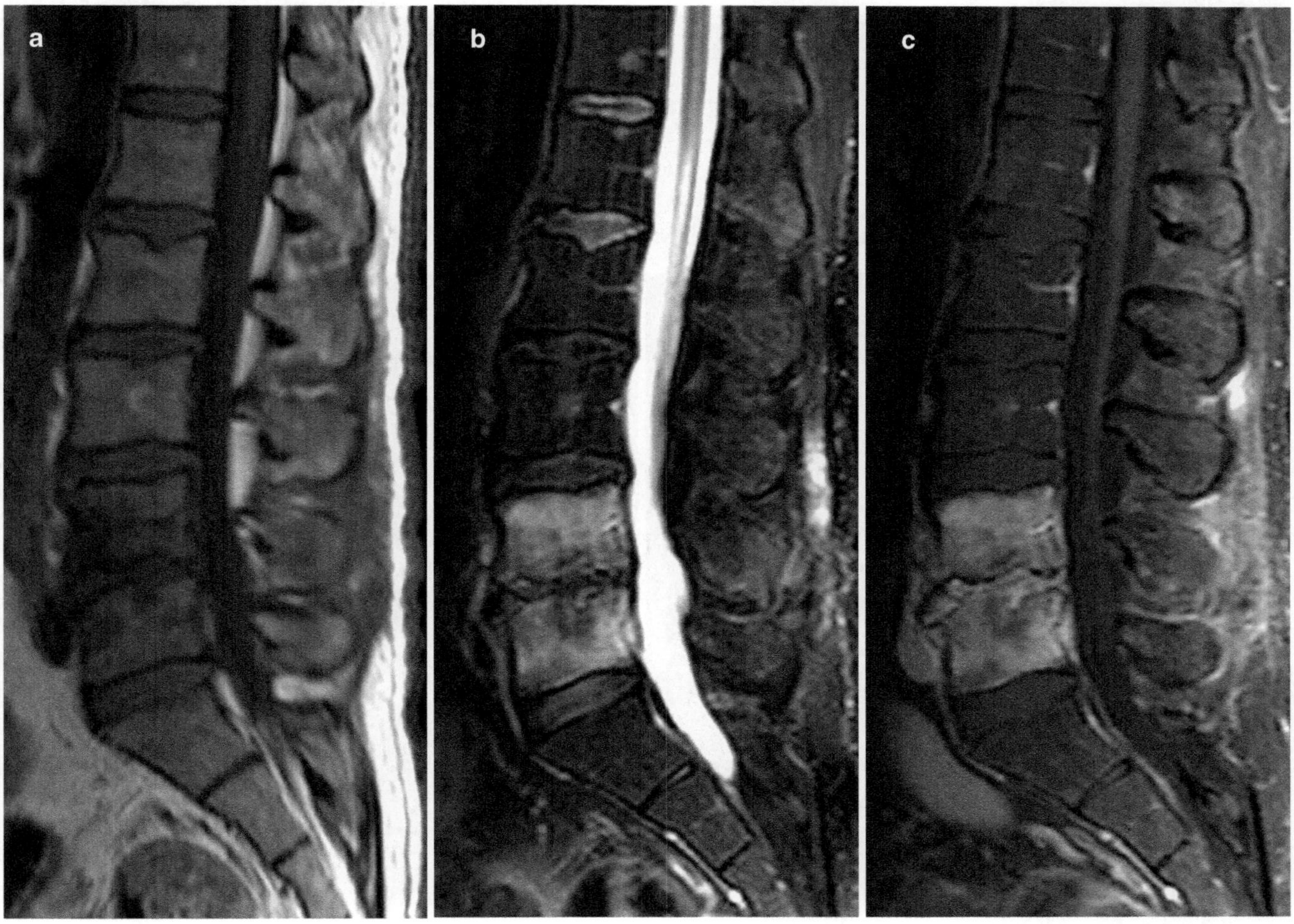

Fig. 8 (**a**–**i**) Sagittal TSE T1-weighted image (**a**), sagittal TSE T2-weighted image with fat saturation (**b**), sagittal and axial TSE T1-weighted images with fat saturation after administration of contrast medium (**c**–**g**), PWI (**h**–**i**). T1-hypointensity (**a**) and T2-hyperintensity (**b**) of the vertebral bodies L4 and L5. Diffuse contrast enhancement of the same vertebral bodies and interposed disc (**c**–**g**). Signs of laminectomy at L4/L5 on the right side (**f**, **g**), with contrast enhancement of the surgical breach and peridural space due to inflammation and scarring phenomena. PWI with diagram intensity/time in ROI inside normal and pathological regions (**h**, **i**). In pathological areas, there is increase of perfusion index. Diagnosis: septic spondylodiscitis

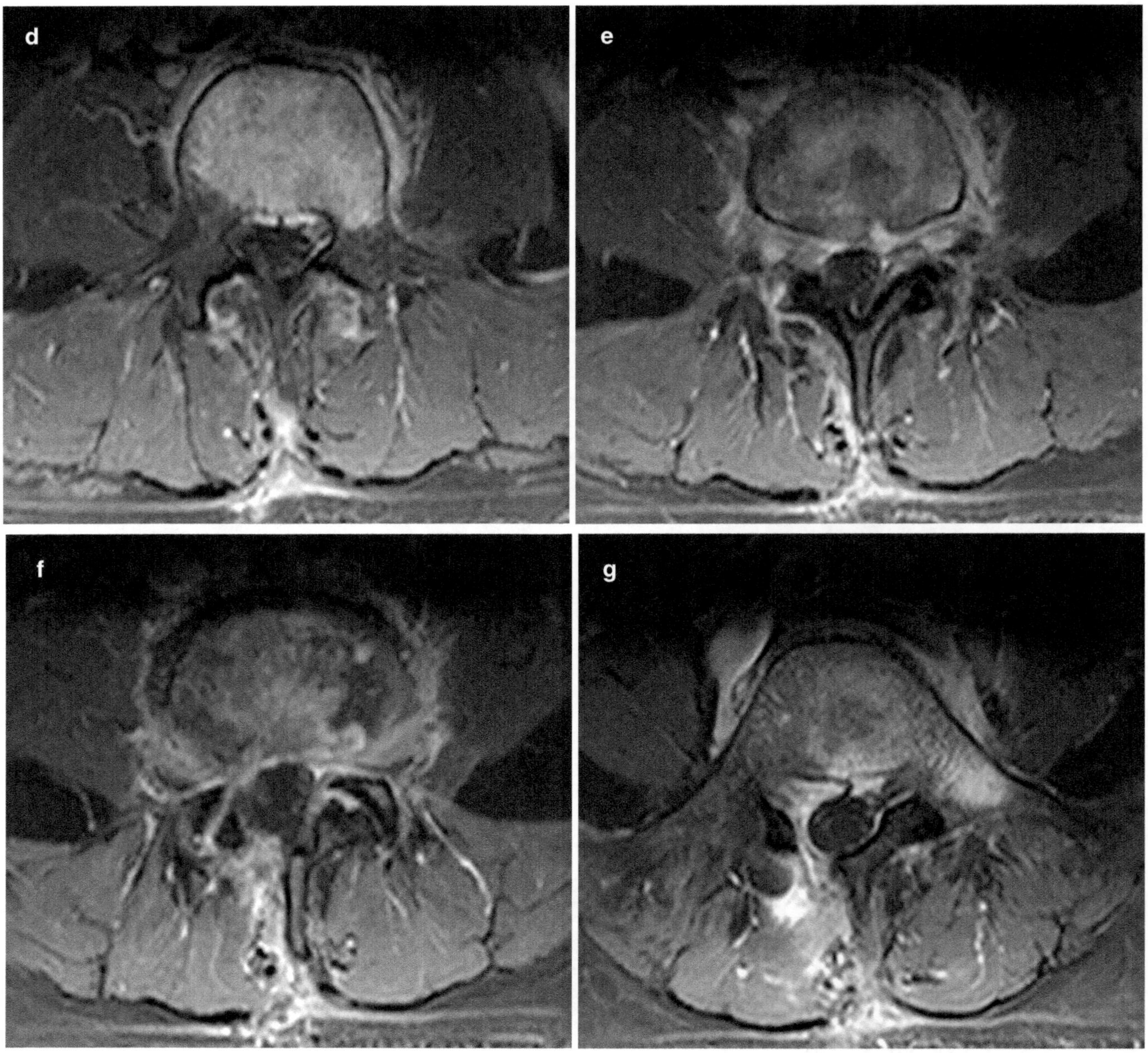

Fig. 8 (continued)

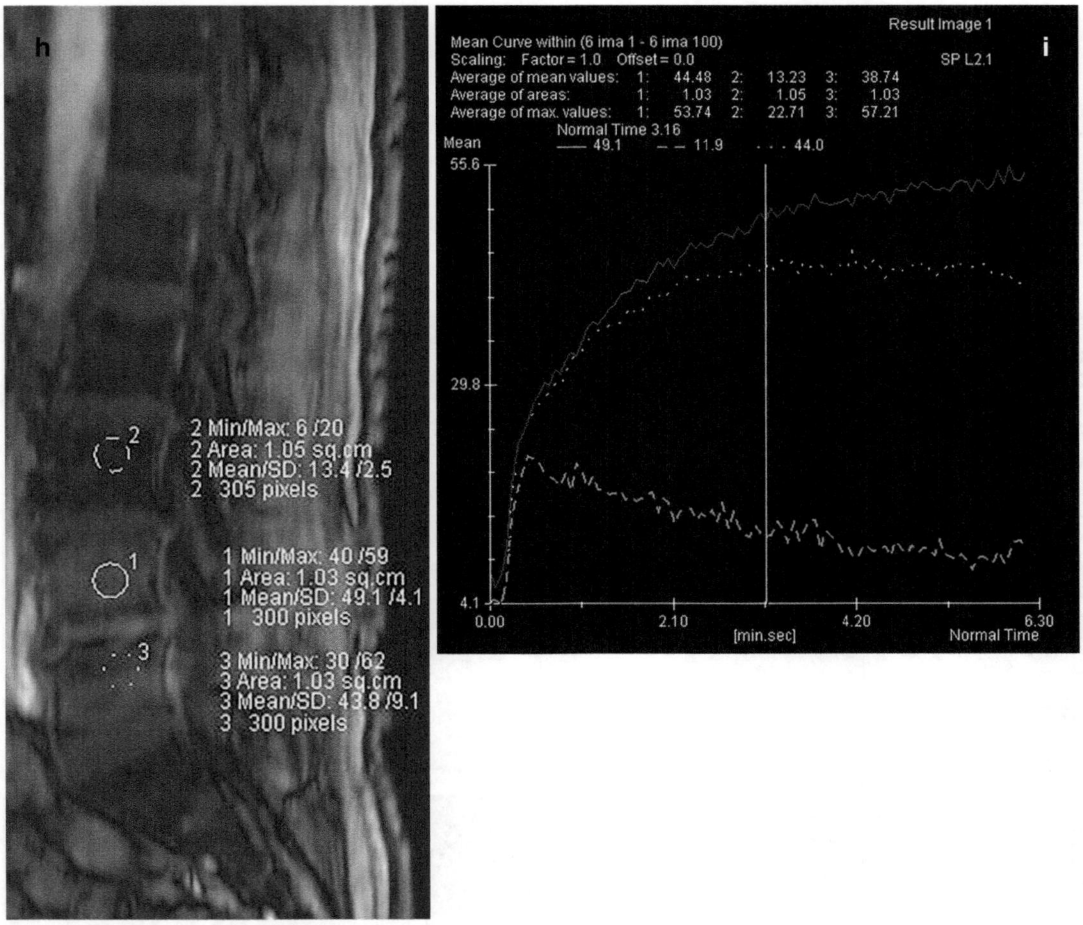

Fig. 8 (continued)

Case 82: Discectomy. Abscess

- A 27-year-old woman
- Left sciatica
- Preoperative MRI

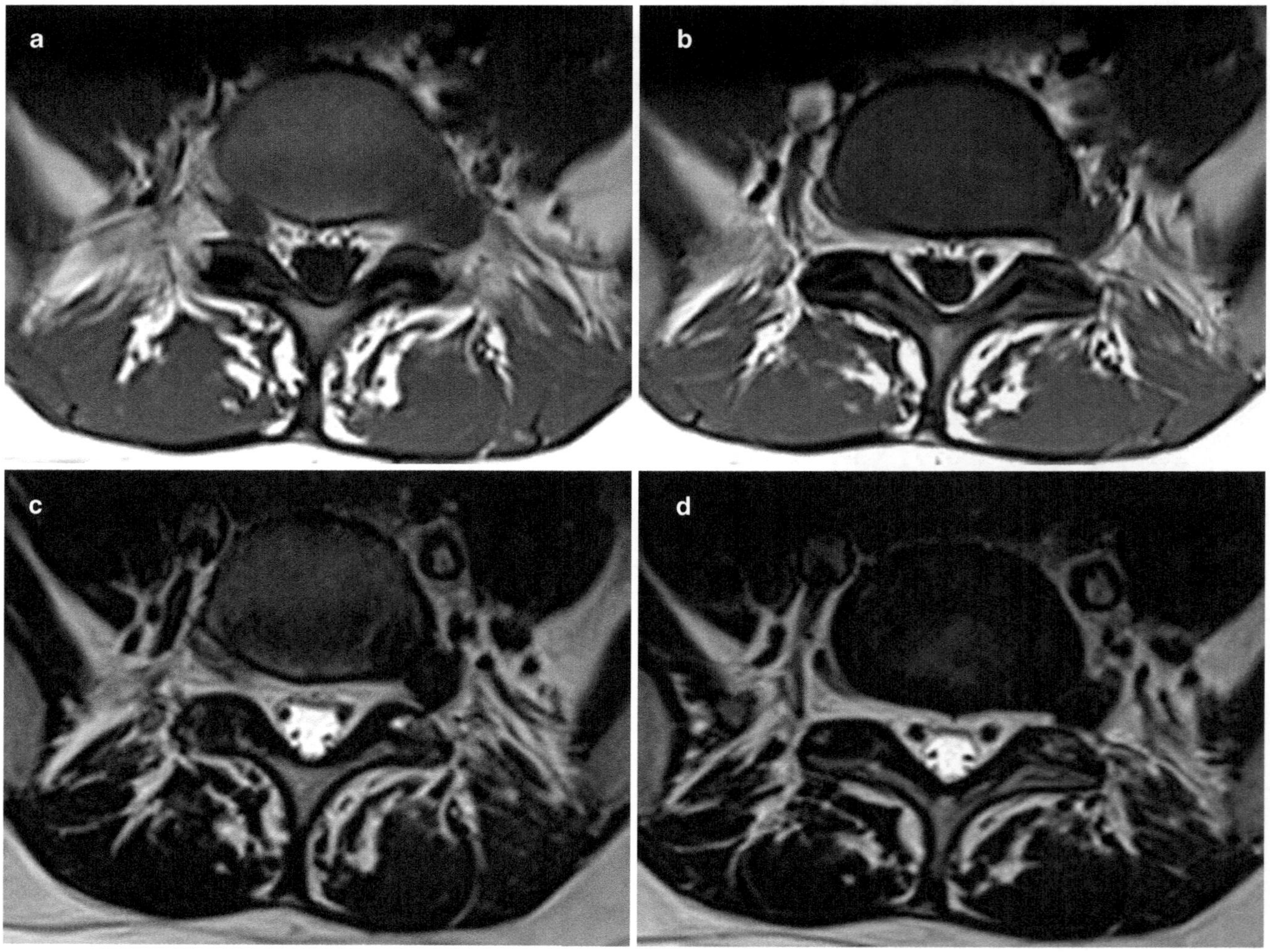

Fig. 9 (**a**–**h**) Axial TSE T1-weighted images (**a**, **b**), axial SPACE images (**c**, **d**), axial TSE T2-weighted images with fat saturation (**e**, **f**), axial TSE T1-weighted images with fat saturation after administration of contrast medium (**g**–**h**). Extraforaminal herniated disc in contact with adjacent nerve root (**a**–**d**). In this case, fat-saturated T2-weighted imaging shows poor spatial definition disc/nerve root (**e**, **f**). Disc material is well delineated after administration of contrast medium, due to peridiscal enhancement (**g**, **h**)

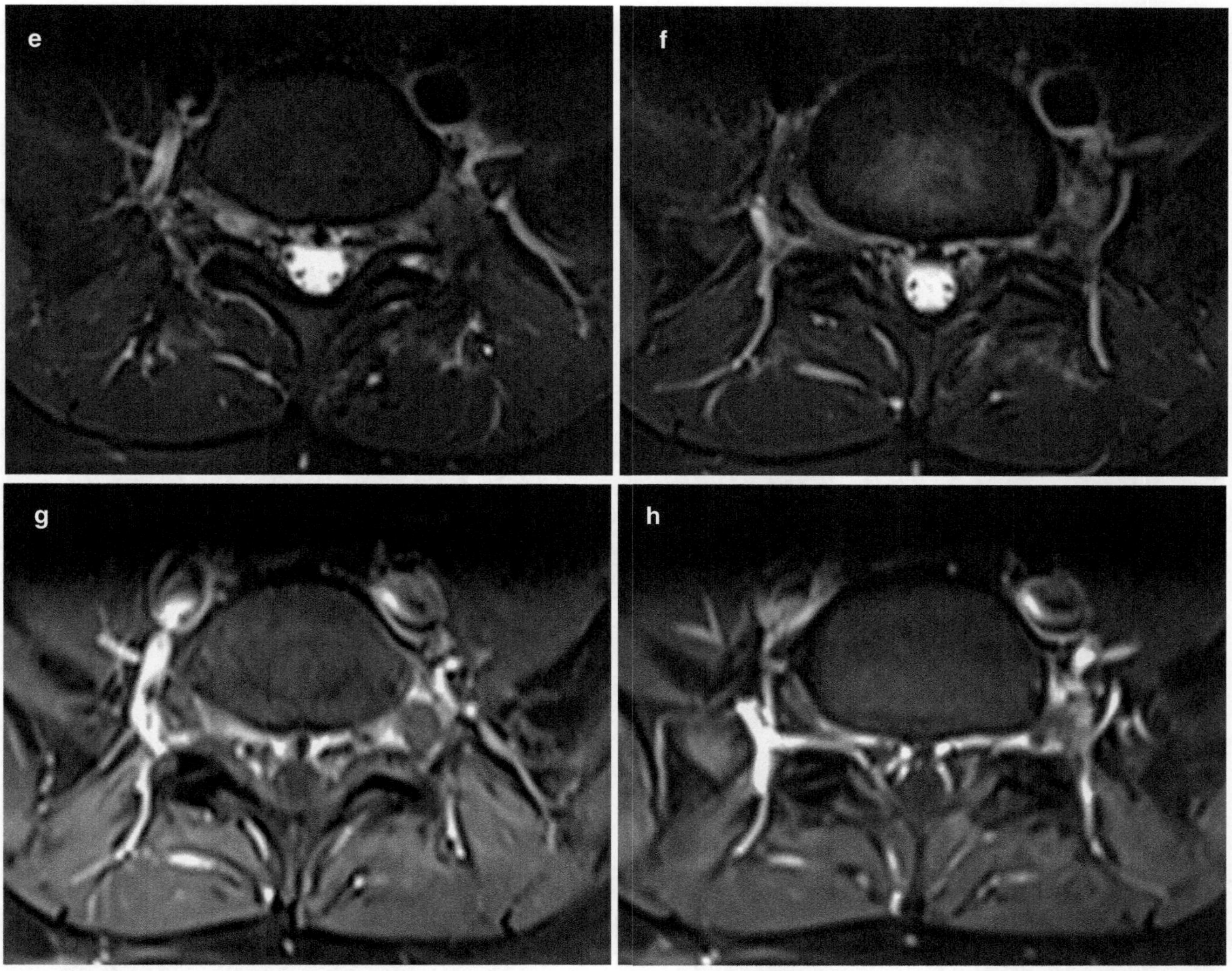

Fig. 9 (continued)

Postoperative MR 3 Weeks After Discectomy

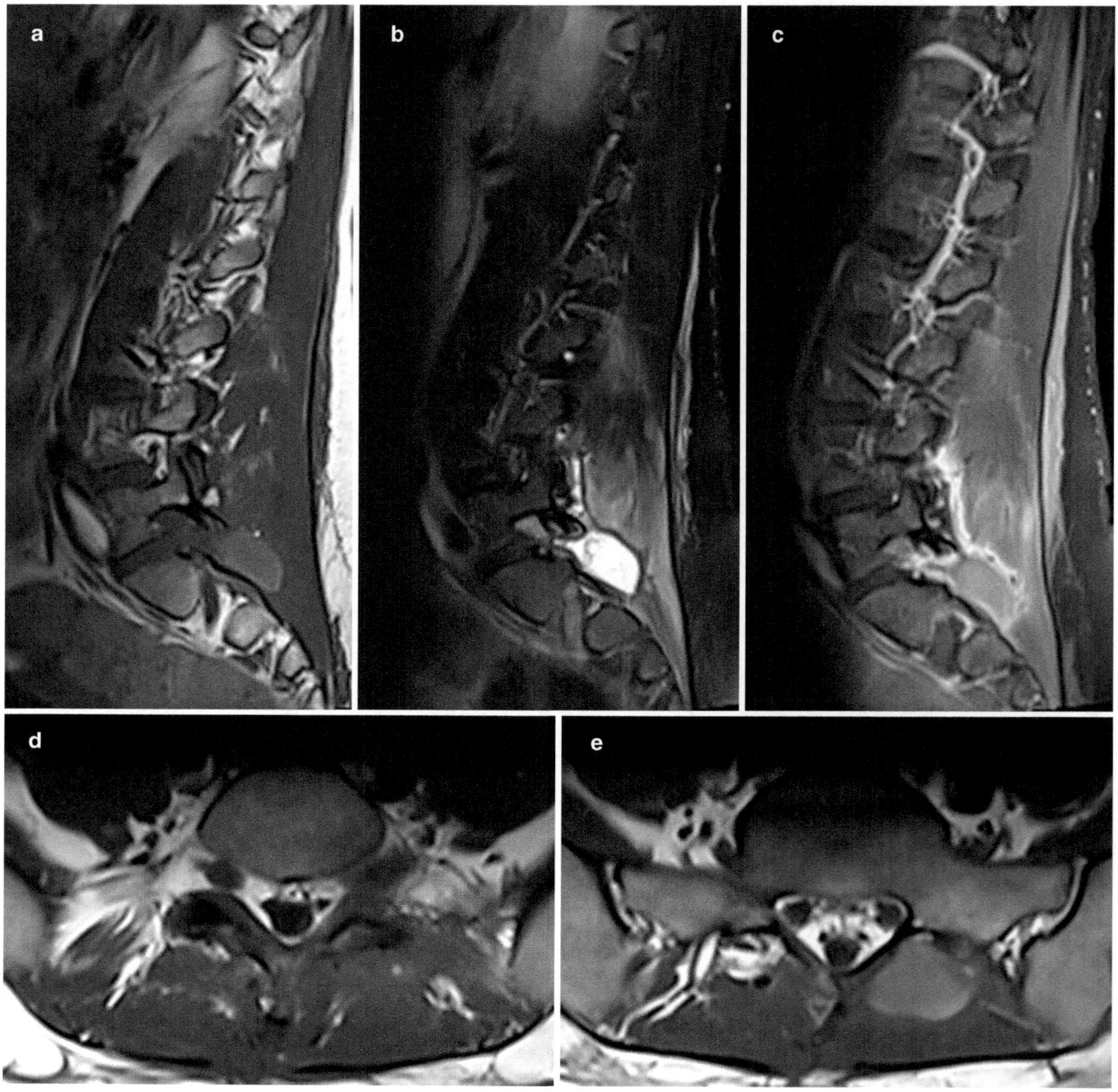

Fig. 10 (**a**–**k**) Sagittal and axial TSE T1-weighted images (**a**, **d**, **e**), sagittal and axial TSE T2-weighted images with fat saturation (**b**, **h**, **i**), axial TSE T2-weighted images (**f**, **g**), sagittal and axial TSE T1-weighted images with fat saturation after administration of contrast medium (**c**, **j**, **k**). Discectomy with laminotomy at L5-S1 on the left (**a**–**k**). Diffuse oedema of the perispinal muscles bilaterally, more marked on the left side and more evident by using T2-weighted imaging with fat saturation (**h**, **i**). Fluid collection in the perispinal soft tissues in the site of laminotomy, hyperintense in T2 (**b**, **g**, **i**), hypointense in T1 (**a**, **e**), with peripheral contrast enhancement (**c**, **k**), due to abscess

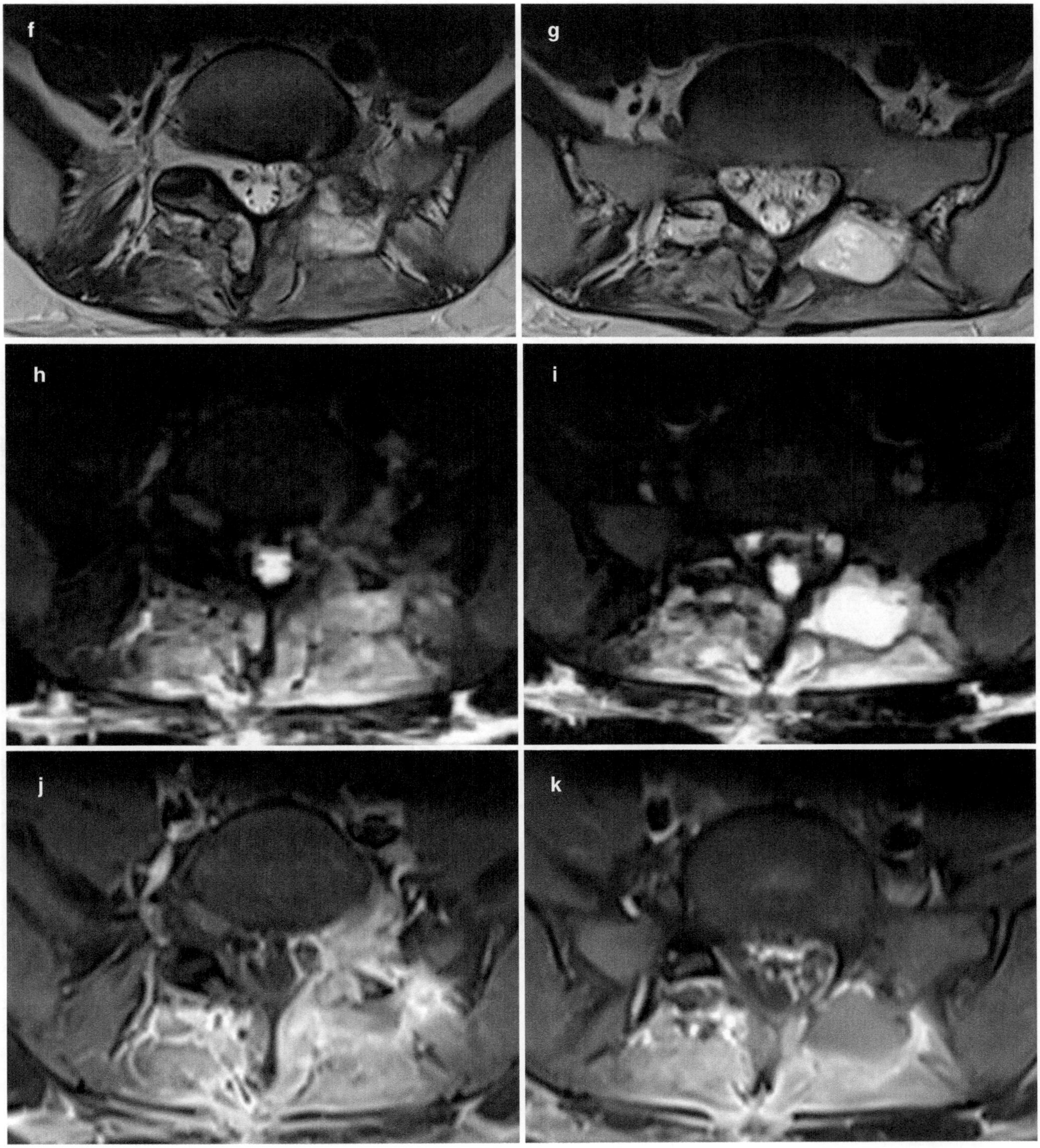

Fig. 10 (continued)

Case 83: Discectomy. Spondylitis. Arachnoiditis. Abscess

- A 49-year-old woman
- Patient with low back pain and high-level flogosis markers after discectomy
- Complete regression of symptoms after antibiotic therapy
- Early MR postoperative follow-up (1 and 5 days) and late (1 year)

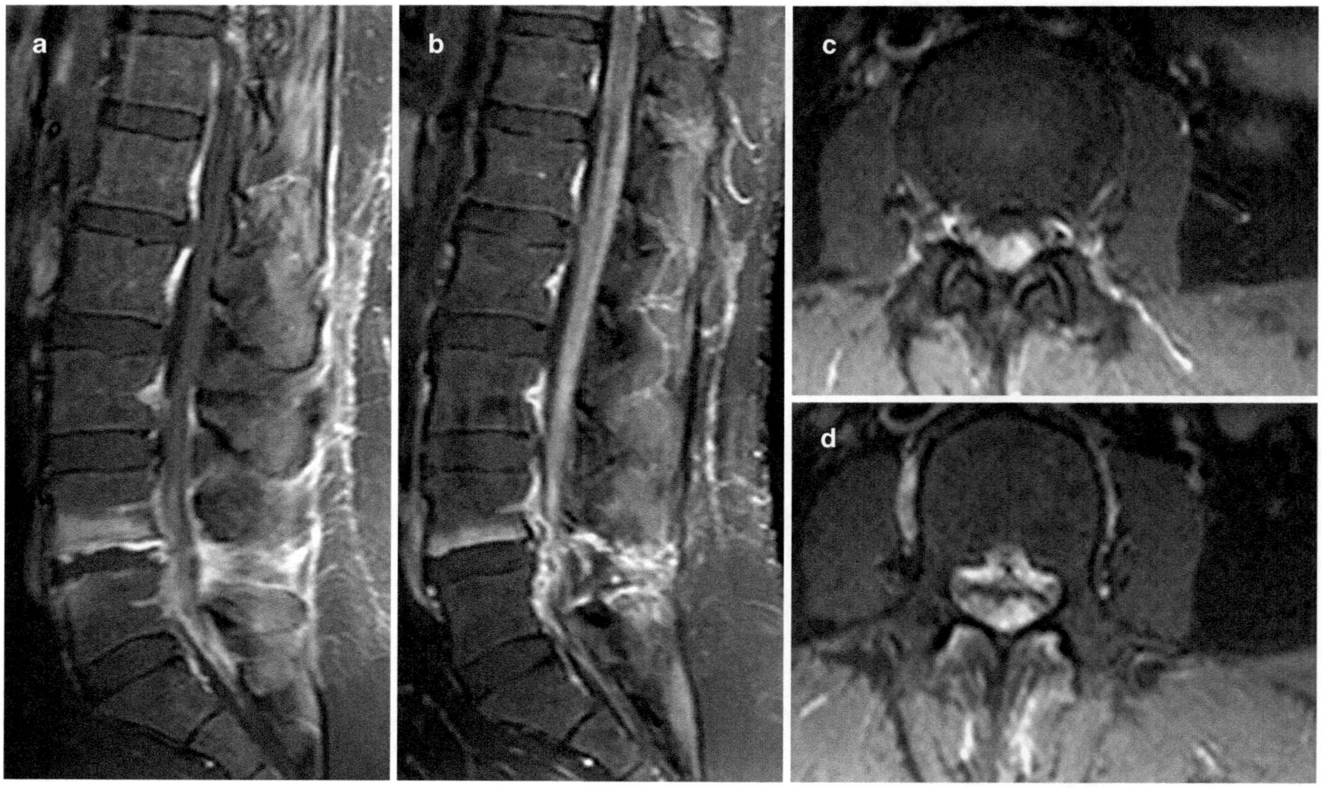

Fig. 11 (**a–d**) Sagittal and axial TSE T1-weighted images with fat saturation after administration of contrast medium (**a–d**). Contrast enhancement of L4 inferior subchondral cancellous bone and subjacent chondral surface, due to spondylitis (**a**, **b**), with associated bundling cauda and contrast enhancement of the nerve roots, due to arachnoiditis (**a–d**)

Postoperative Follow-up After 5 Days

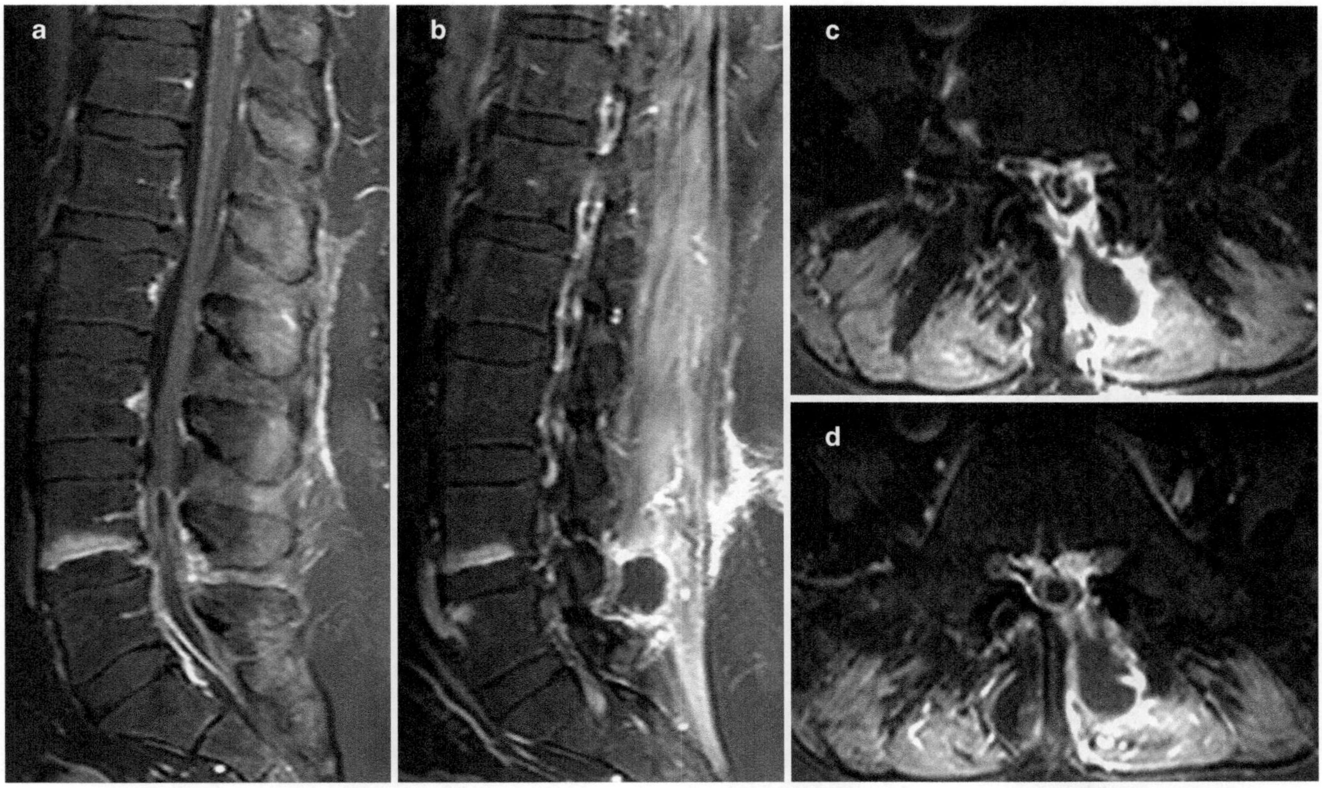

Fig. 12 (**a–d**) Sagittal and axial TSE T1-weighted images with fat saturation after administration of contrast medium (**a–d**). The infection is worsened, with abscess formation in both the intradural space and posterior perispinal soft tissues along surgical breach (**a–d**)

Late Postoperative Follow-up After 1 Year

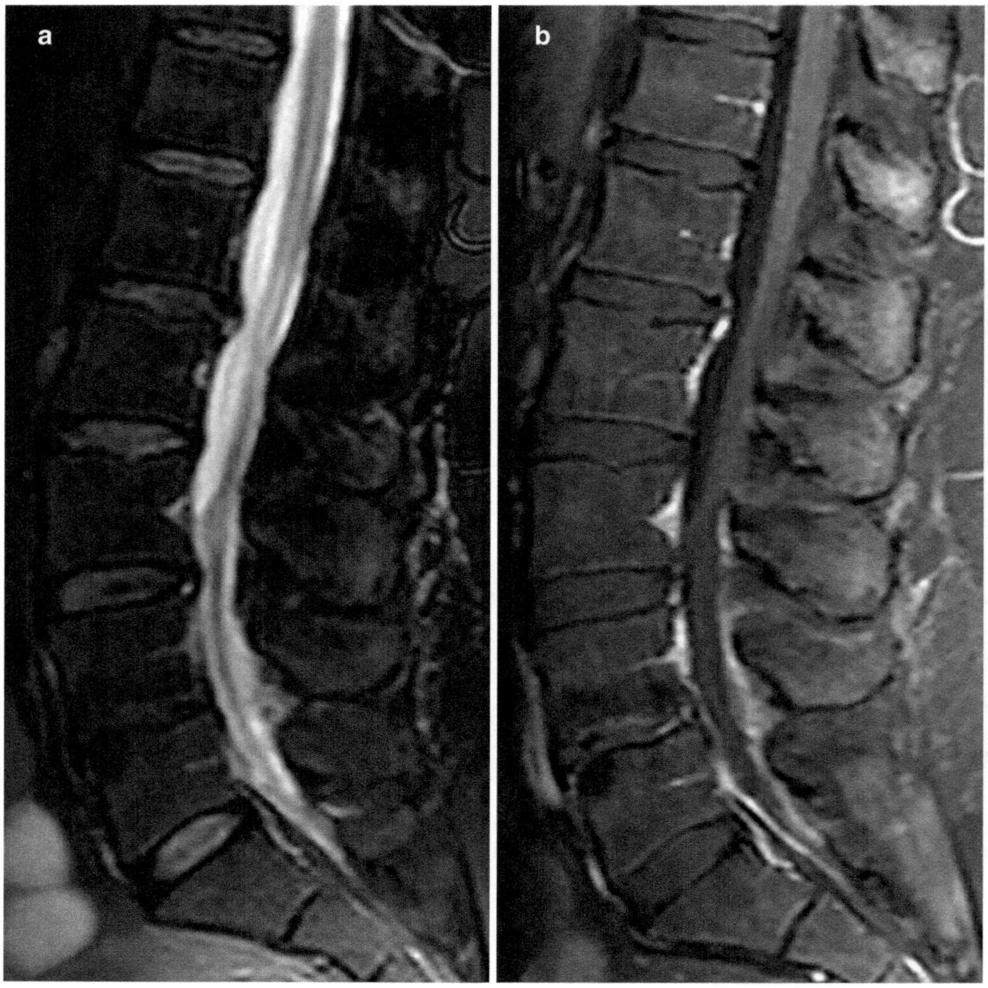

Fig. 13 (**a**, **b**) Sagittal TSE T2-weighted image with fat saturation (**a**), sagittal T1-weighted image with fat saturation after administration of contrast medium (**b**). Regression of the infectious findings (**a**, **b**)

Case 84: Decompression. Stabilization. Fibrous Scar

- A 67-year-old man
- Patient surgically treated for canal stenosis with laminectomy and stabilization
- Persistent low back pain and weakness in the legs
- Preoperative and postoperative MRI

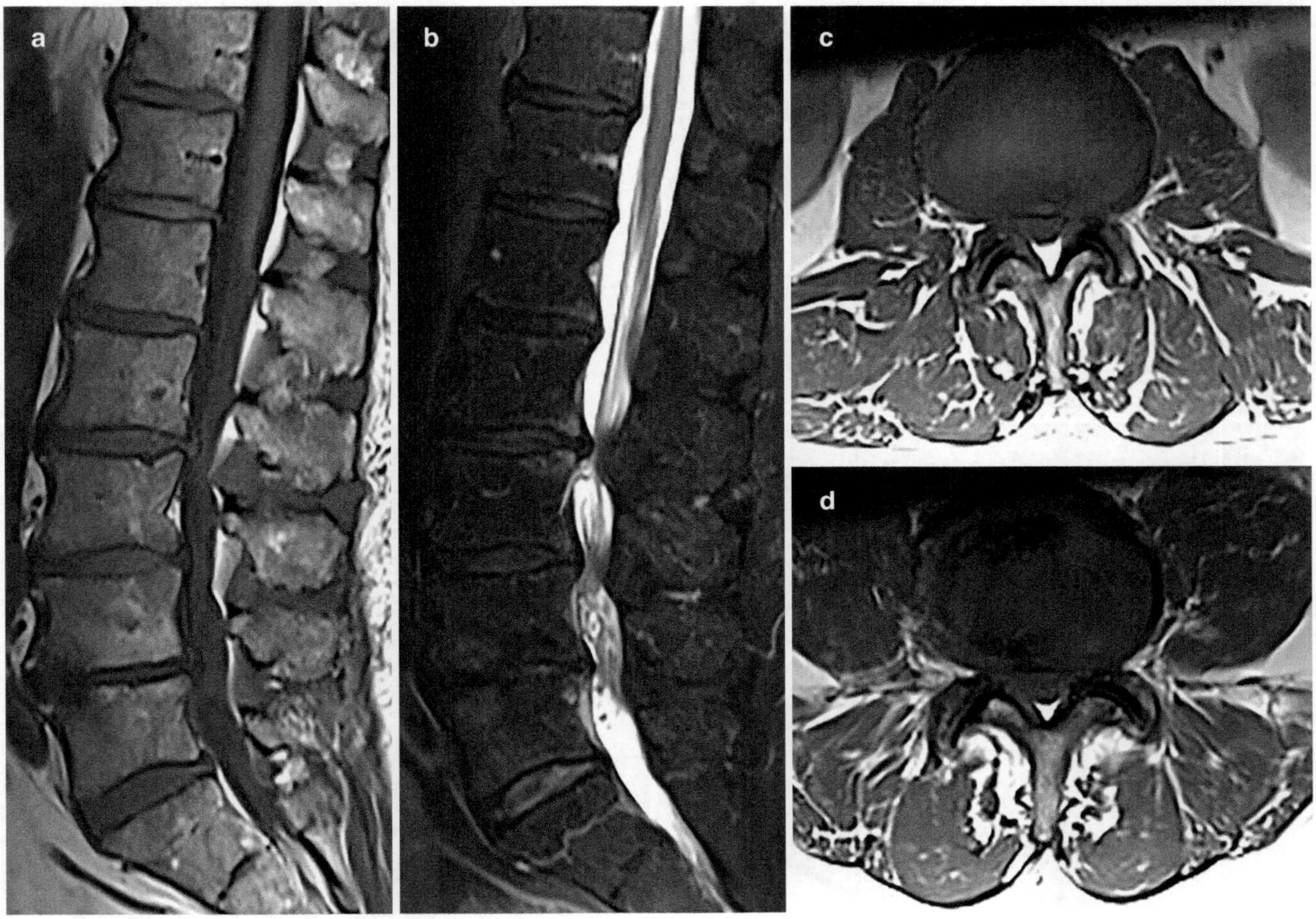

Fig. 14 (**a–d**) Sagittal and axial TSE T1-weighted images (**a**, **c**, **d**), sagittal TSE T2-weighted image with fat saturation (**b**). Small hernia in bulging disc at L2/L3 (**a–c**). Marked bulging disc at L4/L5 (**a**, **b**, **d**). Diffuse stenosis of the central spinal canal between L2 and L5 (**a–d**). Diffuse spondylosis and osteochondrosis, more marked at L4/L5 (**a**, **b**)

Ten Months Postoperative MR Examination

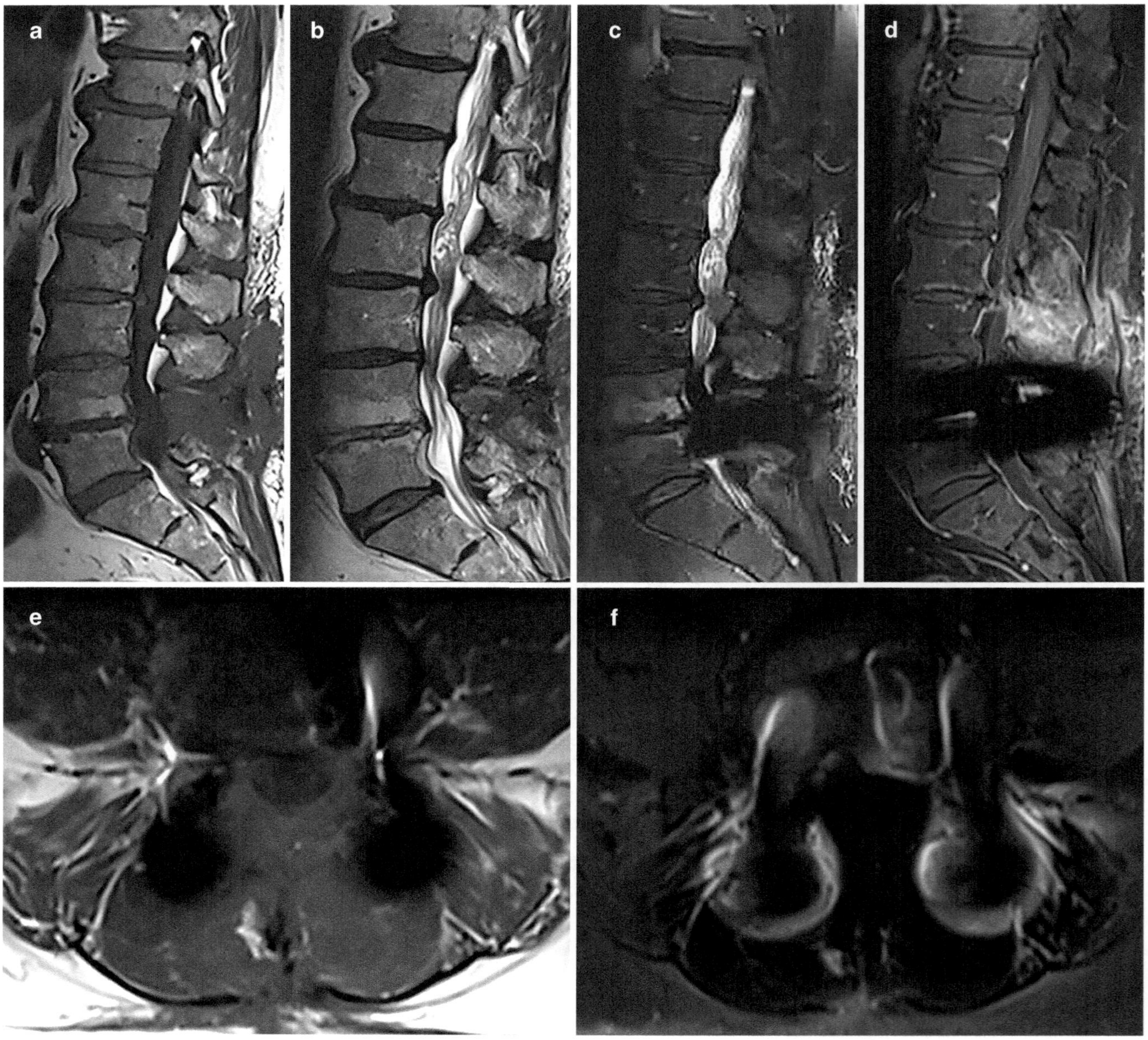

Fig. 15 (**a**–**h**) Sagittal TSE T1-weighted images (**a**, **e**), sagittal T2-weighted image (**b**), sagittal TSE T2-weighted image with fat saturation (**c**), sagittal and axial T1-weighted images with fat saturation following administration of contrast medium (**d**, **f**–**h**). Laminectomy at L4/L5, positioning of intervertebral device, stabilization with metallic device with pedicular screws at L4 and L5 bilaterally (**a**–**f**). Left laminectomy at L2/L3 (**d**, **g**, **h**). Marked artifacts from metallic devices at L4/L5 (**a**–**f**) that are more marked in sequences with fat saturation (**c**, **d**, **f**); in particular, note in this case the impossibility of evaluating the central spinal canal (**c**, **d**, **f**). Contrast enhancement in the site of left laminectomy at L2/L3 due to scarring phenomena (**d**, **g**, **h**). The small hernia at L2/L3 remains (**g**)

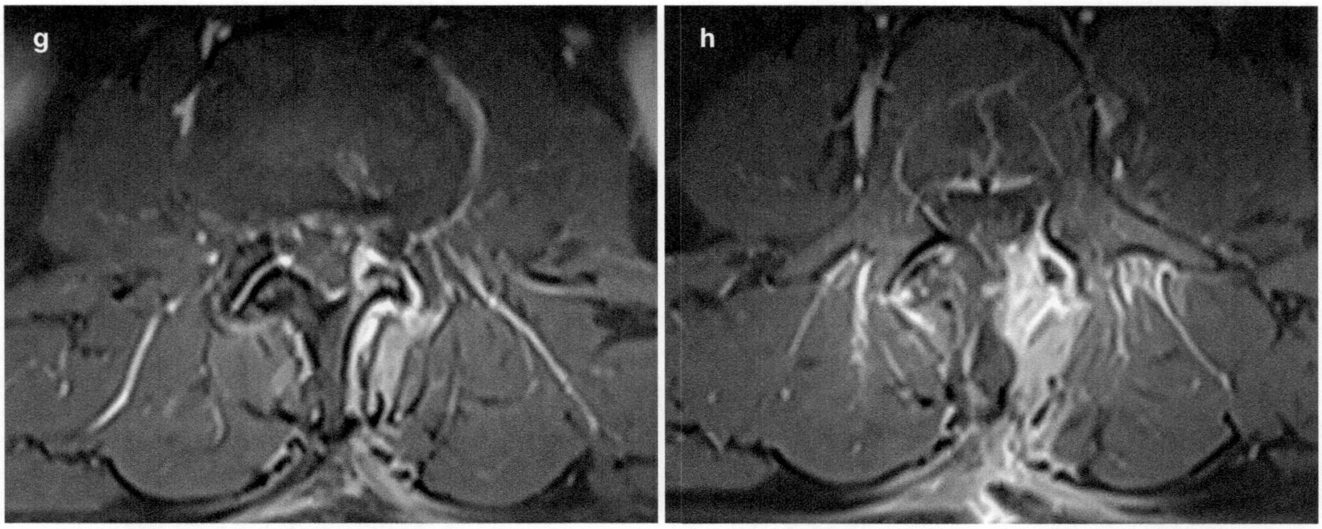

Fig. 15 (continued)

Case 85: Decompression. Stabilization. Stenosis

- A 48-year-old woman
- Patient with low back pain and left sciatica
- Surgically treated for stenosis of central spinal canal
- Late MR postoperative follow-up

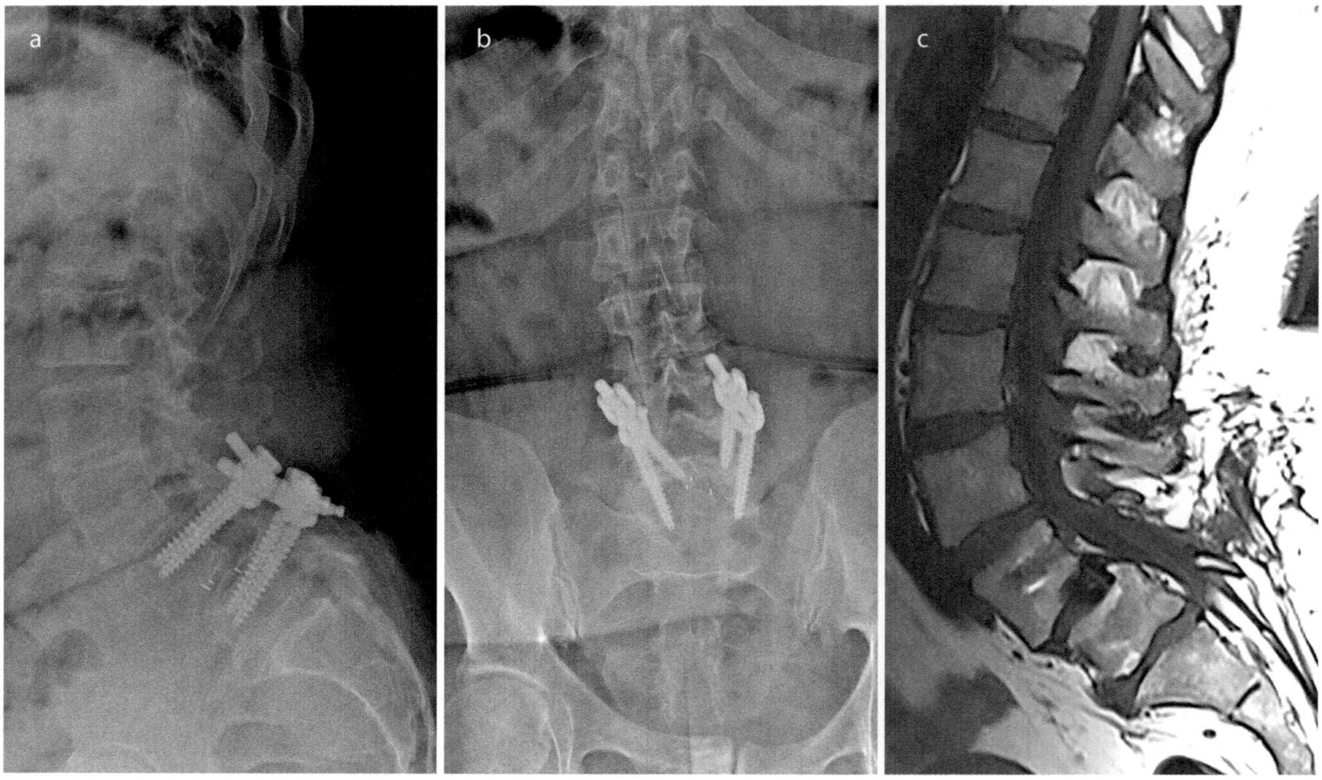

Fig. 16 (**a**–**h**) Lumbosacral XR in lateral (**a**) and anterior-posterior (**b**) views, sagittal and axial TSE T1-weighted images (**c**, **f**), sagittal and axial TSE T2-weighted images (**d**, **g**), sagittal and axial TSE T2-weighted images with fat saturation (**e**, **h**). Intervertebral cage and posterior stabilization at L4/L5 (**a**, **b**). Lumbar hyperlordosis (**a**, **c**–**e**). Laminectomy at L4/L5 (**b**–**h**). MR artifacts from metallic devices (**c**–**h**) that are more marked in fat-saturated sequences (**e**, **h**). Residual mild anterolisthesis of L4 over L5 (**a**, **c**–**e**). Residual stenosis of the left lateral recess of the spinal canal at L4/L5 (**f**–**h**)

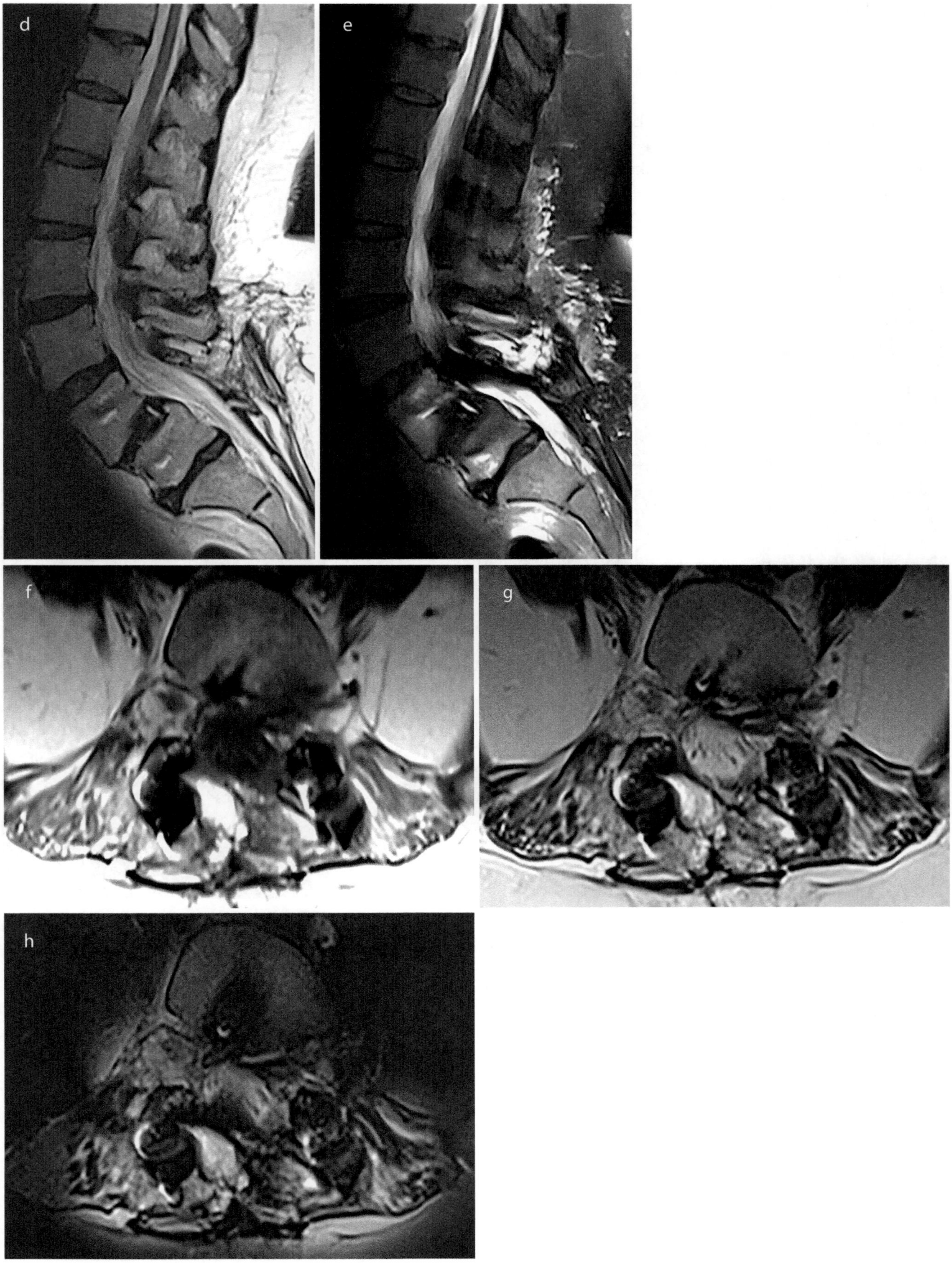

Fig. 16 (continued)

Case 86: Decompression. Stenosis

- A 62-year-old man
- Patient surgically treated for L3–L5 stenosis of the central spinal canal
- Persistent low back pain and weakness in the legs
- MR postoperative follow-up

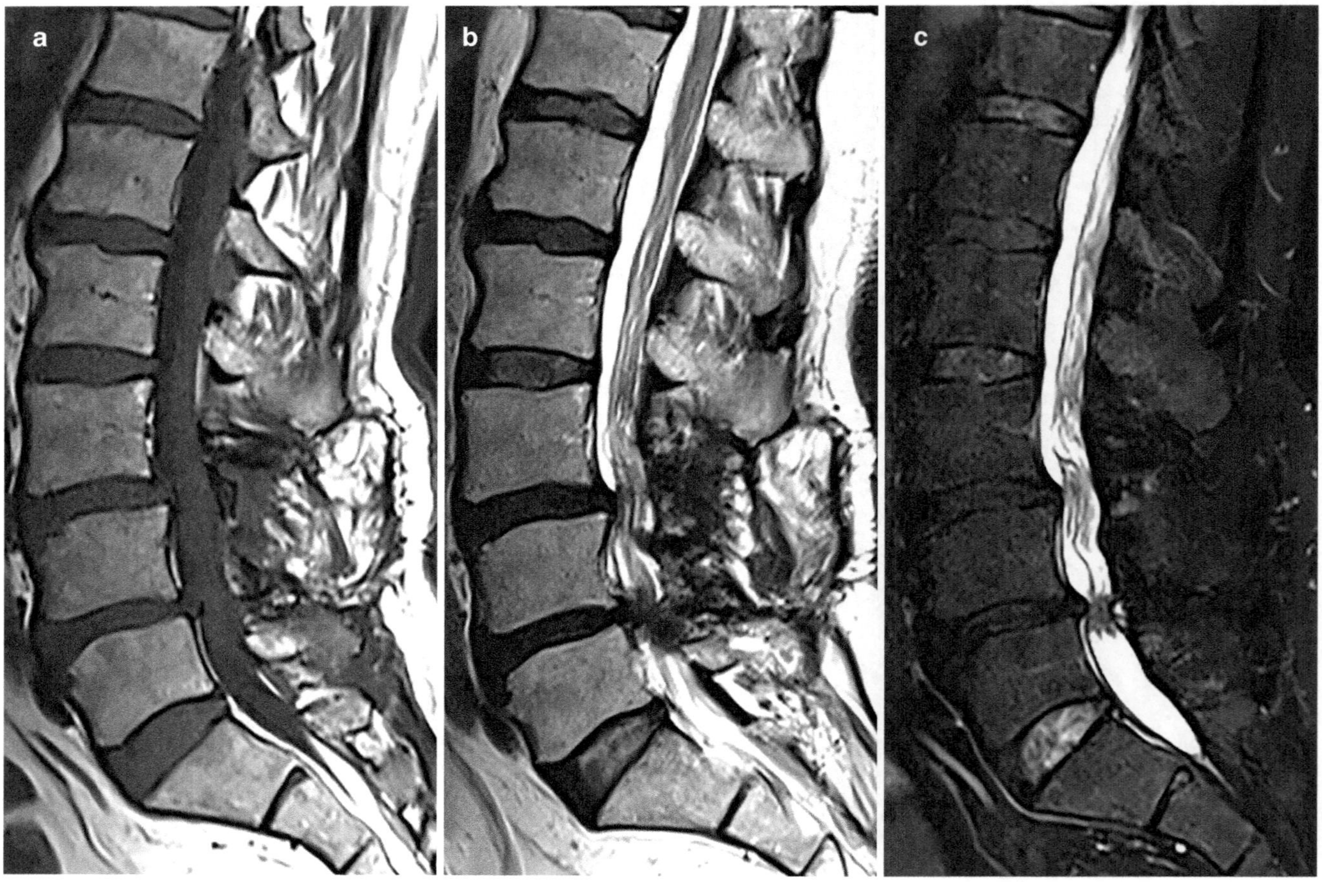

Fig. 17 (**a–j**) Sagittal and axial TSE T1-weighted images (**a**, **d**, **e**), sagittal and axial TSE T2-weighted images (**b**, **f**, **g**), sagittal TSE T2-weighted image with fat saturation (**c**), CT images (**h–j**). Laminectomy and spinousectomy of L4, laminotomy at L3 and L5 (**a–j**), with decompression of the central spinal canal. Residual stenosis of the lateral recesses of the spinal canal (**d–g**). TC examination confirmed bone stenosis of the same lateral recesses (**i**, **j**)

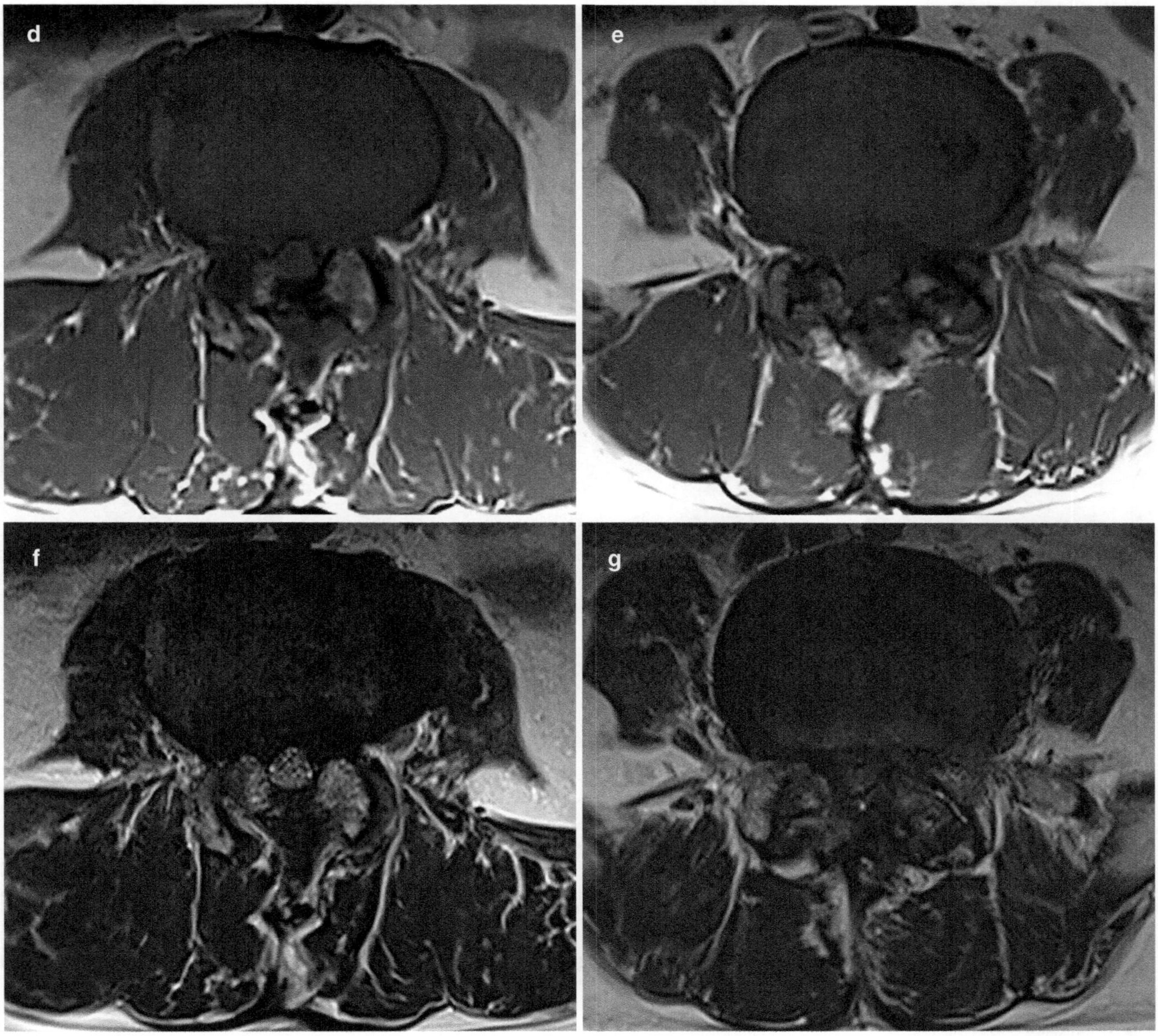

Fig. 17 (continued)

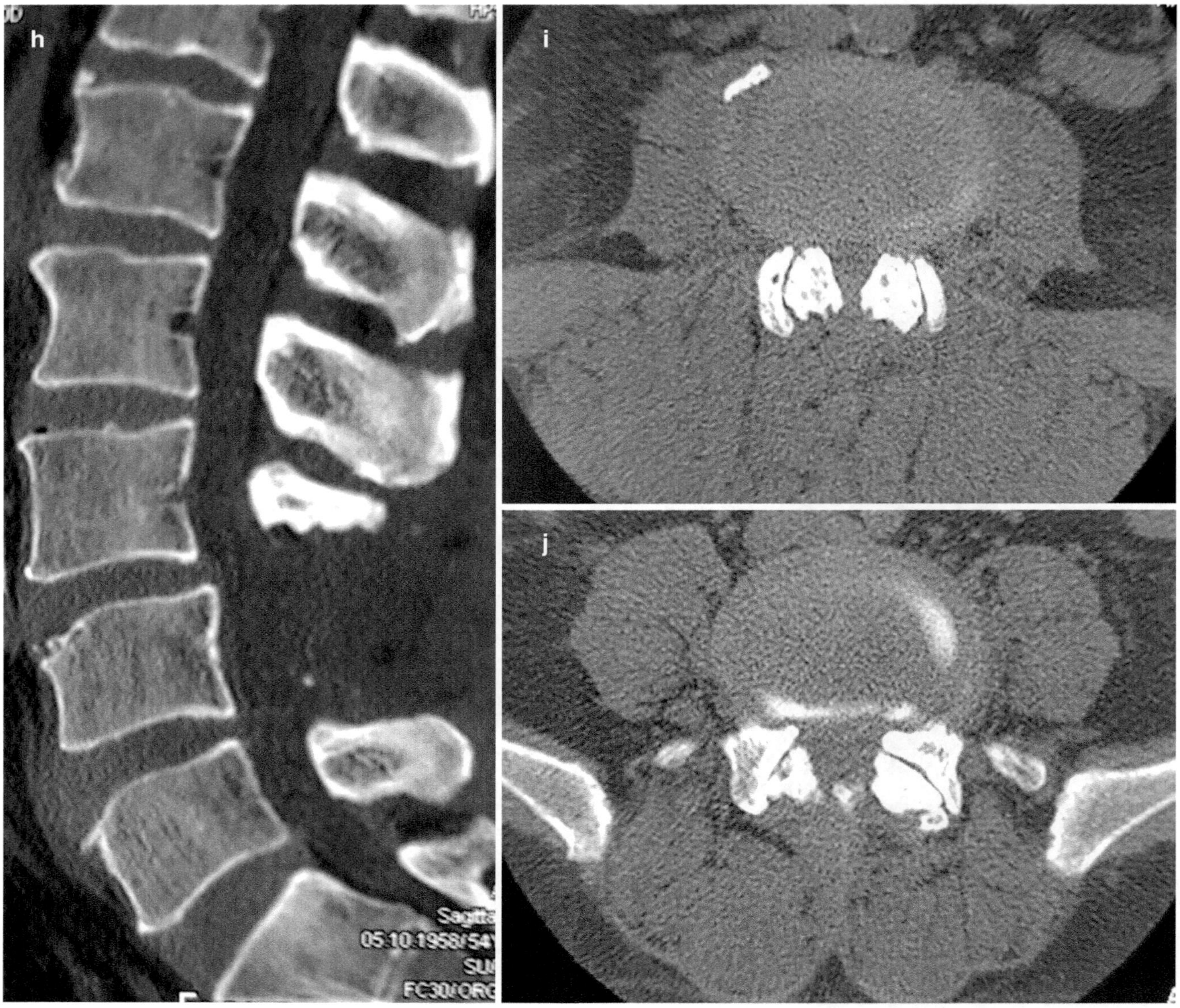

Fig. 17 (continued)

Case 87: Interspinous Device. Perispinal Inflammation

- A 48-year-old man
- Patient surgically treated for L4/L5 and L5/S1 discopathy with double interspinous device positioning (X-Stop)
- MR postoperative follow-up

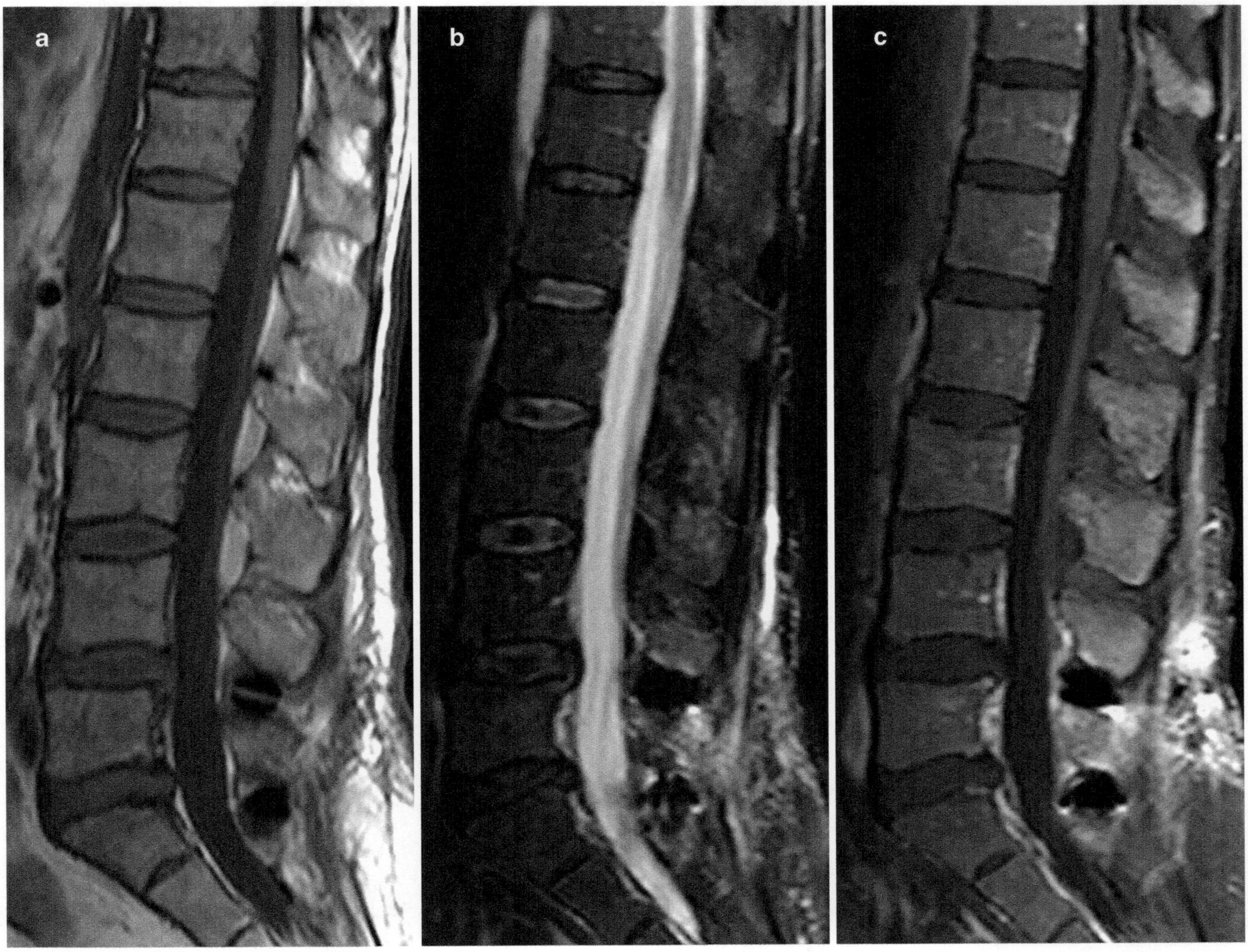

Fig. 18 (**a–e**) Sagittal TSE T1-weighted image (**a**), sagittal TSE T2-weighted image with fat saturation (**b**), sagittal and axial TSE T1-weighted images with fat saturation after administration of contrast medium (**c–e**). Double interspinous devices at L4/L5 and L5/S1 (**a–e**). Contrast enhancement of the perispinous soft tissues, indicating a slight inflammatory reaction (**c**, **e**)

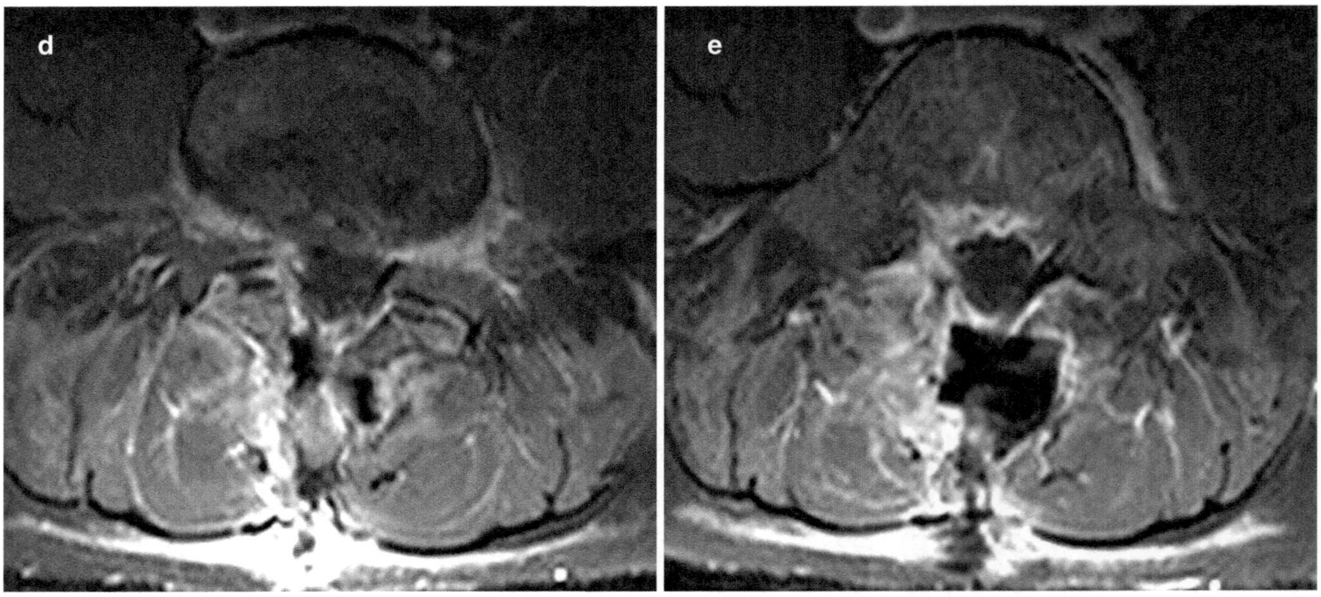

Fig. 18 (continued)

Case 88: Discectomy, Stabilization. Spondylotic Myelopathy

- A 64-year-old man
- Patient surgically treated for cervical discal hernia and central spinal canal stenosis, with anterior cervical discectomy C5-C7, decompressive laminectomy at C6/C7, intervertebral device positioning and posterior fixation
- Quadriparesis more marked in the lower extremities and worsened after surgery
- MR follow-up 18 months after surgery

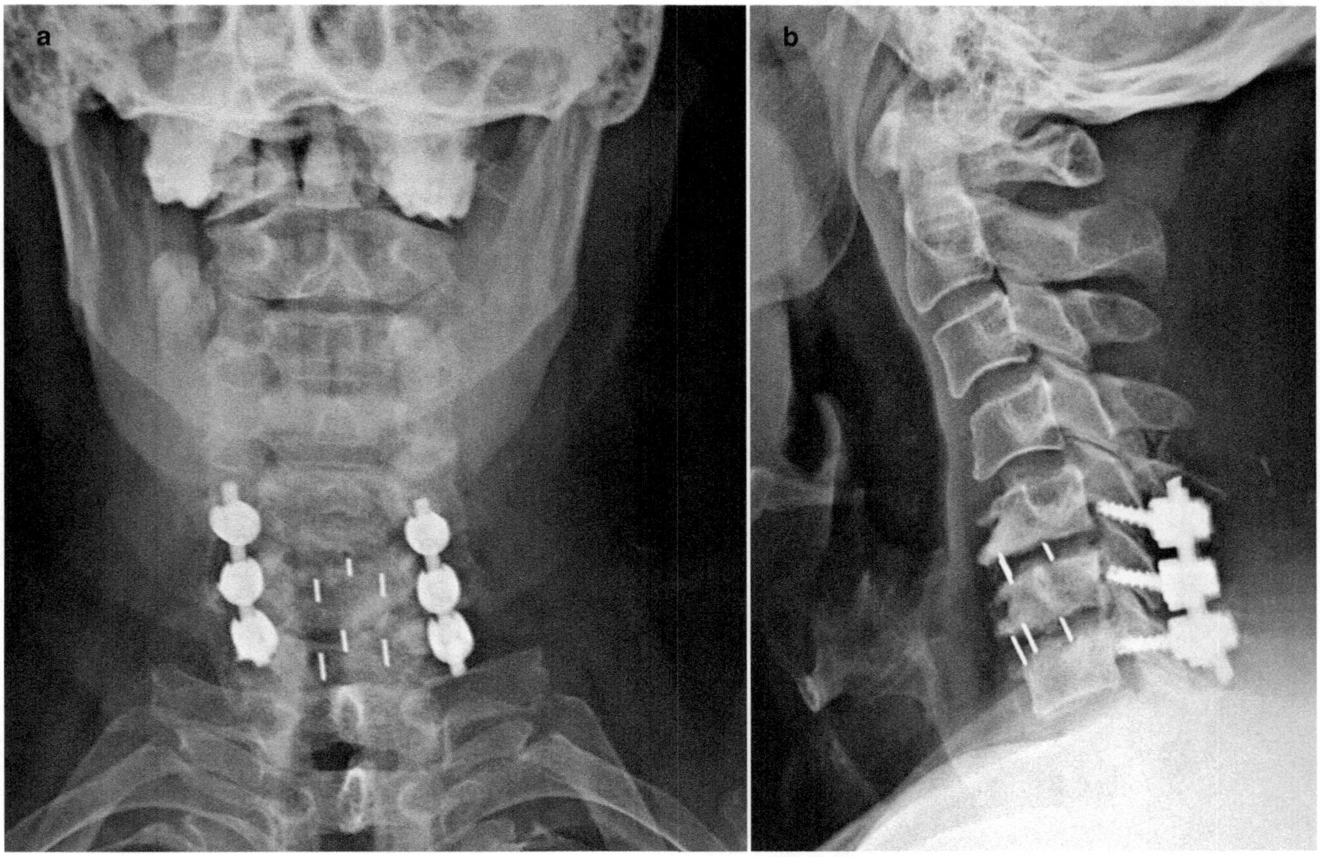

Fig. 19 (**a**–**f**) Cervical spine X-ray in anterior and lateral views (**a**, **b**), sagittal TSE T2-weighted image (**c**), sagittal T1-weighted image (**d**), sagittal and axial TSE T1-weighted images after administration of contrast medium (**e**, **f**). Intervertebral cages at C5/C6 and C6/C7 and stabilization with screws at the same levels (**a**, **b**). Discectomy C5/C6 and C6/C7 and laminectomy C6/C7 (**c**–**f**). Intramedullary high signal on T2-weighted image from C5 to T1, with spinal cord enlargement (**c**). Intramedullary area of persisting contrast enhancement at level C6/C7 18 months after surgery (**e**, **f**). This area of contrast enhancement is localized exactly in the site of preoperative greatest narrowing of the central spinal canal. In these cases, contrast enhancement of the spinal cord may persist many months after surgery. Diagnosis: spondylotic myelopathy

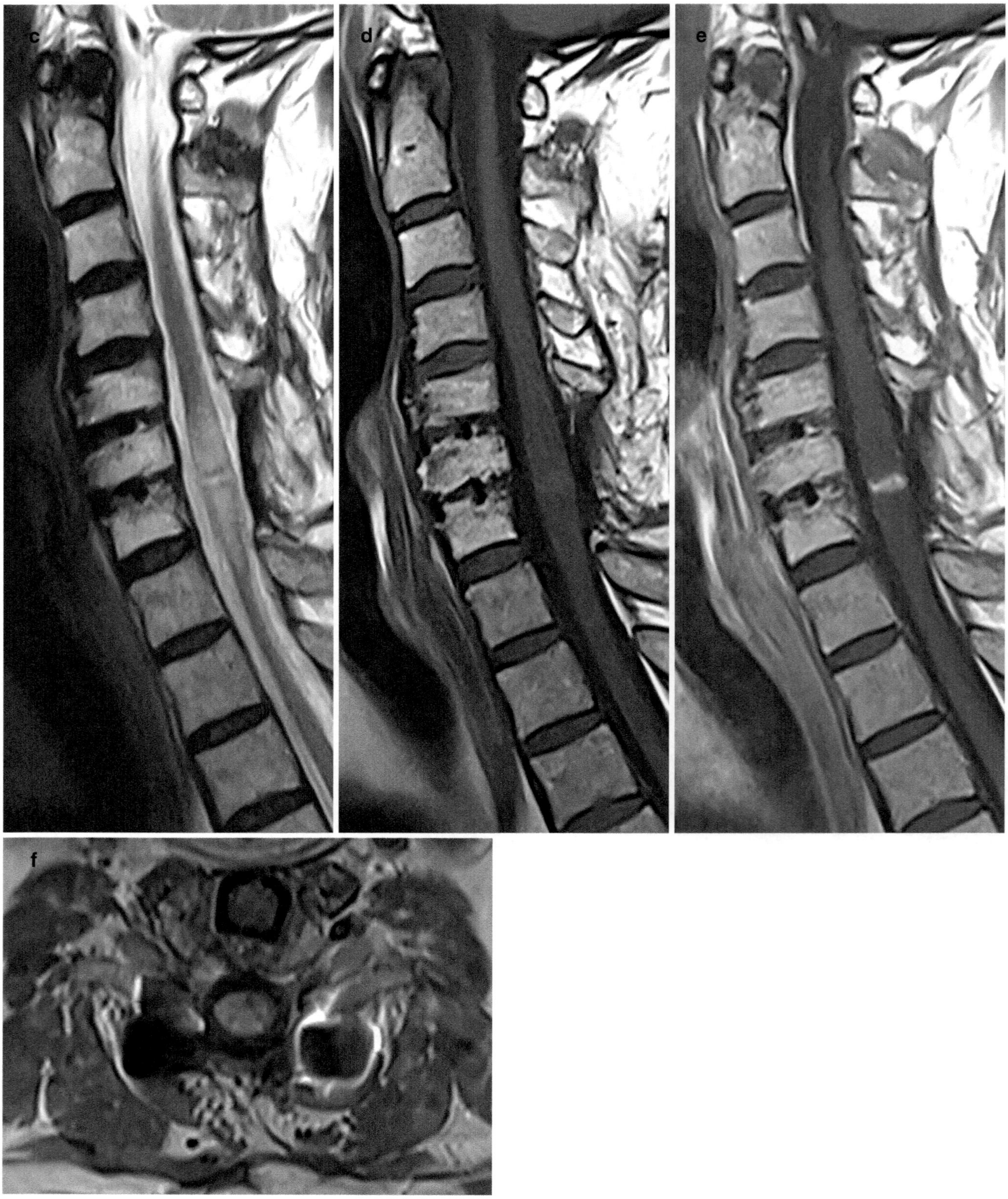

Fig. 19 (continued)

GPSR Compliance

The European Union's (EU) General Product Safety Regulation (GPSR) is a set of rules that requires consumer products to be safe and our obligations to ensure this.

If you have any concerns about our products, you can contact us on ProductSafety@springernature.com

In case Publisher is established outside the EU, the EU authorized representative is:

Springer Nature Customer Service Center GmbH
Europaplatz 3
69115 Heidelberg, Germany

Batch number: 10365229

Printed by Printforce, the Netherlands